Psychosocial Genetic Counseling

OXFORD MONOGRAPHS ON MEDICAL GENETICS

General Editors

Arno G. Motulsky Martin Bobrow Peter S. Harper Charles Scriver

Former Editors

J. A. Fraser Roberts C. O. Carter

1. R. B. McConnell: *The genetics of gastrointestinal disorders*
2. A. C. Kopé: *The distribution of the blood groups in the United Kingdom*
3. E. Slater and V. A. Cowie: *The genetics of locomotor disorders*
4. C. O. Carter and T. J. Fairbank: *The genetics of locomotor disorders*
5. A. E. Mourant, A. C. Kopé, and K. Domaniewska-Sobezak: *The distribution of the human blood groups and other polymorphisms*
6. A. E. Mourant, A. C. Kopé and K. Domaniewska-Sobezak: *Blood groups and diseases*
7. A. G. Steinbert and C. E. Cook: *The distribution of the human immunoglobulin allotypes*
8. D. Tills, A. C. Kopé and R. E. Tills: *The distribution of the human blood groups and other polymorphisms: Supplement I*
10. D. Z. Loesch: *Quantitative dermatoglyphics: classification, genetics, and pathology*
11. D. J. Bond and A. C. Chandley: *Aneuploidy*
12. P. F. Benson and A. H. Fensom: *Genetic biochemical disorders*
13. G. R. Sutherland and F. Hecht: *Fragile sites on human chromosomes*
14. M. d'A Crawfurd: *The genetics of renal tract disorders*
16. C. R. Scriver and B. Childs: *Garrod's inborn factors in disease*
18. M. Baraitser: *The genetics of neurological disorders*
19. R. J. Gorlin, M. M. Cohen, Jr., and L. S. Levin: *Syndromes of the head and neck, third edition*
20. R. A. King, J. I. Rotter, and A. G. Motulsky: *The genetics basis of common diseases*
21. D. Warburton, J. Byrne, and N. Canki: *Chromosome anomalies and prenatal development: an atlas*
22. J. J. Nora, K. Berg, and A. H. Nora: *Cardiovascular diseases: genetics, epidemiology, and prevention*
24. A. E. H. Emery: *Duchenne muscular dystrophy, second edition*
25. E. G. D. Tuddenham and D. N. Cooper: *The molecular genetics of haemostasis and its inherited disorders*
26. A. Boué: *Fetal medicine*
27. R. E. Stevenson, J. G. Hall, and R. M. Goodman: *Human malformations*
28. R. J. Gorlin, H. V. Toriello, and M. M. Cohen, Jr.: *Hereditary hearing loss and its syndromes*
29. R. J. M. Gardner and G. R. Sutherland: *Chromosome abnormalities and genetic counseling, second edition*
30. A. S. Teebi and T. I. Farag: *Genetic disorders among Arab populations*
31. M. M. Cohen, Jr.: *The child with multiple birth defects*
32. W. W. Weber: *Pharmacogenetics*
33. V. P. Sybert: *Genetic skin disorders*
34. M. Baraitser: *Genetics of neurological disorders, third edition*
35. H. Ostrer: *Non-mendelian genetics in humans*
36. E. Traboulsi: *Genetic diseases of the eye*
37. G. L. Semenza: *Transcription factors and human disease*
38. L. Pinsky, R. P. Erickson, and R. N. Schimke: *Genetic disorders of human sexual development*
39. R. E. Stevenson, C. E. Schwartz, and R. J. Schroer: *X-linked mental retardation*
40. M. J. Khoury, W. Burke, and E. Thomson: *Genetics and public health in the 21st century*
41. J. Weil: *Psychosocial genetic counseling*

OXFORD MONOGRAPHS ON MEDICAL GENETICS NO. 41

PSYCHOSOCIAL GENETIC COUNSELING

Jon Weil

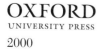

OXFORD
UNIVERSITY PRESS
2000

OXFORD

Oxford   New York

Athens   Auckland   Bangkok   Bogotá   Buenos Aires   Calcutta
Cape Town   Chennai   Dar es Salaam   Delhi   Florence   Hong Kong   Istanbul
Karachi   Kuala Lumpur   Madrid   Melbourne   Mexico City   Mumbai
Nairobi   Paris   São Paulo   Singapore   Taipei   Tokyo   Toronto   Warsaw

and associated companies in
Berlin   Ibadan

Copyright © 2000 by Oxford University Press, Inc.

Published by Oxford University Press, Inc.
198 Madison Avenue, New York, New York, 10016
http://www.oup-usa.org

Library of Congress Cataloging-in-Publication Data

Weil, Jon.
Psychosocial genetic counseling /
Jon Weil.
    p. ; cm. — (Oxford monographs on medical genetics ; no. 41)
Includes bibliographical references and index.
    ISBN-13 978-0-19-512066-0
    ISBN 0-19-512066-3
    1. Genetic counseling—Psychological aspects.
    2. Genetic counseling—Social aspects.
    I. Title. II. Series.
    DNLM: 1. Genetic Counseling.   2. Genetic Predisposition to Disease—psychology.
    QZ   50 W422p 2000]   RB155.7.W45 2000   6169.042—dc21   00-020614

3 5 7 9 8 6 4 2

Printed in the United States of America
on acid-free paper

For Zita

Preface

Traditional Jewish law instructs that if a woman's first two sons bleed to death following circumcision, subsequent sons shall not be circumcised. Similarly, if the first sons of three sisters so die, subsequent sons of all sisters shall not be circumcised (Slotki, 1936). In this ancient religious canon we can identify a number of contemporary issues relevant to clinical genetics and genetic counseling: a recognition of familial patterns of disease, the importance of accuracy in diagnosis, a medically based intervention, the need to reconcile the intervention with prevailing beliefs and practices, and, almost certainly, the stigmatization of those whose lives were saved by this intervention.

This brief example illustrates the central tenet of the present book—while clinical genetics and genetic counseling utilize the remarkable and ever increasing information and technologies of contemporary science, they apply them to human experiences that are age-old in their impact on individuals and societies. The science is contemporary, but the hopes, fears, and anxieties surrounding genetic disorders and birth defects remain, in many respects, unchanged. Genetic counselors serve as gatekeepers between the information and technology of science, on the one hand, and the lives of those individuals for whom the science is applied, on the other. In their role as gatekeepers, genetic counselors must balance attention to the science with attention to the psychosocial concerns of the counselees.

The extent to which psychosocial issues are addressed in genetic counseling varies greatly. At one end of the continuum, an intervention may be as simple as acknowledging the anxiety with which a counselee enters prenatal diagnosis counseling. In such a case, the primary purpose is to set the counselee more at ease and facilitate her ability to understand the technical information presented. At the other end of the continuum lie the extensive discussions, often involving multiple interactions, that may accompany medically positive results of prenatal diagnosis, counseling for presymptomatic testing for Huntington disease, or genetic testing for familial breast/ovarian cancer. Under these circumstances, a careful exploration of beliefs and values, family relationships, and social supports is essential so a potentially life-changing decision may be as appropriate as possible for the individual. Yet, whether the attention to psychosocial issues is brief or extensive, the genetic counselor must be well grounded in the principles and practice of psychosocial assessment and intervention and in the broader social-cultural contexts within which genetic counseling functions and counselees live their lives. Only when this is the case can the relevant issues be appropriately and sensitively addressed in a manner consistent with the often limited time available in genetic counseling. This book is devoted to an understanding of these issues.

The book is intended for all those who practice or study genetic counseling: students in master's degree training programs as well as all practitioners who define themselves professionally as genetic counselors—graduates of master's degree programs, medical geneticists, genetic nurse specialists, and Ph.D. geneticists involved in genetic counseling. The book is also intended to address the needs of the growing number of individuals in other professions who find themselves confronted with genetic issues, as genetics becomes increasingly relevant to broad areas of medicine and public health. These include physicians in many specialties, nurses, social workers, psychologists, and individual and family therapists.

For students and those who teach them, the book will serve as a text in courses covering psychosocial and ethnocultural topics as well as counseling techniques and clinical case review. Case vignettes and examples of clinical dialogue provide opportunities for discussion and suggestions for clinical interventions. For practicing genetic counselors, the book provides a comprehensive approach to addressing psychosocial issues, including an entrée to the relevant literature, and focused discussions on decision making, prenatal diagnosis counseling, cancer risk counseling, and genetic counseling with children and adolescents. The complex issue of nondirective genetic counseling is approached from a broad, historical perspective and there is detailed consideration of the still emerging areas of cross-cultural counseling and ethnocultural competence. For individuals in other professions, the book provides an overview of issues and techniques they may encounter in interactions with genetic counseling and genetic counselors, as well as the opportunity for detailed study in areas in which they are directly involved.

With this breadth of potential readers in mind, the book is designed to be usable at three somewhat distinct levels. First, a general reading provides an overview of the multiple topics relevant to genetic counseling. Second, the various sections, although relatively succinct, present in some detail the complexities of theoretical material and the subtleties of clinical interventions. Thus, a careful reading of any section will support a more expanded understanding of the topic. Finally, insofar as possible, cited references provide more thorough explication of the topic and/or an introduction to the relevant literature. My hope and intention are to present the material in a manner that is useful to all who work directly with individuals and families affected by genetic diseases and birth defects. Although most of the material is drawn from work in the United States, Canada, Great Britain, and Western Europe, the principles presented and the attention to cross-cultural issues should make the book applicable wherever genetic counseling is practiced.

Inevitably, the book reflects my own theoretical training and clinical experience as they relate to understanding human nature and social interactions and the application of such understanding to genetic counseling. Although other theoretical and clinical orientations have value, I believe the book presents a cogent, integrated approach to the practice of genetic counseling. Another constraint of the book involves the disjunction between the linear nature of written text and the multidimensional reality of genetic counseling. In this regard, a major problem relates to ethnocultural issues. Ideally, they would be discussed throughout the book, with respect to both theory and practice. Realistically, it has been necessary to address them in a single chapter. I urge the reader to use the chapter on ethnocultural issues as well as other relevant resources to reassess the theory and practice presented in the rest of the book from a broader, multicultural perspective.

When referring to those who do genetic counseling, I consistently use the feminine gender. In part this reflects the predominance of women among master's level genetic counselors in the United States and Canada. However, it is also intended to make use of the fact that, unfortunately, for many people, myself included, there remains a useful shock of awareness concerning gender issues when the feminine gender is used to refer to both sexes.

A word is also needed concerning the vignettes and clinical dialogues presented throughout the book. While based on clinical cases, they have been altered, both to protect confidentiality and to succinctly elucidate or demonstrate specific theoretical or clinical issues. In general, they probably depict a more insightful, efficient, and effective set of interventions than most of us could hope for on average. Thus, they should be used for their heuristic value but not taken as setting an unrealistically high standard of clinical practice.

No attempt to present the psychosocial aspects of genetic counseling within multiple contexts can overlook the evolving trends in health care reimbursement, managed care, and the commercialization and marketing of clinical genetic testing. All, in varying ways, may promote approaches to genetic counseling that reduce the time and attention given to psychosocial issues. The orientation of this book relates to these developments in several ways. First, it is both an appeal and an assertion that humane, healing medical practice must address the counselee's emotions, coping mechanisms, beliefs, values, social supports, and cultural background. This is particularly important, as genetic counseling involves increasingly complex technical, practical, and ethical issues. Second, I attempt to show at many points that attention to these issues facilitates genetic counseling by increasing the counselee's ability to understand and utilize the technical information and to reach appropriate decisions that may promote client satisfaction and medical compliance. Finally, application of the material in this book should support efficient, appropriate assessment and interventions within the time constraints that apply.

Two general principles underlie the organization of the book: a general progression from more focused to broader perspectives, and the interweaving of theoretical and practical material. Chapter 1 addresses the counselee from a predominantly individual perspective. It discusses issues such as coping and defenses, self-esteem, grief and mourning, guilt and shame, and the personal meanings of pregnancy and childbirth. Chapter 2 presents the counselee in a social context. The main focus is on family and couple interactions. These are the immediate social contexts within which the counselee functions, and members of these social groups are often included in the counseling process. Attention is also given to the roles of social isolation and social support in the counselee's adaptation to the circumstances surrounding genetic counseling. Chapter 3 deals with a variety of genetic counseling techniques, building in part on the more theoretical material of the first two chapters. Chapter 4 describes the structure of genetic counseling interactions, from initial contacts through postcounseling follow-up. While applicable to the individual counseling session, the concepts and sequence are also relevant to the overall organization of genetic counseling when it involves multiple interactions including telephone intakes and follow-up or more than one face-to-face session.

Chapter 5 addresses the complex core issues of nondirective counseling, risk perception, and decision making. Theoretical and historical material provide a basis for discussing the practical aspects of implementing these central elements of genetic counseling. Chapter 6 covers prenatal diagnosis counseling, which is the major, established specialty area within genetic counseling, and cancer risk counseling, an emerging specialty area that is important in its own right and as a harbinger of future expansion to cover other common adult-onset disorders. This chapter also discusses genetic counseling with children and adolescents. This material is presented to promote the importance and feasibility of enhancing genetic counseling so that it better serves the younger members of society, who are often greatly affected by genetic diseases and birth defects in themselves or in family members.

Chapter 7 addresses the essential issue of providing genetic counseling to individuals from a wide variety of ethnocultural backgrounds. The discussion involves both the general areas of ethnocultural beliefs, values, and experiences with which the genetic counselor should be familiar and the process of developing increased ethnocultural awareness, sensitivity, and competence. Finally,

Chapter 8 addresses the vast array of ethical, moral, and social issues related to genetic counseling from two limited but critical perspectives. One involves sociological investigations of the role of genetic counseling as both passive and active agent in the broad social changes being wrought by modern genetics and the Human Genome Project. The other is the viewpoints and voices of individuals with genetic disorders, birth defects, and other disabilities, who bring a perspective of particular relevance to issues concerning the utilization of clinical genetics and genetic counseling.

Berkeley, Calif.   J. W.
December 1999

Acknowledgments

Many people have contributed to the writing of this book through their knowledge, experience, friendship, and support. The manuscript was critically reviewed by Zita Dominguez Weil, June Peters, Margie Goldstein, Vivian Ota Wang, Sabina Morganti, Jean Benward, and Roberta Wise. Each, in her individual way, contributed significantly to its organization, its manner of exposition, and its ideas. In addition, I received valuable assistance with specific sections from Beth Crawford, Laurie Nemzer, Lucille Poskanzer, Marsha Saxton, Diane Beeson, and John Meaney. Jeffrey House, my editor at Oxford University Press, provided guidance, support, and a steadying hand throughout the process of writing and revising.

Underlying the manuscript are the contributions of many colleagues and friends to my professional development in both the theoretical and practical domains over many years. It is impossible to mention all who have played a role, but it is a pleasure to thank those whom I can name specifically.

Charles Epstein has been a friend and colleague through the full arc of my professional career, from the waning days of research in bacteriophage genetics to my current role as clinical psychologist and Director of the Program in Genetic Counseling at the University of California, Berkeley. His personal and institutional support has been helpful throughout and critical at a number of points in this journey, including the contacts that initiated the writing of this book. I thank him for many years of collaboration and support.

Margie Goldstein has been a friend and colleague throughout my tenure with the Program in Genetic Counseling. She has made the work there immeasurably more interesting and enjoyable and has contributed greatly to my understanding of many issues involving the psychosocial aspects of genetic counseling.

Like all genetic counselors, I am indebted to Seymour Kessler for his many contributions to the development of and advocacy for the psychosocial aspects of genetic counseling. I have been fortunate to work with him personally over the years in a number of settings. Thus, I have benefited directly from his continually creative analysis and application of psychological thinking to genetic counseling.

My understanding of genetic counseling has been greatly enriched through the opportunity to work over many years with Judy Derstine, Laurie Nemzer, Lucille Poskanzer, and Beth Crawford. My understanding of ethnocultural issues and their critical importance in genetic counseling has benefited immeasurably from my friendship and long-term collaboration with Vivian Ota Wang, Ilana Mittman, and John Meaney. Having come to genetic counseling from research genetics, a useful and continuing "outsider's" view of the profession has been supported and broadened by thought-provoking conversations with and through the writings of Diane Beeson, Marcia Saxton, and Rayna Rapp.

Sabina Morganti, Jean Benward, Lawrence Diller, and Mary Jane Nunes-Temple, the members of two very supportive peer consultation groups, have contributed a great deal to my understanding of individual and family psychodynamics and to my firm belief in the value of such peer support. I thank Thomas Long, Tracy Trotter, and Allen Obrinsky for many thoughtful conversations and for a long-term association between my private psychotherapy practice and a behaviorally oriented pediatrics practice, from which I learned much about the interactions between psychosocial and medical issues as they affect individuals and families. I also thank the students of the Program in Genetic Counseling at the University of California, Berkeley, with whom I have worked. Their sensitivity, integrity, and courage in addressing psychosocial and ethnocultural issues in clinical work, supervision, and class discussions have contributed greatly to my understanding of these issues and to the clinical material presented in the book.

My wife, Zita Dominguez Weil, has been a source of continual support and understanding during the life-consuming process of writing this book. She trusted, long before I did, that there was a book to be written, and I could not have completed it without her many contributions. To her I give my most heartfelt thanks.

Contents

Psychosocial Genetic Counseling

1

THE COUNSELEE
AS INDIVIDUAL

THOSE who seek genetic counseling, or have the need thrust upon them, represent a broad cross-section of society. Outside the genetic counseling context, most would probably be regarded as reasonably successful and competent, bringing to life's vicissitudes an adequate, if not stellar complement of individual and interpersonal supports and coping mechanisms. Thus, as we address the psychosocial issues relevant to genetic counseling, and as the genetic counselor addresses them with the counselee, a broad presumption of psychological normality is appropriate. While the genetic counselor must be alert to potential dysfunction and psychopathology, counselees should be approached as individuals who have demonstrated substantial competence in their lives, which they now bring to a new set of challenging circumstances. For the most part, counselees experience normal, albeit painful and complex responses to difficult, sometimes potentially overwhelming situations (Butani, 1974).

Under this presumption of normality, the genetic counselor must work with individuals who face life events with the full range of personalities and experiences and who come from a great diversity of social and cultural milieus. From this diversity of human experience and resources, the genetic counselor must attempt to identify the counselee's strengths and weaknesses, hopes, fears, and anxieties, in order to craft helpful responses. Furthermore, although the psychological processes to be discussed are largely normal, they are often un-

1

conscious or suppressed. Thus, to work effectively, the genetic counselor must maintain a level of doubt and inquiry with respect to appearances, behaviors, and self-reports. For this reason, there is a professional obligation to probe more deeply into the counselee's thoughts, feelings, and behavior than is consistent with ordinary social interactions.

A diversity of theories and processes is potentially applicable to genetic counseling. Those discussed here are the most relevant from the perspective of this book. Of necessity, they are initially treated as separate topics, but in reality, they are different facets of the psychological, physiological, and social responses of a single, integrated individual. They are thus highly interrelated, and references are made to their interrelationships. These interrelationships illustrate an ongoing task of clinical work: to construct an integrated understanding of the individual counselee from an unavoidably compartmentalized analysis of his or her situation.

Pregnancy, Childbirth, and the Psychosocial Meanings of Parenthood

Genetic counseling often involves pregnancy and the diseases and disabilities that affect infants and children. Thus, pregnancy, childbirth, and parenthood offer a useful starting point for a discussion of psychosocial issues. In addition, these topics illustrate the complex interplay between personal dynamics and social interactions, and between objective circumstances and individual perceptions and meanings, that are involved in all situations related to genetic counseling.

Pregnancy and childbirth bring major, irreversible changes to the parents' lives, and the transitions they produce are particularly great with the first child. The early physical and physiological changes in the pregnant woman's body produce a sense of integration and "one-ness" with the fetus. Quickening, and visualization by ultrasound, provide early indications of the fetus's separateness. Thus begins a long, perhaps lifelong, dynamic interplay between intense self-identification with the child and the inevitable separateness of the child's life. Hopes and expectations for the new child and his or her impact on the parents' lives are elaborated both consciously and unconsciously, as are fears and fantasies of unfortunate outcomes (Bibring et al., 1961; Butani, 1974; Solnit & Stark, 1961). With the child's birth, the family increases in size and social complexity, parenthood is confirmed, and the long process of parent–child relations and family development begins.

Both parents experience social and emotional transitions as they enter parenthood. There are changes in their relationship to each other, to their parents, and to society. During this time, unresolved emotional issues involving their own parents are often reactivated and can be worked through in new ways. For example, the new grandparent's desire to be involved and helpful with his or her grandchild may bring up old feelings in the parent of being criticized or talked down to. Conversely, the parent's request for assistance or advice may cause the grandparent to feel old, painful emotions from a time when the parent, during adolescence, angrily rejected such help.

Given their profound biological, psychological, and social significance, pregnancy, childbirth, and parenthood inevitably have many psychosocial meanings. To the parent, a child may represent both a deeply experienced extension of the self and an intensely loved separate individual. In both meanings, the child may fulfill intense needs for self-definition and fulfillment. The child confirms the parents' fertility or virility and represents a consummation of their relationship. The child embodies hopes for the roles of parenthood, the formation of a family, the emotional experiencing and re-experiencing of life's developmental stages, and the extension of life beyond the parents' mortality. For the parent, the couple, and society, the birth of the child may represent a step into adulthood that signifies a variety of social roles including emancipation from parents, acceptance of new levels of responsibility, and a contribution to the social order and the growth of the family or community.

However, not all meanings and associations are positive, especially if the pregnancy is unwanted or if the parents' relationship is ambivalent, tenuous, or ended. Even the most desired pregnancy brings fears of the child's possible disability or imperfection and results in changes and losses in each parent's life and in the couple's relationship (Butani, 1974; Kessler, 1979f; Solnit & Stark, 1961).

When the child has a birth defect or is diagnosed with a genetic disease, there is a serious disruption in the meanings and processes just described. Some of the parents' worst fears have come true! They now confront many practical and emotional tasks, and guilt, shame, and uncertainty may cloud their own relationship and that with otherwise supportive family and friends. As Solnit and Stark (1961) so clearly describe, the parents face the dual, conflicting tasks of mourning the lost, hoped for perfect child and addressing the complex needs and the emotional impact of the actual child.

Ambivalent and negative feelings toward one's child are a normal experience of parenthood, evoked by the child's needs and demands and their inevitable conflict with the parent's other obligations, wishes, and desires. When the child has a serious disability, these feelings are often intensified, and they may include conscious or unconscious death wishes. The parent often experiences these feelings with deep guilt and shame, and they may be among the most difficult for the parent to acknowledge (Laborde & Seligman, 1991; Mintzer et al., 1984). One of the critically important roles for parent support groups is to provide a relatively safe place to express and normalize these feelings. Their expression and acknowledgment by other parents in similar circumstances provide a measure of acceptance, and thus self-acceptance, that is very difficult to obtain from people, including genetic counselors, who are not in similar circumstances.

Coping Strategies

The circumstances under which counselees enter genetic counseling differ greatly in the amount of stress and anxiety that is involved. At one point on this multidimensional spectrum we might consider a counselee requesting prenatal diagnosis for maternal age. She has had a previous pregnancy in which amniocentesis gave normal results and a healthy daughter was born. She feels confident in the clinic to which she has returned and, with minimal anxiety, looks forward to the reassurance that is the most likely outcome of repeating prenatal diagnosis in her current pregnancy. At another point on this spectrum, consider a young woman in her first pregnancy. During routine ultrasound at an obstetrics visit to which she has come alone, possible fetal abnormalities are found whose implications are for the present unknown. Unexpectedly and instantaneously, her hopes and dreams for her future child are threatened, and she encounters a new world of unfamiliar terms, medical specialists, and critical decisions. For both of these counselees, and for all who enter genetic counseling, the nature and extent of the resources available for coping with ongoing stresses and new developments are of critical importance.

In broad terms, coping strategies are of two types. They may be problem-focused, directed toward changing the circumstances confronting the individual, or they may be emotion-focused, directed toward reducing emotional distress (Lazarus, 1999). Within each of these categories is an array of possibilities that are determined, in part, by the nature of the situation (Djurdjinovic, 1998; Schneider, 1994). For example, over time the young woman discussed before may use a number of problem-focused coping strategies in response to the ultrasound findings. She may telephone her partner, asking him to join her so she and he can face the situation together. Following discussions with a genetic counselor, additional diagnostic testing may be undertaken to better define the problem and identify available options. If the couple decides to continue the pregnancy and the child is born with a disability, they may obtain medical treatment that improves the child's health and well-being, and either or both may make financial or work adjustments to help meet the added financial obligations they have incurred.

There is a similarly broad range of emotion-focused coping strategies. The woman may seek additional social support from parents or friends. She may find support in her religious beliefs. The couple may take walks in a local park, using physical activity, the experience of nature, and the opportunity to share pleasant experiences to reduce their anxiety and preoccupation with their child's potential difficulties. After the child is born, they may seek further information concerning her disability, knowing from previous experience that this cognitive activity helps reduce their anxiety and sense of helplessness.

As a general rule, when a stressful situation is amenable to change that will reduce its negative or undesirable aspects, problem-focused strategies predominate. When the situation appears unchangeable, emotion-focused strategies predominate, and they may have a critical role in the individual's psychological adaptation to the new set of circumstances. However, as the examples illustrate, the division between problem-focused and emotion-focused strategies is not absolute. The search for information serves both ends, and several of the other strategies discussed also have elements of both. Equally important, the nature of a stressful situation and the coping strategies it elicits are not static, but evolve over time (Lazarus, 1999). Thus, initial anxiety, fear, or shock may lead to an emphasis on emotion-focused coping strategies. As these and other factors help reduce emotional intensity, and as further information identifies practical steps that can be taken, problem-focused strategies may come to the fore.

Individuals differ in the nature and range of coping strategies they use. For example, some people cope by seeking information. For others, however, new information increases fears and anxiety, and they cope by avoiding additional information. Other aspects of personality also influence the manner in which stressful situations are perceived and the extent to which various forms of coping, such as active versus passive approaches, individual effort versus social support, are utilized (Lazarus, 1999). In addition, there are, on average, gender differences, with men tending to adopt more action-oriented approaches and women using more emotion-oriented strategies (Rando, 1985; Rubin, 1983).

Understanding these differences in coping patterns is helpful to the genetic counselor as she assists counselees in developing and strengthening the means for meeting unexpected or undesired situations. However, the most useful clinical approach involves attempting to understand how and to what extent the individual perceives the situation as a threat to his or her well-being and as taxing or exceeding the resources available for coping with it. It is through the counselee's appraisal of the situation and assignment of meaning to it that personal and social factors and the subjective aspects of the circumstances create emotional stress and activate coping responses (Lazarus, 1999; Pargament, 1997). Thus, careful exploration of the counselee's hopes and wishes, fears and concerns, cognitive and emotional responses to the situation, and perceptions of internal and external resources for responding to it is essential to this aspect of genetic counseling.

These issues can be illustrated by examining counselees' differing reactions to the risk of spontaneous abortion following prenatal diagnosis. For example, a professional couple, in their midthirties with two children, may view the risk as minimal when compared to avoiding the birth of a child with a disability, whose needs they believe would interfere with their life plans. Minimal coping is required for them to handle the risk of procedure-induced abortion. By contrast, for a couple in their early forties, who have conceived their first child after several unsuccessful rounds of fertility treatments, the increased risk of spontaneous abortion may threaten the fulfillment of their hopes and dreams. If they are also concerned about having a child with a disability, they may need a variety of coping strategies to manage their anxiety and determine the most appropriate course of action. If the emotional burden of unsuccessful fertility treatments and the recurring decision whether to continue with additional rounds of treatment have left the couple emotionally drained, this new decision may feel overwhelming. In this case, much of their coping may be emotion-focused. However, if they feel relatively strong emotionally, their coping strategies may be primarily problem-focused. It is only by understanding these aspects of each counselee's responses to the circumstances that the genetic counselor can make appropriate interventions.

An important coping mechanism not yet discussed involves reappraisal of the situation so as to put the circumstances or the means for coping with it in a more favorable light. Although the relationship between reappraisal and coping is complex, there is evidence that positive reappraisal is associated with more successful coping and adaptation (Lazarus, 1999). As the following vignette illustrates, the genetic counselor can often assist in this process by broadening the counselee's view of the situation, suggesting additional ways for dealing with it, or helping reduce emotions whose intensity interferes with thinking and planning.

> Following the birth of a child with Treacher Collins syndrome, the parents were upset and depressed by his facial abnormalities and congenital deafness and by the prospect of high medical costs and anticipated stigmatization. After responding empathically to their emotional distress, the genetic counselor discussed the possibilities for reconstructive surgery and explored the resources available to assist families of children with birth defects. At her suggestion, the counselees visited a family who had a four-year-old son born with similar features and severity. They were encouraged by the child's cognitive and social development and by the outcome of surgery. In addition, they recognized the parents' courage and determination and the depth of their love for their child. With the genetic counselor's assistance, the counselees reassessed the medical and social implications for their son. Equally important, they began to appreciate how their own feelings of love and of commitment to family would support them through what lay ahead and would, in all probability, be strengthened in the process.

Much of what follows in this book is relevant to the process of assisting counselees in assessing their situation and in developing and using appropriate coping strategies.

The Search for Meaning

The occurrence of an adverse event also initiates a more fundamental search
for meaning. An unexpected negative experience shatters the belief in an orderly, meaningful world, in which events are comprehensible and outcomes
are related to behavior in some understandable way. This experience of a random, uncaring universe creates psychological pain and disorientation and a
sense of anxiety and emptiness that can be threatening or overwhelming. There
is an urgent need to recreate a sense of meaning within which the event can
be understood. This often leads to the existential question, "Why did this happen to me (and my family)?" It may involve attempts to understand the event
within a larger religious or spiritual framework. There may be an intense search
for an agent of responsibility, even if this involves assuming personal blame or
guilt (Pargament, 1997; Shapiro, 1994). This search can include a driven need
to understand, at a personally meaningful level, the "cause" of a birth defect
or genetic disease.

The explanations of etiology provided in genetic counseling may help meet
this fundamental need for meaning, especially for counselees who have a predominantly scientific orientation toward understanding the world. However,
counselees often draw on other beliefs and belief systems as well. These beliefs may be held in addition to scientific explanations, from which they may
be psychologically compartmentalized or held in a hierarchical relationship
(Panter-Brick, 1992; Weil, 1991; Rokeach, 1960). As an example of compart-
mentalization, a father may rationally accept the autosomal recessive explanation for his child's cystic fibrosis while emotionally feeling very strongly that it
is due to his adolescent use of recreational drugs. Hierarchically, a mother may
understand trisomy 21 as the mechanistic explanation for her child's Down syndrome, but draw emotional support and comfort from her firmly held belief
that it is God's will. In both cases, the genetic explanation is accepted at one
level, but the personal meaning of the situation comes in large part from other
beliefs. Thus, in the process of presenting and explaining scientific information, the genetic counselor must be respectful of alternative beliefs because of
their potential importance in the search for meaning.

The search for meaning may underlie many of the questions and actions of
counselees. As just discussed, questions about etiology, including possible causes
that seem unlikely or farfetched to the genetic counselor, may be an attempt to

resolve the existential question, "Why did this happen to me?" Questions about what the counselor would do or what other counselees have done may involve a search for clues to how others have ascribed meaning to a similar situation. Willingness to participate in research may involve the desire to impart a larger, more positive meaning to the individual or family misfortune. Furthermore, the search for meaning may play a role in counselee's feelings of guilt and responsibility (Chodoff et al., 1964; Kessler et al., 1984; see later under Guilt and Shame). Thus, the genetic counselor must keep in mind the central importance of the search for meaning and be alert to its many possible manifestations.

Psychological Defenses

Psychological defenses, commonly referred to simply as "defenses," are related to coping strategies yet differ in significant ways. Emotion-focused coping involves conscious activities that attempt to reduce emotional distress. By contrast, psychological defenses are *unconscious* mental processes by which painful, unacceptable, or threatening emotions, wishes, or fears are kept from reaching consciousness. These threatening emotions and thoughts may arise internally, as from unresolved childhood experiences with one's parents, or they may be evoked by external events (Gabbard, 1995). Often, the two sources are interconnected. For example, the birth of a child with a severe birth defect may engender anger. This in turn may activate anxiety that originated in childhood experiences with the expression of anger.

There is no universally agreed upon list of psychological defenses, which reflects the fact that the actual mental processes are complex and multidimensional. Nevertheless, a number of defenses are well defined and commonly accepted, and several of these, discussed below, are particularly relevant to genetic counseling (Gabbard, 1995; Schneider & Marnane, 1997).

Repression, in which feelings, perceptions, or memories are lost to consciousness. While repression is a defense in its own right, it is also a component of all other defenses.

Denial, in which the reality of a situation or perception is not consciously experienced or recognized.

Intellectualization, in which the emotional responses to a situation are repressed and the situation is addressed through rational, cognitive processes.

Displacement, in which the expression of an emotion to the appropriate recipient is unacceptable or anxiety producing, and the emotion is thus expressed to a more socially acceptable recipient. For example, anger felt toward a partner who has transmitted a dominant allele to a child is redirected to the genetic counselor who has explained the genetics.

Sublimation, in which wishes or drives that are deemed unacceptable are channeled into more socially acceptable activities. For example, pain and anger over a child with a serious disability are channeled into committed, thoughtful work for a parent support group.

Reaction formation, in which the individual utilizes the *opposite* action or emotion to ward off unacceptable emotions or wishes. For example, compliance and agreement are used to avoid awareness of and the expression of anger.

Projection, in which repressed or unacceptable emotions or wishes are perceived as residing in others. For example, a counselee who is feeling deep but unacceptable shame perceives that his or her partner is ashamed.

Projective identification, in which the individual's behavior induces a repressed or unacceptable emotion in another person. For example, a parent who is angry over a child's disability, but who in childhood learned to repress anger because of his own parent's responses to it, acts toward the genetic counselor in a manner that makes the counselor feel angry.

This last example allows us to look more closely at the psychological complexity that often underlies defensive processes. By inducing anger in the genetic counselor rather than expressing it himself, the parent obtains emotional protection and relief in three ways: First, he can deny his unacceptable and anxiety-producing anger because it is not he who is expressing it. Second, his projected perception of anger in the genetic counselor, as well as any actual expression of anger by her, can be disapproved of or condemned in a manner similar to that which he experienced from his parents when he was a child. Thus, he continues a defensive pattern established in childhood and, rather than being conscious of the pain and dysfunction it has caused, identifies with those who induced it. Finally, the genetic counselor's perceived or actual anger allows the parent to express and experience his own anger, albeit vicariously.

There are implications for the genetic counselor as well. If she is unaware of the induced anger, she may act it out with an angry or unsupportive comment or through more long-term responses such as failing to provide full follow-up after the session. If this happens, her countertransference has resulted in therapeutically inappropriate actions. However, if she is aware of the induced anger, she can avoid such inappropriate responses. In addition, she may be better able to perceive and respond appropriately to the parent's repressed anger. In this case, her countertransference has played a positive role in the counseling process (see Chapter 3 under Countertransference).

Because they distort perceptions of reality and reduce the individual's range of emotions and potential behavioral responses, defenses are commonly thought of as contributing to psychological dysfunction or pathology. Indeed, when unduly strong or rigid, defenses do have this role. However, psychological defenses are also critical to healthy mental functioning. When defenses are inadequate for the internal and external stressors an individual faces, he or she is psychologically vulnerable to anxieties and fears, to the experience of emotions that threatened the sense of self, and to the potential for more serious psychological decompensation. Thus, defenses are most functional when operating at a midlevel of intensity, with a flexible, adaptable repertoire (Chodoff et al., 1964; Falek, 1984).

The role of defenses in supporting healthy psychological functioning can be illustrated with the example of denial of one's own mortality. On the one hand, inappropriately strong denial can lead to life-threatening recklessness or inattention to physical health. On the other hand, a variety of situations, such as the death of a loved one or the experience of a natural catastrophe, may temporarily overwhelm this denial, leading to an acute awareness of one's own eventual death. This may cause intense anxiety, fear, or hopelessness, and it can significantly interfere with the ability to function in everyday life. When this occurs, the return to psychological equilibrium usually involves a re-strengthening of denial. It may also involve other defenses. For example, intellectualization may allow one to think through aspects of the experience without reliving the full emotional impact. In addition, philosophical or spiritual acceptance may reduce the need for denial.

Psychological defenses are related to coping strategies (Kroeber, 1964). For example, the defense of denial, in which emotions or information are unconsciously repressed, is related to the more conscious coping strategy of concentration, in which one intentionally sets aside emotions or thoughts in order to facilitate thinking or acting. Similarly, as the example discussed earlier in Coping Strategies illustrates, the defense of intellectualization is closely related to the coping strategy that involves seeking information. The relationship between defenses and coping is continuous, with no clear-cut demarcation, and is yet another indication of the role of defenses in supporting healthy psychological functioning.

The continuum of dysfunctional defenses, functional defenses, and coping strategies is illustrated in the following example, which also shows the interrelated involvement of several different defenses.

Immediately following the diagnosis of Hurler syndrome in his son, a father made a driven search for information about the disorder and displayed virtually no emotion. This helped him through the acute pain of the first few days. Had this driven search persisted, it would have interfered with his relationship with his wife and child as well as his own emotional accommodation to the situation. However, within a few days he expressed more emotion, was able to comfort his wife, but still had an intense desire to obtain information. After two months, he had acknowledged and worked through some of his initial feelings. At this time, he used his knowledge and understanding to help plan for his son's treatment. In addition, he consciously recognized that reading and thinking about the disorder helped calm him when he experienced periods of fear and hopelessness.

Although psychological defenses, strictly defined, are unconscious, they are an established and well-recognized concept in contemporary society. Thus, they are not always, in reality, entirely unconscious. For example, people often have some awareness that they are being "defensive" or are redirecting their anger toward a safer or more socially acceptable target. This broad awareness of defenses influences the thinking of genetic counselors as well, and it can lead to overattribution or misattribution of defenses, particularly denial. Lubinsky (1994) has shown that what is commonly labeled "denial" can actually involve a variety of other processes. He identifies three of these "mimics of denial" and describes appropriate interventions for each:

Disbelief occurs when the information provided is heard but not accepted, because it does not appear to make sense. For example, the signs and symptoms on which a diagnosis of Down syndrome is based when an infant does not have major medical problems may not appear serious or convincing to the child's parents. The child appears normal, the signs and symptoms are individually not outside the range of normality, and it goes against the parents' hopes and expectations that the child has a major disabling syndrome (Applebaum & Firestein, 1983) When the genetic counselor recognizes the characteristics of disbelief, as opposed to applying the more general assessment of denial, she may intervene in a more appropriate and empathic manner. Responses of disbelief are best addressed by prioritizing and promoting necessary treatments or interventions, while allowing time for the information and its implications to be understood and accepted through repetition and experience.

With *deferral,* the information is accepted but the implications are not. This defense helps prevent the impact of the information from exceeding the counselee's psychological or physical resources. It allows time for adaptation and coping before the full impact is felt. Canceled or missed appointments at the time of a potential or recent serious diagnosis are an example, in which the counselee acts to defer the time at which the new information must be faced. Deferral is a relatively common situation in cancer risk counseling. The primary danger of deferral is that essential diagnosis or treatment will be forgone or delayed. Deferral is best addressed by empathically acknowledging that the information is scary or difficult to face while helping the counselee obtain or mobilize social or psychological resources for coping.

Dismissal involves devaluing or attacking the legitimacy of the professional or the profession from which bad news is received. This is often accompanied by anger, which may be a defense against fear or shame. Dismissal may be addressed by acknowledging the anger, emphasizing aspects of diagnosis or treatment that the counselee does accept at least tentatively, carefully exploring areas of disagreement, and maintaining a nonjudgmental stance that does not return the counselee's anger or dismissive judgments. However, dismissal, especially if coupled with anger, can evoke strong emotions in the genetic counselor. If unrecognized, these emotions may interfere with the counselor's ability to maintain an empathic, nonjudgmental stance, or they may lead to a retaliatory dismissal of the counselee as "in denial." Thus, as with other aspects of genetic counseling, attention to countertransference issues is essential.

In the short-term work of most genetic counseling, counselees are often best helped when the counselor supports the development of a variety of defenses, of midrange intensity, that are flexible and adaptable to evolving circumstances. In many instances this involves strengthening functional defenses. In other circumstances it involves attempting to reduce rigid or overly utilized defenses. An individual's use of specific defenses can sometimes be engaged to help develop useful coping mechanisms. Lubinsky's (1994) emphasis on careful analysis of defenses, empathic understanding of the counselee's psychological situation, support for appropriate coping and defenses, and appreciation of the value of the passage of time are examples of this approach.

The Coping Process

When a highly negative or stressful event occurs, such as the birth of a child with a birth defect or the diagnosis of a genetic disorder, a sequence of psychological responses is initiated. These involve the psychological processes discussed above as they evolve and interrelate over time.

The initial response to bad news is shock and a rapid mobilization of defenses (Falek, 1984). The individual often experiences a sense of disbelief, numbness, or unreality, with the commonly expressed feeling, "I can't believe this is happening." This is an involuntary psychophysiological process that buffers the emotional impact and prevents potentially more serious psychological disorganization. During this phase, the ability to understand and utilize information is very limited. Often the initial information, such as "Unfortunately, I have to tell you that your daughter has Prader-Willi syndrome," is all that registers before numbness and withdrawal set in. While numbness and disbelief may persist, the acute stage of this phase may be relatively brief.

With the passage of time, and confronted by the ongoing reality of the situation, the initial shock and numbness partially subside and the individual's intellectual acceptance increases. There is a beginning attempt to understand the meaning of the event and its implications, which leads to consideration of possible courses of action. The person is more open to receiving and discussing information. When decisions must be made, the individual can begin to muster the psychological resources to do so. The initial stages of the coping process and the value of understanding them is illustrated in the following example.

A couple was informed by telephone in the evening that amniocentesis indicated their fetus had trisomy 18. The conversation was brief and the genetic counselor expressed sadness and compassion concerning the news. A counseling session was scheduled for the following day. By the time of the session, the initial shock had begun to subside and the couple had begun to process the information and discuss what they would do next. The evening timing of the call was chosen because both parents would be at home and thus the initial phase of shock and numbness would occur when the couple were together.

The passage of time and the demands of reality also lead to an initial breakthrough of emotions (Chodoff et al., 1964; Kubler-Ross, 1969). Anxiety, a sense of increased vulnerability, and a great sense of loss may be the first emotions experienced. In a very deep sense, the expected, hoped for, "normal" outcome and life course have been irrevocably lost. Anger is common—outrage at what fate has wrought. It may be displaced onto specific individuals, including the genetic counselor, or toward the self (Benkendorf, 1987). Guilt and shame are common. Depression may result from several sources. It may be a direct result of the experience of loss or it may derive from guilt, shame, or anger directed toward the self. It may be preparatory, in anticipation of future losses, such as a child's severe future limitations or eventual death. Although it may be less consciously experienced, there is often a deep sense of narcissistic injury.

The shattered expectations of normality can themselves lead to a number of emotions and psychological defenses. There may be magical thinking—something will intervene and it will all turn out all right (Falek, 1984). There may be "bargaining" with God or fate: "If only I (we) are given another chance, I will do such and such" (Kubler-Ross, 1969). When a child is born with an observable or diagnosable disorder, a complex process of mourning the loss of the hoped for normal child must be carried out at the same time as the realities of the actual child's condition are confronted (Solnit & Stark, 1961).

Again, with time, a new phase occurs in which there is a renewed sense of psychological equilibrium. The transition to this phase depends on several factors. These include adequate expression and subsequent reduction of the various emotions, the evolution of defenses appropriate to the new situation, the development of coping mechanisms sufficient to address both the individual's emotions and the requirements of the situation, and mourning coupled with psychological and spiritual adjustment so that the new situation can be experienced as the real, if difficult, course of events. As discussed earlier, under Coping Strategies, changes in the perceived meaning of the event or situation are an important component of this process (Lazarus, 1999).

As the preceding discussion indicates, there is an expectable pattern or "natural history" to the coping process. However, for any given individual, the specific course is influenced by many factors (Lazarus, 1999). These include the person's repertoire of defenses and coping mechanisms and, more generally, the psychological resources and previous experiences that he or she brings to the situation. The nature and extent of family, social, and spiritual resources are major determinants, as are the specifics of the situation the individual must confront and the medical, financial, and other external resources that are available. In addition, the coping process is highly cyclical, and several elements may be experienced simultaneously. Emotions break through to consciousness, ebb, and then recur, repeatedly. Coping mechanisms and defenses strengthen, then weaken in response to the underlying emotions and to the sustained realities that must be confronted, and then strengthen again. Often, specific events or situations play a role in this cycling. Furthermore, there may be incomplete processing of any of the emotions. Thus, greater or lesser elements of denial, grief, mourning, guilt, and shame may persist and become part of the new reality (Falek, 1984).

Much of the critical work of genetic counseling can be understood in terms of this coping process. In the initial phase of shock and numbness, the genetic counselor's empathy and respect for the necessary withdrawal, even if brief, are critical. If information must be provided, it should be limited in scope and primarily designed to set the stage for further discussion at a later time.

As the individual emerges from shock, the need to address the ongoing situation, the coping mechanisms of intellectual activity and rational thought, and the related defenses all promote the acquisition of information and the attempt to make rational decisions. Thus, the counselee becomes more receptive to and desirous of the informational content of counseling and the process of decision making. At the same time, the intense, fluctuating emotions that are repeatedly experienced require the empathic, knowledgeable interventions of the genetic counselor. The counselor must be alert to emotions or psychodynamic issues around which the counselee appears to be "stuck," whose intensity or longevity appear to seriously compromise functioning. These require that an effort be made at referral for appropriate professional assistance and/or group support.

From a broader psychosocial perspective, eliciting the counselee's emotional responses is critical to reaching decisions that will serve the counselee's long-term needs, resources, and values. Finally, the complex process of psychological accommodation that marks the final phase of the coping process provides additional opportunities for the information of genetic counseling to be incorporated into the counselee's new world view.

Because of individual variability, spouses or partners frequently have different primary defenses and coping mechanisms, and they may proceed at different rates through the phases and cycles of the coping process. Although there may be great strength in this complementarity, it can also be a source of pain and misunderstanding. In addition, family, friends, and acquaintances may fail to recognize the intensity of emotions and may express a more optimistic view than the counselee feels. This can contribute to a sense of social isolation and place an additional burden on interactions with others.

Self-esteem and Narcissistic Injury

Efforts to maintain one's feelings of self-esteem play a central role in psychological functioning. A sense of ethical and moral consistency, of the ability to adapt effectively to life's challenges, and of self-worth and dignity all contribute to the experience of self-esteem. It is further enhanced by social standing and acceptance, by one's achievements and possessions, and by the personal and social validation one receives from various relationships. Unfavorable events, the judgments of others, and failure to maintain one's own sense of achievement and integrity work to undermine self-esteem (Baumeister, 1993; Elson, 1987).

Underlying the relatively conscious experience of self-esteem is a more fundamental, often largely unconscious experience of innate self-worth and ability to love oneself. Although the term *narcissism* is commonly thought of as involving dysfunctional self-centeredness, it is also used to describe this healthy, functional feeling of self-worth. This usage is illustrated by the phrase "narcissistic injury," which implies that something of value has been injured. When appropriately integrated into the adult personality, narcissism provides a "healthy enjoyment of our own activities and successes . . . an adaptively useful sense of disappointment tinged with anger and shame over our failures and shortcomings . . . [and] a healthy sense of direction and [a] beacon for our activities and pursuits" (Kohut, 1966, p. 254).

Functional adult narcissism (as well as its dysfunction and pathology) has its origins in infancy and early childhood. The infant, who cannot yet distinguish self from others, experiences physical comfort and well-being, and his mother's empathic care, as due to his central place in the world: "When I am hungry and cry, I get fed." The toddler, who is still developing a sense of independent psychological existence, feels fundamentally loved and valued when her parent applauds her achievements or provides comfort and shelter when the enlarging world she is exploring feels scary. With its origins in the empathic responses of others and in feelings of well-being and achievement, narcissism is vulnerable to the loss of loved individuals and relationships, to feelings of failure or shame, and to the sense that events are spinning out of control. Furthermore, given its origins in the earliest stages of life, narcissistic injuries are experienced as deeply painful and often difficult to describe in words. They can involve a sense of having lost part of one's self, of disorientation and disintegration, and of a debilitating, pervasive loss of control (Elson, 1987).

Many of the experiences and situations surrounding genetic counseling can cause narcissistic injury and loss of self-esteem. Genetic disorders and birth defects shatter hopes and dreams, at least initially, and their diagnosis can produce profound feelings of loss of control. A sense of defectiveness and stigmatization may result from one's own illness or disability, from that of one's child, or from knowledge of a familial disorder or one's own genetic contribution to a child's disorder. Infertility, fetal demise, abortion for genetic reasons, the death of a child or adult, the loss of the hoped for perfect child, or the loss of body parts in the treatment or prophylaxis of cancer may all evoke a deep sense of personal diminution and the severing of deeply valued relationships to self or others (Kessler, 1979c, Chapters 6–12). Thus, it is essential that the genetic counselor support and enhance the counselee's self-esteem and respond empathically to narcissistic injuries.

Much of the material in this book supports these efforts by promoting informed, empathic understanding and responses. However, the genetic counselor can also make specific interventions (see Chapter 3 under Empathy, Genuineness, and Unconditional Positive Regard and Promoting Competence and Autonomy). Counselees frequently have limited or primarily negative perceptions of the situation they confront or of their own actions and responses. Direct affirmation of the counselee's skills, integrity, insights, fortitude, and courage, both regarding the issues relevant to genetic counseling and the broader aspects of the counselee's life, can be very helpful and are often gratefully received (Kessler, 1997b). Such affirmations provide direct support, recapitulate positive formative interactions from childhood, and mobilize positive self-images (Spencer et al., 1993). But beyond specific interventions, the empathic attention to detail and the relatively generous allotment of time involved in much of genetic counseling may also be perceived by counselees as affirming their inherent self-worth.

Grief and Mourning

The intense, often agonizing pain of grief and the complex process of mourning are responses to loss. The death of a beloved person is the paramount cause of grief and mourning. Among such situations, parental grief and mourning are among the most intense and devastating, owing to the multiple hopes, attachments, and sources of meaning involved in the parent–child relationship (Rubin, 1993; Shapiro, 1994). Other forms of parental loss or loss of potential parenthood also cause grief and mourning: miscarriage and stillbirth, abortion following prenatal diagnosis, fetal reduction for multifetal pregnancies, and infertility (Dallaire et al., 1995; McKinney et al., 1996; Meyers et al., 1995b; Seller et al., 1993). Grief and mourning may also result from the loss of current or future capabilities by oneself or by others to whom one has strong attachments, as in the birth and life of an affected child or the loss of one's own abilities due to a progressive genetic disease. Thus, the genetic counselor will encounter grief and mourning caused by the circumstances that lead to or arise from genetic counseling. However, grief may also occur in genetic counseling when memories and emotions related to old losses, such as spontaneous abortions, are evoked in obtaining medical and family histories.

Two major tasks confront the individual who has suffered such a loss: There is "a crisis of attachment and a crisis of identity" (Shapiro, 1994, p. 14). The initial intense grief and the welter of other emotional responses such as shock, anger, and guilt resulting from the loss may be overwhelming, cause great pain, and interfere with effective functioning. There is thus an intense need to regain emotional control. At the same time, the death of a loved person or the loss of a significant capability restricts the context in which life is lived, affecting relationships, activities, and meaning . Thus, there is a concurrent need to redefine the nature and meaning of one's life. Ultimately, this involves reestablishing one's own identity; finding meaning in the circumstances that led to the loss; and developing a new relationship to the lost individual, or in the case of pre- or perinatal loss, to the individual who might have been.

Clinical lore, cultural attitudes, and some commonly cited references have perpetuated a number of beliefs about mourning: that it involves a sequence of more or less distinct stages related to those of the coping process; that it can be completed with some form of final resolution within a relatively limited period of time; that full expression of emotions is always healing; and that "normal" mourning can be clearly distinguished from that which is abnormal or pathological. However, a significant body of evidence, encompassing all the causes of mourning listed above, suggests that mourning is in many cases a more complex, cyclical, protracted, and individualized experience than these beliefs imply. Thus, uncritical acceptance of these common beliefs, whether by professionals, friends and family, or the mourning individual, can create misunderstanding, social isolation, and incorrect assumptions of pathology (Shapiro, 1994; Wortman & Silver, 1989). A more complex understanding is required.

There are undoubtedly different phases of grief and mourning. The gasping shock of the initial moments or days differs in many ways from the pain and loss that remain when emotional fluctuations and daily functioning have returned to a more familiar pattern. The stages of grief that have been identified by various authors are descriptive of some of the sustained experiences of mourning and of their temporal relationships. However, the various elements of mourning are interrelated, there are shifts back and forth from one set of emotions and thoughts to another, and the process is cyclical at the same time as it evolves. In addition, some individuals do not show intense distress, depression, and emotional working through after major loss. Available evidence suggests that these individuals do not have poorer long-term emotional or adaptive outcomes than those individuals whose responses are more openly emotional (Wortman & Silver, 1989).

Although most people reach a state of relative resolution and adaptive functioning, mourning may continue for years. For some people, the remainder of life is deeply affected by the loss or losses of loved ones. Prenatal and perinatal loss can result in continuing, low-level grief decades later. After such an interval of time, individuals who report only occasional thoughts of the loss may nevertheless have strong emotions when the issues are again raised (Rosenblatt & Burns, 1986; Seller et al., 1993).

Grief and mourning can be reactivated by a variety of expected and unexpected experiences. For example, when a child has died or a pregnancy has been lost, encounters with children, parents, or childhood situations may have this effect. This can involve memories of the child who was and thoughts of whom he or she would have become. When a child has mental or physical disabilities, grief and mourning may arise at the time of missed developmental milestones, such as when other similarly aged children are learning to walk or are entering college, or when milestones such as talking or playing simple games are reached at a very delayed age (Marshak et al., 1999). Grief and mourning may also be reactivated at specific times, such as the due date for a lost pregnancy or the anniversary of a loss. The mind's unconscious ability to track and respond to such dates is remarkable. Counselees may be unaware that such a time point is the cause of renewed grief. Recognition of the cause may help alleviate both the grief and concern that its reactivation is unpredictable and out of control.

Social support, from within and outside the family, plays an important role in mitigating the pain of grief and in facilitating healing. However, the mourning individual faces several sources of potential social isolation and loss of support. The person who is grieving may attempt to avoid reminders of the loss, such as friends who have children of a similar age. Friends, relatives, and acquaintances may feel unclear about how to approach the grieving individual or threatened by the feelings of vulnerability that the grieving individual's loss and pain raises (Rando, 1985; Shapiro, 1994). Not infrequently, partners, family members, professionals, and others who could provide support minimize the effects of perinatal loss or assume that grief for a given loss should be completed after some discrete period of time. If the grieving individual accepts the belief that perinatal losses are insignificant or that grief is time-limited, contrary experiences can lead to feelings of being abnormal or fears of mental illness (Kolker & Burke, 1993). For those who have experienced prenatal loss or infertility, the lack of rituals for acknowledging the loss and expressing grief can compound feelings of social isolation (Seller et al., 1993).

Given the diversity of experience among those individuals whose overall adaptation appears adequate, there is no professional consensus regarding "normal" as opposed to abnormal or pathological grief and mourning. It does appear that the hoped for adaptation should involve a return to adequate day-to-day functioning, relative emotional stability, and emotional resources that allow joy and enthusiasm for life and relationships; not, it will be noted, the end of grief. Concern regarding pathology should be based on long-term failure to achieve these adaptations or on other more definable problems such as continuing depression or somatic complaints (Middleton et al., 1993; Shapiro, 1994).

The genetic counselor can have an important role in helping grieving counselees. To do so, she must identify the nature of the loss, its emotional impact, and the possible role of previous losses in the counselee's current grief (Raphael et al., 1993). The genetic counselor can provide guidance by explaining the diversity of grieving responses and giving emotional support during recurring painful periods of mourning. Although expressions of grief are often helpful, the counselor must also honor situations in which the counselee feels the need to control emotions either individually or within the family (Shapiro, 1994). Counselees should also be assisted in identifying and addressing sources of social isolation. Referral to support groups or to other professionals may be helpful. However, referrals should be presented as a response to the specific needs of the counselee, not on the basis of presumed or implied pathology (see Chapter 3 under Mental Health Referrals).

It is important to recognize that even the brief interventions of a single genetic counseling session may be very helpful, at least in part because they relieve the sense of isolation (Rosenblatt, 1988). However, follow-up phone calls or sessions may be important in providing continued support for the recurring and long-term aspects of mourning.

Guilt and Shame

Guilt and shame are normal responses to adverse events over which one has little or no control, as well as to aspects of life such as sexuality and bodily functions that have guilt- or shame-related social connotations. Thus, many situations relevant to genetic counseling inherently evoke guilt and shame. These include the birth or diagnosis of an affected child, the state of being at increased risk of having an affected child, identification as a heterozygous carrier or the transmitter of a dominant or X-linked mutation, being a nonaffected member of a family with affected individuals, and abortion following prenatal diagnosis or detection of abnormality by ultrasound (Chapple et al., 1995; Kessler et al., 1984; Suslak et al., 1995). A parent's normal, ambivalent feelings toward an affected child, which sometimes include anger and death wishes, may result in intense guilt and shame (Laborde & Seligman, 1991). Issues of sexuality, reproduction, and infertility may evoke long-standing feelings of guilt or shame, in which attitudes developed in childhood or adolescence underlie responses to the circumstances involved in genetic counseling (Kessler et al., 1984). Many other interactions with genetic counselors and other health care providers, if not handled thoughtfully by the professional, may also evoke or exacerbate feelings of guilt and shame.

The terms "guilt," or more accurately, "guilt feelings" or "sense of guilt," and "shame" are sometimes used interchangeably, or with one subsumed beneath the other. However, the two emotions are distinct, although interrelated, and an understanding of their differences is essential for correct identification and effective intervention. In addition, their roles differ among cultures. In the dominant culture of the United States, guilt is more readily acknowledged and acceptable than shame (Kessler et al., 1984). There is, as Kaufman (1996, p. 4) states, "shame about shame." However, shame is a central, acknowledged experience in many other cultures (Wang & Marsh, 1992).

In the dominant culture of the United States, the emotional distress of guilt is well known. Feelings of guilt often include rather detailed thoughts, memories, or internal dialogue. These may involve the event or situation that produced the guilt, personal actions or inactions that are thought to have contributed to what happened, and feelings of being punished for one's transgressions. Because of the high ideational content and relative social acceptability of guilt feelings, individuals may, under appropriate circumstances, acknowledge and describe their experience of guilt in considerable detail. In contrast, shame has limited ideational content. It is primarily experienced physiologically, in reactions such as blushing, and emotionally, with feelings of failure, inadequacy, helplessness, and exposure. Whereas guilt involves a sense of the self as a responsible agent *in* the world, shame involves feelings of exposure and judgment *by* the world. Individuals may certainly be aware of feeling shame. However, the experience is often internal, unexpressed, or unconscious (Kaufman, 1996; Kessler et al., 1984).

A brief description of theories concerning the origin and manifestations of guilt and shame will assist the genetic counselor to accurately identify and respond to these emotions. Psychoanalytically derived theories relate guilt to a sense of failure with respect to internalized standards of social, moral, and ethical responsibility. Both the internalized standards and the fear of punishment originate in the growing child's interactions with parents and are elaborated and strengthened by broader social interactions and cultural values. In many cultures guilt plays a major role in developing, defining, and maintaining a person's relationships to others and to society. Thus, in addition to the internal, self-monitoring dynamic, guilt may be induced by interpersonal interactions and by a sense of responsibility to larger groups (Baumeister et al., 1994; Kessler et al., 1984).

Guilt also serves as a psychological defense against the powerful feelings of helplessness and meaninglessness in the face of a random, uncaring world, as was discussed earlier under The Search for Meaning. Guilt implies responsibility, which in turn implies that one *might* have changed the outcome, even if one has failed to do so. This often unconscious chain of reasoning substitutes the personal pain of guilt and responsibility for the greater existential void of a random, uncaring universe. It also provides a sense of control over recurrence: One's failure last time implies that one might do it differently, and thus control the outcome, next time (Nixon & Singer, 1993).

The relationship between the sense of guilt and "objective causality" is complex. In many genetic counseling situations, the counselee bears no responsibility for the guilt-inducing event or situation. This is true of the individual's genotype and the occurrence of new mutations, chromosomal abnormalities, or recombination events. It is equally true of many instances of genetic transmission to offspring, although the biological mechanism may contribute to a sense of responsibility (Chapple et al., 1995). However, in some situations the individual's behavior or decisions may have influenced an outcome or limited the available options. Fetal alcohol syndrome is an example of the former; declining prenatal diagnosis or carrier testing or withholding relevant genetic information from a partner are examples of the latter. In addition, other belief systems may imply culpability, as in the belief that a pregnant woman's contact with scissors causes cleft lip or that evil spirits cause Down syndrome (Lee et al., 1988; Mittman, 1988) (see Chapter 7 under Cultures and Cultural Differences: Health Care Beliefs and Practices).

The medical-genetic explanation for a disorder may reduce the sense of culpability, and thus feelings of guilt, and the genetic counselor's knowledge and authority in presenting such information are very important. However, this situation is also complex. The mechanistic, statistical nature of such explanations may evoke a sense of randomness and meaninglessness that induces guilt as a defense. This may be exacerbated if the genetic counselor indicates that the probability of the outcome was very low, as with a new dominant mutation or a rare autosomal recessive disorder for a nonconsanguineous couple. Furthermore, counselees' beliefs or concerns about medically noncontributory actions or situations, such as medication taken during pregnancy as a cause of neurofibromatosis, may support belief in orderly causality and ability to control recurrence that is eliminated when the genetic explanation is given. Finally, routine questions asked by the genetic counselor while taking a medical history, such as about alcohol use during pregnancy with a child who has Down syndrome, may induce guilt that alcohol played some role in the occurrence of the disorder (Kessler et al., 1984).

It is essential to recognize the complex interplay of internal self-assessment, deeply ingrained social experiences and roles, health care beliefs relating to causality, psychological defenses, and responses of others that influence the individual's sense of guilt. *Simple reassurance that the counselee is not responsible is often insufficient.* Exploration and clarification of internal dialogue and beliefs should be coupled with the opportunity for "confession" and the experience of continued acceptance by the genetic counselor despite the revelation and confession of "guilt." This need not be a lengthy process. However, it should be carried out before the genetic counselor invokes her knowledge and authority to reassure the counselee that he or she has not contributed to the occurrence of the disorder or condition (Kessler et al., 1984). This is discussed further in Chapter 3 under Addressing Guilt and Shame.

In psychoanalytic terms, shame is conceptualized as occurring when one fails to attain the performance or expectations of internalized standards for the self. These standards originate in idealized, internalized images of parents or parent-figures, but may be greatly expanded by broader social interactions. In this formulation, shame is experienced as the world watching and judging. However, this is actually a projection of the internal process of watching and judging oneself (Kaufman, 1985).

There are, however, major interpersonal aspects to the induction and experience of shame. Formative shame experiences occur when the individual's hopes and expectations concerning a valued relationship are dashed, through unintentional lack of empathy or attention or by active shaming responses. When this happens, a wished for interpersonal connection is broken and one is left feeling unworthy and inadequate. Furthermore, Kaufman (1985) argues that such experiences have particular impact when the other person fails to acknowledge or validate the feeling of shame that has occurred.

One may also feel shame for the impact of one's actions or perceived failures as they affect one's family or larger social units. Furthermore, family members may concur with or induce these feelings. This is an intentional component of the socialization process in some cultures (Kaufman, 1996; Toupin, 1980). However, it also occurs at a more subconscious, less acknowledged level in other cultures. For example, a couple with an affected child may feel ashamed that they have let down their parents by failing to produce a "normal" grandchild. Depending on how the grandparents deal with their own disappointment, narcissistic injury, and shame, their responses may either reduce or reinforce the parents' sense of shame.

Shame is often masked or unconscious. However, the resulting sense of failure and exposure undermines core aspects of the sense of self. Thus, shame, even when unconscious, often causes the individual to feel that his or her failures are obvious and self-evident to others. Furthermore, as discussed earlier, when shame is not acknowledged in an interaction, or when the other person responds unempathically, the feelings of shame are reinforced. Thus, it is essential that genetic counselors be alert to indications of shame and respond in a knowledgeable manner that alleviates, rather than reinforces, the experience (Kaufman, 1985; Kessler et al., 1984).

2

THE COUNSELEE IN A
SOCIAL CONTEXT

F AMILY issues are inherent in genetic counseling. Even with a single counselee, the process of eliciting and evaluating the pedigree brings family issues into the session, as do considerations of why the individual is attending
genetic counseling alone. When multiple family members are present, family
issues and dynamics are, to greater or lesser extent, expressed and enacted in
the session. Beyond the counseling session, families play a crucial role in counselees' responses to genetic counseling, their approach to and degree of success in coping with the genetic counseling situation, and the process and outcome of decision making.

Several concepts are basic to understanding the family. The family is a social system in which the individual's behaviors and emotions influence and are
influenced by other family members in a reciprocal, ongoing manner. These
interactions are guided by a set of transactional rules that are largely unconscious and thus "invisible" to the family members. The rules include those gov-
erning power relations within the family, expectations of support and nurturance, and deeply embedded expectations and prohibitions concerning
communication patterns and expression of emotions. These rules are in part
socially determined and in part the outcome of the family's individual history
and evolution. The family is also influenced by outside individuals, institutions,
and events. Thus, the family evolves in response to both internal and external

factors. Finding appropriate compromises between stability and continuity, on the one hand, and flexibility, on the other, and between family expectations and values as opposed to social necessities and expectations is one of the essential elements for healthy family functioning (Minuchin, 1974; Walsh, 1993a).

Family Structure

The concept of subsystems and their boundaries is critical to understanding family dynamics. In principle, each individual and possible grouping of family members represent a subsystem, and any such subsystem may be useful in understanding a specific family. In practice, however, three subsystems are commonly considered, based on the relative consistency of membership, roles, and importance they have across the wide diversity of actual families. The Couple Subsystem consists of the husband and wife, or the partners in an unmarried relationship. The Parental Subsystem includes those individuals who have primary responsibility and authority for the support, nurturance, guidance, and protection of the children. The Sibling Subsystem includes the children in their relationships to one another. Subsystem boundaries define subsystems and characterize the relationships among individuals in different subsystems (Hand-Mauser, 1989; Minuchin, 1974).

These concepts reflect the fact that a given individual has a qualitatively different relationship with a family member who shares a subsystem than with one who is outside the subsystem. For example, with respect to the responsibility and authority of child rearing, one parent has a very different relationship to the other parent than to a child. Furthermore, individuals have different roles and relationships as a function of their membership in different subsystems. Thus, although it is common for the same two individuals to make up the couple subsystem and the parental subsystem, designation of the two subsystems highlights the very different roles, responsibilities, and expectations of the couple's intimate relationship and their shared activities as parents.

Interactions across subsystem boundaries vary from enmeshed to disengaged (Minuchin, 1974), or in less pathological terminology, show varying degrees of cohesion (Walsh, 1993a). With very low cohesion, there is limited communication or awareness of the emotional experiences and needs of family members. This may lead to a diminished sense of emotional support, and family members may be unaware of or inattentive to interpersonal issues until they reach high intensity or dysfunction. In the case of high cohesion, there is intense emotional involvement between family members, and this may interfere with the autonomy of individuals in different subsystems.

The presence of a child with a serious disability influences family interactions. In a problematic example, the mother may have a high level of emotional involvement with the affected child, perhaps due in part to feelings of guilt. This may lead to an emphasis on the child's needs that inhibits the child's autonomous development, leaves siblings feeling deprived of maternal attention and emotionally distant from the affected child, and limits the father's role in decision making and his emotional closeness with his wife. In analyzing such a situation, one must keep in mind that the wife's sense of guilt may arise in part from her husband's words, actions, or beliefs concerning the cause of the child's disability, which may in turn be due to his attempts to deal with his guilt, shame, and pain. Furthermore, her emotional involvement with the child may be a defense against marital problems that predated the child's birth or disability. As this example illustrates, enmeshment and disengagement may occur within the same family, and linear analysis is insufficient for understanding the complex interactional nature of family dynamics.

Family functioning is enhanced when boundaries are clearly defined yet allow effective communication and emotional support (Minuchin, 1974). In an example of well-functioning boundaries, the parents exercise appropriate authority and responsibility for their children's behavior, but they are attentive to the children's emotional needs, wishes, and developmental stages and there is communication in both directions. For example, if a child attempts to exert inappropriate parental authority over a sibling, through criticism, tattling, or direct action, the parent briefly explains to the tattling child that this is inappropriate and then addresses the situation with the sibling independently of the tattling child. Thus, appropriate parental authority is reasserted and the integrity of both the parental subsystem and the sibling subsystem is reestablished.

Family functioning is also enhanced when boundaries are flexible with respect to differing situations and changing circumstances (see next section). Thus, following the diagnosis of serious medical problems in a newborn infant, a relatively rigid parental boundary may be necessary so the parents can devote their time and energy to critical decision making. As the medical crisis resolves and the family accommodates to its new circumstances, the parents' relationships with the older children can return to their previous levels of interaction. However, even during the acute period, some time should be set aside for the parents to communicate with and comfort the other children. In a related example, the demands for parenting due to the child's acute needs may impinge upon the parents' time, energy, and sense of support in a manner that significantly affects their couple relationship (Hand-Mauser, 1989). While they may understand and accept this in the short run, a long-term shift in this direction may have a serious impact on their relationship and thus on family functioning.

The concept of boundaries is also applicable to the extended family and to interactions with the larger society. The couple's relationship involves support and intimacy that excludes, to greater or lesser extent, other individuals, including the couple's parents, siblings, and friends. Establishing and maintaining an appropriate boundary are critical and ongoing. The family boundary describes the extent to which the family functions as an integral unit and the nature of interactions with individuals and institutions outside the family. Family boundaries vary greatly because of social and cultural differences, over time as the family's composition and circumstances change, and with respect to the specific situation, individual, or institution.

An example of shifting family and subsystem boundaries involves the hospitalization of a child for an acute or life-threatening illness. New interactions of high emotional intensity may be established with hospital personnel and with the hospital or clinic as institutions. One parent, or alternating parents, may spend much time at the hospital including overnights, stressing the couple and parental subsystems. The sibling subsystem must respond to the absence and jeopardy of one of its members, to the reduced availability of the parents, and to possible increased involvement of extended family members or family friends. And all this occurs as each person struggles with his or her fears, anxiety, and other emotions, and as family members attempt to support and sustain each other.

Minuchin (1974) has stressed that the quality of boundaries, not subsystem composition, is the critical element in family functioning. Thus, many family problems or dysfunctional interactions may be usefully analyzed and addressed in terms of boundary issues. Furthermore, as the examples given previously illustrate, the circumstances of families involved in genetic counseling frequently contribute to boundary issues. Hand-Mauser (1989) provides a useful discussion of these and other concepts of family dynamics as applied to genetic counseling.

However, care must be taken in utilizing these concepts. As will be obvious from consideration of one's own family, a one-dimensional continuum from enmeshed to disengaged is clearly inadequate to describe the complexity of actual family interactions (Hoffman, 1981). Communication and emotional involvement have many qualitative dimensions and differ depending on the issue, circumstances, and specific individuals involved. In addition, the genetic counselor will usually observe the family under a very limited, often stressful set of circumstances. A greater understanding of the family's structure and dynamics can often be obtained from information relevant to the family's functioning over time and its relationship to the extended family and the larger society.

There is also a great diversity of family structures in contemporary society. These include unmarried, single parent, divorced and remarried (blended), grandparent–grandchild, multigenerational, foster, adopted, gay, and lesbian families. Each has specific social and structural complexities associated with it, some of which are directly relevant to genetic counseling. It is essential that genetic counselors have an understanding of the variously structured families with which they work and recognize the potential sources of strength and support as well as the particular issues confronted by families with different structures (Carter & McGoldrick, 1989; Fuller-Thomson et al., 1997; Guerin et al., 1987; Minuchin & Fishman, 1981; Walsh, 1993b). Some relevant issues are illustrated in the following example.

> A routine question during prenatal diagnosis counseling for advanced maternal age revealed that the couple, both previously married, had different feelings about a potential diagnosis of Down syndrome. The husband was sure he would wish to terminate while the wife was equally certain she would want to continue the pregnancy. The emotional intensity of their responses alerted the genetic counselor to the importance of further exploration. The husband's first marriage had involved a traumatic late miscarriage of a trisomy 13 fetus. This led to great anxiety about the implications of a chromosomal abnormality for his wife, his future child, and himself. Early in her first marriage, the wife had had a therapeutic abortion at her husband's insistence that she now bitterly regretted. This led to great emotional investment in the current pregnancy and a strong need to feel empowered regarding any reproductive decision. Although they each knew of the other's reproductive history, they were unaware of the intense emotions that each had experienced with another partner. The sequelae were potentially destructive to their relationship until the genetic counselor opened a discussion that led to more empathic understanding between them.

It is important not to exaggerate the two-generation nuclear family in terms of its functionality and representativeness or to view the diversity of family types as unique to contemporary Western society. Worldwide, there are a variety of accepted, functional family structures. Historically, families in Western society have adopted a variety of structures in response to economic hardship and poverty, to high adult mortality rates that resulted in frequent spouse/parent death while children were young, and to the need to integrate the family into the social and economic fabric of society (Carter & McGoldrick, 1989). It is important to keep in mind Minuchin's (1974) observation, cited previously, concerning the importance of boundaries as opposed to subsystem composition. Or, as Walsh (1993a, p. 16) has succinctly stated, "The critical difference between well-functioning and dysfunctional families is found not in their form but, rather, in the quality of their relationships and their adaptive processes."

The Family in a Temporal and Social Context

As family members are born, develop, mature, age, and die, the family undergoes inevitable, profound changes. Periods of relative equilibrium are interspersed with times of major transition, both anticipated and unanticipated. Intergenerational relationships change and expand. The nature and direction of responsibility and authority between parent and child shifts, is tested, and may be reversed. The parent–child and sibling relationships of one period form a basis for the cohesions and fissures of the extended family and for multigenerational interactions at later times: grandparent–grandchild, aunt/uncle–niece/nephew, cousins, and so forth.

One of the principal tasks of the family is to provide support for the biological, emotional, and social development and individuation of each member (Hand-Mauser, 1989; Minuchin, 1974). This task unavoidably involves a compromise between structure, guidance, and obligation, on the one hand, and flexibility and independence, on the other. The family faces changes as a result of the growth and development of its members and as a result of the family's interactions with the larger society. This, too, requires a balance between structural continuity and flexible adaptation.

Over substantial periods of time, growth and change may occur in a rather smooth, incremental manner. During these times family structure is relatively stable, a sense of continuity and shared experiences develops, and the ongoing growth and maturation of individual members is accommodated with *relative* ease. The interval between the birth of the last child and the first child's entry into adolescence frequently has these qualities if other life events do not unduly interfere. However, periods of transition also occur during which the family undergoes major reorganization. Some transitions are usual and normative, whereas others are relatively unique to the individual family.

One formulation of the family cycle, which is based on a normative model of the intact middle-class American family, identifies six transition stages (Carter & McGoldrick, 1989). Each involves expansion or contraction of the family, with changing roles for family members. Thus, each requires that the individuals, subsystems, and entire family redefine their roles and interactions.

Launching: The first stage involves the separation of the young adult from his or her family of origin. To greater or lesser extent, the development and individuation of adolescence have occurred and the young adult assumes greater personal responsibility and independence. The remaining family members must adjust to the reduced involvement of this previously integral family member.

Marriage or formation of the couple: A new family is begun. The couple commits to forming a union in which their mutual interests, attraction, and love support the complex task of incorporating their different backgrounds, friendships, interests, psychological makeups, and families of origin. A couple's boundary is formed to provide the protected intimacy for these tasks, which alters relations with the extended family and broader society. Parents and siblings acquire in-laws and must adjust to the new family member and to the new couple's boundary.

Parenthood: The birth of the first child dramatically alters the family structure. The gratifications and obligations of parenthood impinge on the couple's relationship and a new, distinctive parental boundary is formed. In the extended family the generational roles shift: children become parents, parents become grandparents. Additional children increase the complexity of structures, boundaries, and interactions.

The children reach adolescence: With the growing, yet conflicted independence of adolescence, the parent–child relationship changes qualitatively. Parental authority declines and the task of providing guidance and control, tempered with opportunities for independence and responsibility, becomes more complex. The parental boundary changes, and the family boundary may be altered as adolescents actively bring their friends and their generational interests and values into the family. The parents, reaching new stages in their own lives, may face crises of identity involving their relationships to each other, to work, and to other values and goals.

The family at midlife: In this transition, children leave home. Their marriages or partnerships bring in new family members, who may come from very different social, cultural, or family backgrounds. The parents must continue to redefine their individual lives and their parental and couple relationships in the face of more dramatic structural changes than occurred in the previous transition. This transition involves the launching of the next generation. It thus brings us full circle, demonstrating that the family's developmental course cycles forward through successive generations. In so doing, the family incorporates members from other families and contributes to the formation of new families. Because of contemporary low birth rates and long life spans, the life stage initiated by this transition may span a substantial portion of the parents' lives.

Later life: Although they may occur over the course of many years, a number of events in this stage represent major transitions. Grandchildren may enrich interactions at all the intergenerational boundaries. Retirement provides new opportunities as well as adaptive challenges to the individual and the couple. If the parents experience extended illness or incapacity, the roles of the generations may be further reversed. The deaths of the parents are often times of particular stress for the adult children and thus for their families. With the parents' deaths, the cycle of the generations has completed another turn, and the children become the oldest, parental generation.

There are other formulations of family transitions based on finer subdivisions of the family life cycle, different theoretical orientations, or consideration of families with other structures (Carter & McGoldrick, 1989; Duvall, 1977). However, the family life cycle as just described illustrates the general features of normative transitions. Each involves multiple generations and substantive changes in the composition and organization of the family. Thus, even when anticipated and desired, these transitions test the family's ability to negotiate a complex, dynamic compromise between the need to retain continuity of structure, with its history of familiar interactions and emotional supports, while adapting to unavoidable structural changes and altered self-definitions (Hand-Mauser, 1989).

Transitions are times of family stress. Patterns of enmeshment or disengagement may exacerbate the transition. Furthermore, attempts to negotiate the transition may strengthen enmeshment, disengagement, or a combination of the two, as when a parent's escalating attempts to maintain earlier patterns of authority and emotional involvement lead an adolescent or newly married "child" to initiate a break with the family.

The transitions just discussed are generally recognized as involving normal although challenging periods in family life. Social and institutional supports are often available, and these help buffer family members from feeling isolated or stigmatized by the difficulties they encounter. Some but not all of these transitions are associated with well-established rituals, such as weddings, funerals, and a variety of formal and informal activities surrounding childbirth. Rituals provide a time-honored, but time-limited situation in which the transition is formally acknowledged, strong emotions may be expressed, and there is a sense of family cohesion and continuity and of connection with the larger society.

Unexpected life events may greatly affect these normative transitions. In addition, families experience transitions that, due to timing or nature, deviate from the expected and normative. Some of these events or transitions are largely positive in their impact. For example, the family undertakes a major geographic move that is desired, even though it separates members of the extended family. However, many such transitions are experienced, at least initially, as negative and highly stressful. These include a variety of situations relevant to genetic counseling: They may initiate a transition (e.g., the death of a child or young parent or the onset of chronic illness in a family member), radically alter a normative transition (the birth of a child with a genetic disease or birth defect), or impede a desired transition (miscarriage, stillbirth, genetic abortion, infertility) (Imber-Black, 1989).

These situations share with normative transitions the need to retain structure and continuity while also responding flexibly to the new circumstances (Hand-Mauser, 1989; Rolland, 1994). However, many factors in addition to the overt emotional, social, medical, and financial stressors contribute to the complexity of the family's response. These factors include the grieving of wished for outcomes and definitions of the family while at the same time requiring new definitions of the family's tasks and meaning, for example, when there is infertility or the birth of a child with a serious disability. Unlike normative transitions, there may be a lack of social supports, rituals, and previously utilized or anticipated individual and family responses. These deficiencies increase the likelihood that family members and the family as a whole will feel stigmatized and isolated (Imber-Black, 1989).

In studying the impact of illness on families, Rolland (1994) identified five relevant disease characteristics that relate to the family's tasks and adaptation over time.

The *onset* may be acute, or gradual to varying degrees. This influences the intensity and rapidity with which practical, emotional, and structural accommodations must be made.

The *course* may be progressive with respect to severity, relatively constant, or relapsing and episodic. Each of these patterns presents different challenges, which are also affected by rate of change or frequency and pattern of relapses. Among the many consequences of the course are the extent to which the family can reach a stable accommodation or must continually adapt, the extent of structural adaptation required, and the length of time over which the family's "staying power" is tested.

Outcome refers to the impact, if any, on life span and the likelihood or predictability of death. This affects family members' anticipation of structural change and loss and influences their attitudes toward the affected individual.

The extent and nature of *incapacitation* affects the specific impact on the family and influences the extent of stigmatization, isolation, and loss.

Affecting each of these characteristics is the degree of *uncertainty* or *predictability*. This is determined by the specificity and certainty of the diagnosis, the available information concerning the disorder, and the disorder's inherent variability or heterogeneity.

Roland's integrative model of families and disease contains much of value that cannot be reviewed here. However, this brief discussion demonstrates that genetic disorders such as sickle cell disease, cystic fibrosis, muscular dystrophy, spina bifida, Marfan syndrome, familial cancers, etc., vary greatly with respect to the above factors and thus with respect to the nature, intensity, and timing of their impact on the family. As Rolland points out, a typology of disease and illness relevant to psychosocial impact differs greatly from that used in medicine or genetics and requires a different orientation toward diseases.

The genetic counselor's knowledge of a disorder, when coupled with information about a family's structure and stage in the family life cycle, supports counseling related to management and coping, anticipatory guidance, and decision making (Hand-Mauser, 1989; Rolland, 1994).

Family Belief Systems

Every family functions with a complex set of beliefs, perceptions, values, and rules concerning the nature of the world, appropriate responses to situations and problems that are encountered, and the resources and degree of control that are available to meet life's challenges. For brevity, I shall in general refer to these collectively as "beliefs." Their scope extends from the broadest views of human nature and the individual's place in the universe to the details of interpersonal interactions that have been discussed earlier. They include beliefs about health and illness, the appropriateness of human intervention and utilization of technology in natural processes, the sharing of information and expressing of emotions, and the roles of individuals within the family (family scripts). Commonly, family members do not have identical beliefs, and one component of family beliefs involves the acceptability of and means for resolving differences among its members. As in other aspects of individual and family life, an appropriate degree of flexibility and openness to alternatives enhances the family's ability to respond to stressors and transitions (Minuchin, 1974; Rolland, 1994).

A family's beliefs develop from its sociocultural history and milieu, religious and spiritual values and practices, accumulated experiences, and continually evolving structure and responses to life's challenges. Stories and myths, experiences of success and failure, the meanings assigned and developed to explain events, and the powerful conscious and unconscious emotions experienced by family members all contribute. Many of the beliefs, rules, and perceptions are unconscious, and much of their power comes from the fact that they are experienced unconditionally as lived reality. By the same token, they provide a sense of continuity and guidance for negotiating transitions and responding to new stresses (Imber-Black, 1986; McGoldrick, 1993).

Several aspects of family beliefs are particularly relevant to genetic counseling. These include:

Beliefs concerning the normal and acceptable range of human variability. For example, whether the birth of a child with Down syndrome is perceived as personally and socially acceptable or as an unacceptable burden that may include social disapproval for the failure to use prenatal diagnosis and elective termination.

The personal and social meanings of the particular situation or disorder, including its specific characteristics and symptoms. A major variable is the relative and absolute importance given to cognitive abilities, physical abilities, and physical appearance as they influence social acceptability, life goals, and definitions of success (Rapp, 1993a).

Beliefs concerning the ability to affect the course of life events, including the appropriateness of and responsibility for so doing. This includes fundamental beliefs and values concerning humankind's place in the natural world and the appropriateness of using technology to alter natural events; the perceived impact of the disease or condition; the perceived availability of personal, social, financial, and medical resources; and the degree of openness to accepting or seeking out these resources including issues of privacy, vulnerability, and shame (Rolland, 1994). Beliefs and values concerning abortion for a given disorder can affect decisions about whether to use carrier testing and prenatal diagnosis, as can religious beliefs and emotional attachment to an affected family member (Varekamp et al., 1992; Wertz et al., 1992). Belief in romantic love as the basis for choosing a partner may preclude carrier testing prior to making a marital or romantic commitment (Beeson & Doksum, in press).

Beliefs concerning the cause of genetic disorders, birth defects, and other situations relevant to genetic counseling. Such beliefs span a broad spectrum and include natural, religious, and supernatural causes; personal attributes including guilt and punishment; fate and chance. Different members of a family may have different beliefs. Furthermore, a given individual may hold apparently disparate or conflicting beliefs, such as deeply held religious beliefs combined with acceptance of a genetic etiology (Rolland, 1994; Weil, 1991). Beliefs may be based on medical genetic information obtained in genetic counseling or from other sources. However, misinformation or misunderstanding may arise because of the quality of the source, a misunderstanding concerning information and its significance, or the process of genetic counseling itself (Fanos, 1996; Richards, 1996). For example, reports in the popular media concerning the effects of environmental contaminants may lead to concern that a child's Down syndrome was caused by chemical exposure in the home or workplace. Alternatively, routine medical history questions concerning alcohol and tobacco use may lead to a belief that these are causal agents. Careful inquiries concerning sources of guilt and shame provide one way to identify and address such misconceptions (see Chapter 3 under Addressing Guilt and Shame).

Kessler and Bloch's (1989) discussion of patient preselection in families with Huntington disease illustrates the role of family beliefs in the complex interactions between family process and individual psychodynamics. In patient preselection, family members collude, often unconsciously, to identify one of the asymptomatic children as the presumed presymptomatic carrier of the mutant allele. The assignment of this "sick role" to one individual helps reduce family anxiety concerning the uncontrollable elements of the disease, allows ambivalent feelings toward the affected individual to be projected elsewhere, and helps organize the family's experience and the meanings they give to it. Often, the process of choosing the preselected individual is based on family myths concerning the inheritance of Huntington disease or on superficial similarities between the affected and the preselected individuals. Although the process has a defensive role that partially supports the functioning of the family and some of its members, the presumption of impending illness and disability with an accompanying withholding of family resources can have a profound, lifelong negative impact on the preselected individual. Fanos and Johnson (1995) have also reported preselection for cystic fibrosis carrier status, with psychological effects that include attitude toward carrier testing.

The beliefs, values, and perceptions held by a family and its members play a significant role in many genetic counseling situations. Thoughtful questions concerning beliefs about the cause of the situation that led to genetic counseling will help identify misinformation, misunderstanding, disagreement among family members, beliefs that are contrary to the medical genetic explanation, and issues that are of particular concern or are sources of guilt or blame. Inquiry concerning beliefs and values is particularly important when counselees have difficulty with decision making or when there is reason to infer that these issues interfere with effective coping and adaptation. Irrespective of the level of inquiry, it is essential that the genetic counselor show respect for the family's beliefs, values, and perceptions. A counselee's sense that his or her individual and family beliefs are not valued and accepted by the genetic counselor, or that they are discounted or denigrated, may lead to anger, withdrawal, or resistance to the explanations and recommendations that are provided (Rolland, 1994).

Communication

Communication among family members is integral to the process of genetic counseling and to the coping and adaptation of the family and its members. It affects the quality and utility of information obtained in a general pedigree or relevant to the specific disorder or situation that is of concern to the counselee. Communication is critical to identifying and notifying extended family members who may be at increased risk or whose present or future children may be at risk. Beyond the counseling situation itself, open communication is, in general, associated with more effective coping, including greater emotional support, the sharing of relevant information, and effective, informed planning (Fanos, 1996; Rolland, 1994).

The few available studies on genetic counseling confirm what is apparent from clinical experience, that communication within nuclear and extended families varies greatly. Within some families or among certain family members there is open communication with free sharing of information and ideas. At the other extreme, communication among family members or contact by genetic counselors is explicitly resisted or rejected (Green et al., 1997).

Fanos (1996) conducted in-depth interviews with adults whose sibling had died of cystic fibrosis (CF) when they were children or adolescents. She found that approximately 20% came from families with good communication concerning the severity and lethality of the disorder, 30% were from families with "veiled" communication, and in the families of 50% CF had been a "family secret." She thus confirmed Turk's earlier observation that for many such families there is a "web of silence" (Turk, 1964, p. 71) "in which communication serves to conceal as much as it reveals" (Fanos, 1996, p. 45). This concealment led to anger, confusion, worry about the sibling, anxiety for themselves concerning CF and their parents' apparent lack of trust or sense of their importance, and the burden of maintaining the secret from the outside world, and contributed to the lifelong emotional sequelae experienced by some of these surviving siblings. Other relatively systematic studies of families with genetic disorders have identified 20%–50% in which there is little or no communication (1) with siblings concerning positive presymptomatic Huntington disease carrier status, (2) among extended family members concerning the hereditary nature and availability of carrier testing for cystic fibrosis, (3) within nuclear and extended families concerning the hereditary nature of hemophilia, and (4) among extended family members concerning balanced translocations and other karyotype abnormalities (Ayme et al., 1993; Tibben et al., 1993; Varekamp et al., 1992).

Many factors may limit or block communication. The defenses of denial and suppression as well as more conscious coping mechanisms such as the desire to avoid stigmatization, pity, "undeserved" sympathy, a sense of guilt and shame, or surveillance (after positive presymptomatic Huntington disease testing) may all be involved. While these may be thought of as "individual" issues, their origins and dynamics involve family interactions. Family issues are evident in the wish not to become a burden or to cause alarm or distress to others, and in the desire to avoid denial, blaming, anger, and other hurtful or dysfunctional responses of family members (Bloch et al., 1992; Green et al., 1997). More generally, the family's interactional patterns, including family rules, roles, beliefs, and geographical and emotional distancing, are major determinants of communication.

This discussion of the limitations to communication is not meant to underestimate the occurrence of effective communication, which is also clearly documented. Family members are an important source of information about the nature and inheritance of genetic disorders (Fanos, 1996; Green et al., 1997). Furthermore, once barriers to communication are overcome, unexpected emotional support may be found (Bloch et al., 1992). However, given the medical and psychosocial value of such communication, genetic counselors should be aware of the factors that inhibit it and assess relevant individual and family dynamics (Eunpu, 1997b).

As the genetic counselor explores communication patterns, it is critical to respect the defenses, coping mechanisms, and family dynamics that influence them. Counselees may need assistance reconciling the advantages and obligations of communication with the fears and anxieties that accompany it. A problem-solving approach, including role play (Chapter 3) and scenarios (Chapter 5) may be helpful. A discussion of the mode, time, and place of communication may help the counselee identify a pace and circumstances that are sufficiently comfortable. The genetic counselor may assist the process with educational materials designed to meet the needs of extended family members, medical letters written with extended family members in mind, and appropriate offers to make initial contacts. However, it is by addressing communication issues as an integral part of the counseling process that the most general and knowledgeable assistance can be provided.

When counselees are resistant to communicating with family members who are potentially at risk, difficult ethical issues develop around counselee confidentiality and autonomy, on the one hand, and the duty to inform, on the other. Several published guidelines list criteria that must be met prior to breaching counselee confidentiality to inform at-risk relatives. These include a high probability of serious harm to identifiable individuals if the information is not provided, the relevance of the information to preventing this harm, precautions to limit the nature and extent of breach of confidence, and failure to elicit consent from the counselee for voluntary disclosure (Baumiller et al., 1996; American Society of Human Genetics, 1998). As the preceding discussion indicates, I believe the last criterion can be considered met only after psychosocial concerns as well as technical issues have been addressed with the counselee.

Couples

Couple issues are intimately related to two of the most common elements of genetic counseling: reproduction and parenting. Aspects of a couple's interactions are inevitably expressed in the counseling session, whether one or both members are present, and in the presence or absence of other family members. Thus, the genetic counselor has the opportunity to observe and evaluate a couple's dynamics and to make interventions that are helpful in the moment or as interpretations and guidance (Eunpu, 1997b).

The intensity and centrality of an intimate, dyadic relationship carries with it the potential for comfort, satisfaction, and joy as well as for pain, struggle, and loss. Any such relationship must balance the deeply felt need for joining and intimacy with the opposing need for autonomy and independence. Those involved in a couple relationship must attempt to balance these competing needs, which relate as much to unconscious desires, fears, and expectations as to those that are conscious (Hof & Treat, 1989; Scharff & Scharff, 1991b). The degree of psychological differentiation and autonomy achieved developmentally by each partner plays a central role. To the extent that there are deficits in psychological differentiation, differences and disagreements between the partners and the inevitable emotional ebb and flow in a relationship may produce anxiety, anger, rage, or fear of abandonment. Conversely, emotional and sexual intimacy may be experienced as involving a frightening loss of autonomy or sense of psychological fusion with the partner.

Each partner brings many things to a relationship. These include the interactional patterns and expectations learned during childhood; emotional deficits and traumas that each hopes will be compensated for by the other; and social, cultural, and religious norms and expectations concerning sexuality, reproduction, social relations, and marriage. Furthermore, members of the extended families affect a relationship both through their present interactions and expectations and by their role in maintaining previous patterns of interaction. Thus, what often seems like the most unique and personal of interrelationships is heavily laden with personal, family, and social meaning. Furthermore, because of the intense unconscious processes involved, psychological defense mechanisms such as projection and projective identification are readily activated and may become fixed elements in the couple's interactions (Guerin et al., 1987; Scharff & Scharff, 1991a).

Several aspects of contemporary society have increased the social isolation of the couple in terms of responsibility for defining and maintaining their relationship. The relatively common geographic and emotional isolation of the nuclear family reduces the role of the extended family in mediating issues that arise in the couple's relationship and in assisting with child rearing and response to stressors. The growing frequency with which both parents must work outside the home places additional responsibility on one (most commonly the mother) or both members of the couple to provide for the economic, homemaking, and emotional needs of the family. Marriage is now commonly conceptualized as an individual and contractual relationship as opposed to one based on social or religious expectations and duties. Both this concept and the practice of living together without marriage place primary responsibility for evaluating and maintaining the relationship on the couple itself, with reduced social supports and fewer legal, cultural, or religious norms or expectations for the continuity of the relationship (Carter & McGoldrick, 1989; Guerin et al., 1987).

Similarities and Differences

The formation of a couple relationship involves the complex process of partner selection combined with the development and negotiation of those aspects of the couple's interactions that are to be distinct from interactions with family, friends, and society. The latter, as discussed previously under Family Structure, is conceptualized as the formation and maintenance of the "couple boundary." Partner selection is based, at conscious and unconscious levels, on both similarities and differences. Similarities provide the basis for shared interests, enjoyment, sense of identity, goals, social roles, and social responsibilities. They also support the deeply desired feelings of acceptance, self-worth, and self-esteem. Differences, which are often complementary, provide a sense of interest, excitement, and broadening of experience. These differences play a central role in the attempt to find support for one's own deficiencies and limitations as well as comfort and healing of previously experienced emotional deficits and traumas (Black, 1991; Guerin et al., 1987).

A useful example of complementarity is the pairing of a lively, emotionally expressive, outgoing person with one who is more quiet and introspective. For the expressive person, the partner's thoughtfulness and apparent inner calm may provide a much needed sense of grounding and solidity. For the quiet person, the expressive partner may provide a sense of excitement, emotional responsiveness, and social interaction that is equally important. At a deeper level, the expressive person may feel listened to and understood in a way that was lacking in the family of origin. The quiet person may feel that a long-standing sense of isolation and depression is being alleviated.

As a relationship develops, similarities and differences may form the basis for deeper, richer interactions. However, they may also become problematic, and much of this may be experienced at an unconscious level. What were initially experienced as supportive, enlivening differences may come to feel irritating or rigid. In addition, any deficits that underlie the differences may become more evident, resulting in a reduced sense of support and complementarity and an increased sense of neediness or dysfunction in the partner (Guerin et al., 1987; Scharff & Scharff, 1991b). Thus, in the previous example, depressive qualities underlying the quiet partner's demeanor and a lack of secure emotional groundedness in the expressive partner may become more clearly manifest.

Stressful situations such as infertility, reproductive loss, or the diagnosis, care, or death of a child affect the couple's relationship through their impact on both partners. At the individual level, these and other stressors lead to anxiety, strong emotions, and a natural tendency to utilize more rigid, less mature psychological defenses. As a consequence, each partner is likely to wish for or demand increased emotional support from the other. However, the same factors may decrease the ability of each to provide such support to the other (Rando, 1985; Rosenblatt, 1988). These paired responses increase the probability that differences between the partners will be experienced as uncaring and as emotional abandonment. They also increase the likelihood that projection and projective identification will occur, thus reducing each partner's ability to empathically perceive the other's pain and ways of attempting to cope with it. Thus, personality differences that had been largely complementary or at least tolerable may become sources of anger, despair, or bitterness. Furthermore, in the inevitable ebb and flow of emotions and degree of coping that are part of grieving and adaptation, the two partners may experience brief or extended periods of time when they are out of phase with respect to their degree of vulnerability and/or ability to comfort the other (Meyers et al., 1995b; Shapiro, 1993).

Returning again to our example, increased emotionality in the one partner and/or increased depression in the other may lead to a situation in which one or both feels severely unsupported, emotionally abandoned, or helpless in attempts to comfort the other. This may be experienced at particular times or as a relatively constant aspect of the relationship.

In addition to these individual personality differences, there are gender-related differences in responses. While it is important not to stereotype, a substantial number of systematic and anecdotal reports indicate that there are, on average, differences between men and women in their responses to stress and their processing of loss and grief. In general, women tend to wish to discuss and express their feelings more than men, they are aware of and are consciously affected by grief over a longer time period, and in the case of reproductive loss they are more likely to have an increase in grief at the time the birth would have occurred. In general, men tend to express anger as well as or instead of grief, to be less open to expressing or discussing their emotions, and to return more quickly to involvement in work or other activities. These differences, which are often reinforced by societal expectations, can also be a source of anger, misunderstanding, feelings of emotional abandonment, and a sense, on both sides, that each is carrying an undue portion of the burden of pain and adjustment. These issues are particularly significant when gender-related differences are already a source of stress in the relationship (Fanos, 1996; Kolker & Burke, 1993).

Many couples empathically support each other through such stressful situations, and they may draw closer as a result. This support is promoted by psychological individuation sufficient to allow each partner to separate his or her own responses from those based on the other's perceptions and ways of coping. It is facilitated by a relationship in which personal differences are recognized and valued in their complementarity and there is sufficient communication to allow an understanding of each other's experiences. However, even in such circumstances, there may be periods of blame and pain. Many couples struggle repeatedly to address these issues.

To return to our example, the expressive individual may understand that the quiet partner's increased silence and withdrawal is not a lack of caring, but a way of coping. The quiet individual may recognize that the expressive partner's emotions are not something "to be gotten over," but are deeply felt, necessary responses. With this understanding, they may each be able to comfort the other. In addition, they may both recognize that the quiet partner's ability to study and understand the medical information, despite partial withdrawal, and the expressive partner's ability to actively engage necessary resources, despite temporary difficulty thinking clearly, are important in helping them address the practical issues and improve their situation.

I have emphasized the role of individual differences in couple relations because I believe this is one area in which genetic counselors can have a direct, helpful role. Differences in defenses, coping, and expressions of grief, as well as their impact on the relationship, may be expressed in the session or identified through limited but focused inquiry. Questions such as, "How are each of you handling this?" "How does his (or her) way of coping compare to yours?" "Are you able to discuss the differences in how you are responding?" can initiate further discussion and exploration. Both current and anticipatory guidance can be implemented by normalizing such differences, reframing in terms of complementarity, and discussing the difficulties of perception and empathy under such circumstances (Black, 1991). Sometimes the genetic counselor's empathic engagement with a withdrawn or angry counselee provides the first opportunity for a more open expression of grief. This can have a salutary effect for both members of the couple. The angry or withdrawn member may experience emotional relief and a new sense of being understood, thus freeing emotional energy for more functional interactions with the partner. The partner may, for the first time, or more clearly, perceive the pain behind the withdrawal or anger. Thus he or she can be more empathic and more receptive to support in subsequent interactions.

Inquiries regarding differences are also useful with respect to assessment and referral for marital or couple counseling. The manner in which each partner responds to the other's coping and defenses is indicative of critical elements in their relationship: extent of psychological individuation, quality of communication, occurrence of projection or projective identification, and existence or extent of anger and bitterness (Guerin et al., 1987). When there is evidence of serious dysfunction, the reported and observed dynamics can be used as the basis for an empathically based referral. For example, the genetic counselor might say, "I know, from past experience and what you have told me, that you are both experiencing a lot of pain. However, your ways of expressing it are very different, so it's not surprising that it's hard for each of you to understand the other's feelings and actions. Each of you feels misunderstood and rather abandoned, and it's reached the point of anger and even bitterness. This is the sort of normal, but difficult couple's issue where a professional could be of help."

Triangles

The couple's interactions are naturally and profoundly influenced by the relationships of each partner with other individuals both within and outside the family. These interactional triangles, which develop from responsibilities, activities, and choices related to family, work, and social relations, have many positive functions. They provide emotional and social support for each partner and for the couple's relationship. They create interests and activities that increase the vitality and attractiveness of each partner for the other. They provide essential buffering for the inevitable tensions and cyclic interactions that grow out of the opposing needs for intimacy and autonomy. Thus, as alternate sources of emotional support and intimacy, they fulfill some of these needs outside the relationship, thereby reducing the demands on the other partner. Viewed conversely, they provide each partner with opportunities to function autonomously outside the relationship (Guerin et al., 1987).

However, these triangles may also be sources of tension and conflicting loyalties, and they may involve dysfunctional defenses against the couple's emotional problems. One way this occurs is in unresolved issues with the couple's parents. This type of problematic triangle is encountered in genetic counseling around issues of reproductive decision making and the parenting of children with disabilities. The couple's parents have natural and legitimate concerns regarding their children's well-being, their desire for grandchildren, and their grandchildren's well-being. However, if a partner has not adequately resolved issues of autonomy and communication with a parent, or if he or she turns to the parent in an attempt to resolve tensions with the partner, the parent's involvement may be intrusive, disruptive of the couple's relationship, and detrimental to the couple's ability to function autonomously (Guerin et al., 1987). A familiarity with these dynamics is essential to the genetic counselor's understanding and exploration of couples' coping and decision making. On occasion, direct interventions can support the couple's relationship, even though the larger systemic issues remain (Eunpu, 1997b).

> The parents of a child with severe developmental delay were accompanied to genetic counseling by the father's parents and the mother's sister. It was clear that the extended family members provided much needed support and assistance in the care of the child. However, the father's mother was somewhat demanding and intrusive regarding her perceptions of the child's needs. This angered the mother, and the father appeared anxious and withdrawn due to conflicting loyalties to his wife and his mother. When the genetic counselor gave a 5% empiric recurrence risk the child's mother said, "I can't imagine facing these problems again." Almost simultaneously the father's mother said, "We can help you manage." The father appeared to withdraw further and seemed incapable of contributing to the discussion.
>
> Anticipating intergenerational issues and as a matter of routine clinical practice, the genetic counselor had stated early in the session that she would want some time alone with the couple. She now invoked this privilege. In the ensuing discussion three important issues were identified and briefly explored. First, both

parents were torn and confused by the support coupled with intrusiveness of their extended families. Second, both had unresolved autonomy issues with their parents that caused conflict within the marriage. Finally, the fact that their first and only child had severe disabilities had disrupted their hopes and plans for forming a family, and this had added to the difficulty in defining their relationship independent of their parents.

Discussion of these issues helped the couple better understand the confusing, intense emotions they had been experiencing and provided the basis for a preliminary suggestion that they might find value in couple counseling. The clarification and validation they experienced with the genetic counselor led to the father's active involvement in the discussion, to a lessening of the mother's anger, and to a general reduction in tension. This allowed the counselees to begin to address the meaning of the recurrence risk to each of them and to their plans for a family. They also considered ways in which to continue this discussion as a couple in order to reach an autonomous, if potentially difficult decision.

This case allows the following more general observations. First, it can be analyzed both in terms of the couple boundary and in terms of triangles. These are complementary formulations; each has relative strengths and limitations and is more or less useful with respect to different aspects of the complex reality. Second, the genetic counselor's decision to meet alone with the couple was an active therapeutic intervention. It altered the individual experiences and interpersonal interactions of all the counselees in a manner that supported the couple's autonomy and, at least in the session, enhanced the couple boundary. In a reasonably well functioning family, it might provide some impetus for more long-term structural change, as it appeared to do in this case, or demonstrate the value of further professional assistance in addressing these issues. Finally, although the issues evoked while meeting with the couple are complex and may appear daunting, relatively simple empathic comments may open them for discussion. For example, for the three major issues confronting this couple, the genetic counselor might say, respectively:

It must be confusing to have such loving support come with some pretty strong strings attached. [confusion over parental support coupled with intrusiveness]

I would guess, based on my experience, that you had feelings like this even before the baby was born. [unresolved autonomy issues with parents]

It sounds like having a child was an important part of defining yourselves as independent adults. Your child's problems must have made that much more complicated than you had expected. [child's disabilities disrupted hopes and plans for forming a family]

Due to their proximity and continual emotional involvement, children are readily drawn into dysfunctional triangles that originate in their parents' relational problems (Minuchin, 1974). A common dysfunctional pattern is the emotional overinvolvement of one parent with the child and the underinvolvement of the other, with anger and bitterness on both sides regarding this difference. The induction of the child into the conflict externalizes the underlying dysfunction regarding intimacy versus autonomy. It may stabilize the relationship by preventing direct, more disruptive conflict over this issue. Thus, a wife who desires greater emotional intimacy than her husband can provide seeks substitute intimacy with the child. She can more safely vent her anger at her husband's emotional distance by displacing it into anger about his emotional distance from the child. The husband, by expressing anger at his wife's "overinvolvement" with the child, maintains the desired emotional distance from her while displacing his anger onto a less potentially disruptive target (Guerin et al., 1987). The child may experience confusion, torn loyalties, and depression, and these may lead to withdrawal, behavioral problems, or academic problems. Furthermore, the wife's overinvolvement may inhibit appropriate development of the child's autonomy. Nevertheless, the child may play an active role in maintaining the triangulated dynamics because he or she recognizes, consciously or unconsciously, that this avoids the potentially more frightening and disruptive possibility of direct parental confrontation.

Parental triangulation with a child may arise under diverse circumstances. However, the birth, diagnosis, and care of a child with a disability or chronic disease provide a variety of situations and stressors that may foster these dynamics. They include the legitimate and unavoidable attention and care required by the child; the practical and emotional stresses of caring for the child; the potential for guilt, blame, and anger at oneself or one's partner for the child's condition; sexual problems arising from emotional issues or anxiety about recurrence risk; and unresolved anger and bitterness related to different ways of coping and grieving. In most instances, assistance in the resolution of these issues lies beyond the scope of genetic counseling and requires a referral to an appropriate mental health professional. However, substantive opportunities to discuss such issues may arise in ongoing, long-term follow-up involving families of children with chronic disorders such as hemoglobinopathies and metabolic diseases. In either case, it is essential that the genetic counselor recognize the potential complexity of issues such as parental overinvolvement with a child who has a disability or chronic disease. Education and guidance with respect to a single issue, such as parental guilt, may be ineffective or rejected if the possible additional complexities have not been explored and acknowledged.

Sex

Since sex and sexual relations are at the core of both reproduction and the couple relationship, they are a potentially significant issue in many genetic counseling situations. Sex may be a central element in the couple's sense of commitment, intimacy, and well-being. It may also be a focus of discord and conflict, either as a primary area of disagreement and dysfunction or when it is secondary to conflicts involving power and control or intimacy versus autonomy (Guerin et al., 1987; Scharff & Scharff, 1991a). Stress, emotional pain, and loss may increase or decrease a person's desire for sexual intimacy. Thus, when a couple is stressed or grieving, the partners may find comfort and closeness through their sexual relationship, may agree in reducing their sexual involvement, or may diverge with one desiring sex and the other finding it undesirable (Rando, 1985; Shapiro, 1993). This divergence of desire may grow out of previous issues in the couple's relationship, it may add to the pain and loss that accompanies differences and asynchrony in the partners' coping and grieving patterns, or it may grow out of anger and bitterness engendered by such differences.

In addition, many genetic counseling situations affect the couple's sexual relationship directly. Infertility, infertility evaluations and treatments, and assisted reproductive technologies all directly affect sexual interactions. To greater or lesser extent, the spontaneous and emotional aspects of sexuality and intercourse are subjected to observation, planning, and instrumentality (Meyers et al., 1995a). Older couples who desire a child, especially after reproductive loss or abortion for genetic causes, may also find that their sexual relations become oriented toward conception. Reproductive loss, the birth of a child with a genetic disorder or birth defect, or the death of a child can lead to reduced sexual desire due to anxiety that sex will lead to a recurrence of the painful situation or loss. This anxiety may be based on the actual recurrence risk or on a more general cognitive and emotional association between sexuality and the previous outcome or loss (Black, 1991; Shapiro, 1993). Sexual desire may also be reduced by feelings of guilt or shame evoked by infertility, reproductive loss, or an affected child that expands to include guilt or shame regarding sexuality (Kessler et al., 1984). Hormonal and surgical cancer treatment or prophylaxis may affect sexual drive, physical appearance, and the sensitivity of erogenous areas. As with other emotional issues, the partners may also differ in the nature or timing of their sexual needs and desires in response to any of these situations (Rando, 1985).

The discussion of sexuality with counselees must be undertaken with care. For some couples it is threatening because of a lack of experience or trust in discussing sex in their relationship. For some it is so central to issues of power in the relationship that it may elicit anger or bitterness that is difficult to address and contain in the limited, short-term format of genetic counseling (Guerin et al., 1987). Other couples are open to some discussion or find it helpful when the genetic counselor provides assistance in overcoming inhibitions and anxieties regarding these issues.

It may be relatively easy to raise this topic in the context of coping, grief, or reproductive decisions and problems.

Genetic Counselor: When couples are at this stage of grieving for a child, it often affects their sexual relationship. It's normal and understandable, but it can certainly add to the stress they feel. Are the two of you experiencing this?

Another approach, when there is a child with a chronic disease, involves inquiring about the parents' sleeping arrangements. Not infrequently, they are sleeping in separate rooms, with one parent sleeping with the child. This may interfere with or be an attempt by one or both to deal with difficulties in their sexual relationship.

When issues of this sort are identified, guidance and normalization or referral for counseling may be helpful. Whatever the approach, it is critical that the sexual issues be addressed within the broader context of the couple's relationship and the stresses that they are experiencing.

Social Isolation and Social Support

Many factors contribute to the potential for social isolation among individuals, couples, and families who are involved in genetic counseling. When an individual has a disability, demands on time and resources plus medical procedures or limitations may constrain the social activities of the affected person and other family members. For the parents of a disabled child, and for counselees who have experienced infertility, perinatal loss, or the death of a child, common social interactions and situations may evoke painful reminders of their loss and grief. These can lead to an understandable avoidance of such interactions or, when confronted by them, voluntary or involuntary responses of distancing and withdrawal (Miezio, 1983; Suslak et al., 1995). Individuals with disabilities and the parents of affected children may also experience shame and a sense of stigmatization in social situations. The parents of children with a disability that affects appearance or behavior often confront inappropriate, hurtful responses from strangers in the course of routine shopping or other public activities (Marshak et al., 1999; Darling, 1991).

In lectures and workshops with parents of children with disabilities, my use of the term "supermarket syndrome" routinely evokes wry smiles of recognition and pain. Stares, inappropriate comments, and assumptions of poor parenting when a visually normal child exhibits severe behavioral problems are unavoidable experiences in the life of these parents.

The actions and responses of friends, colleagues, or the parents of other children may contribute to social isolation. There is the common problem of uncertainty and ineptitude about how to respond to those who have suffered a loss. Failure to recognize the extent of loss or the time required for grieving may lead to comments that inappropriately minimize the loss or attempt to cheer the individual. Furthermore, loss or tragedy experienced by others threatens one's own sense of invulnerability, and this may result in defensive distancing or overt avoidance (Rando, 1985; Seller et al., 1993).

The counselee's own emotions may also contribute to social isolation. Depression or grief can lead to withdrawal. There may be a sense that the loss or tragedy lies outside normal experience, setting one apart from the majority of people. Ambivalent or angry feelings toward a child with a disability or an adult who has died, and particularly death wishes toward a child, may lead to a deep sense of guilt and shame. Guilt may also be experienced following abortion for a genetic disorder or birth defect. Finally, normal, highly intense emotions early in the grieving or coping process may lead to concern that one's responses are outside the normal range, that one is "crazy," or that one must prevent others from seeing how one is reacting (Laborde & Seligman, 1991; Suslak et al., 1995).

Not infrequently, counselees must decide who should be given information related to genetic counseling. This situation occurs with infertility, prenatal diagnosis findings, and abortion following medically positive ultrasound or prenatal diagnosis results. Parents of newly diagnosed children and adults with newly diagnosed disorders face similar decisions. Clearly, there can be advantages to withholding or limiting information. It may reduce the anxiety or pain of others, and it helps set limits to the problematic interactions discussed immediately above and under Communication. However, it also limits potential sources of support, including from those who have experienced similar circumstances, and it may also contribute to the overall sense of social isolation (Marshak et al., 1999).

The relevance of social isolation extends beyond its direct social and emotional impact. Social support has been identified as a major factor related to positive coping and adaptation after stressful or deleterious experiences. The extensive research literature includes evidence for the positive effects of social support on parents of children with disabilities, women who have experienced reproductive loss, and parents during the terminal illness of their child (Black, 1993; Darling, 1991; Rando, 1983).

Wills (1985) has identified a number of functions of social support that, in the course of actual social interactions, are often highly interrelated: Self-esteem is improved through the opportunity to discuss one's situation with others and through acceptance by others despite one's difficulties. Participation or membership in socially sanctioned relationships, organizations, and activities provides evidence of acceptance and the ability to function in interactions with others. Individuals outside the immediate situation may provide helpful information, advice, guidance, and independent assessment. Practical or instrumental support takes innumerable forms, including assistance with daily needs or obligations, gifts or loans of helpful items or resources, respite care, financial assistance, etc. Social companionship may provide opportunities for desirable social, recreational, and leisure activities and increase opportunities for the other forms of social benefit. Social interactions may provide motivation to persist in efforts to meet and overcome the practical and emotional consequences of the situation. An additional function must be added to these: Through the sharing of feelings, experiences, memories, values, and beliefs, social interactions play an important role in the process of finding meaning in the situation and the pain and loss that follow (Rosenblatt, 1988).

Interactions with others who confront or have confronted similar situations may be of particular value. These individuals can provide help through information, advice, and problem solving. They may serve as role models or offer motivational support. Furthermore, it is among such individuals that the counselee may feel most understood and accepted. The sense of isolation, of being singled out by fate, and of having frightening or unacceptable feelings and thoughts may be alleviated. For example, when other parents of children with disabilities acknowledge ambivalent feelings or death wishes, it may lead to a sense of normality and relief from guilt that is unavailable in any other setting. As "Rose Green" (1992, p. 67) has poignantly stated concerning her experience following an abortion for Down syndrome, "The advantage of going to the support group is that the other people there are also struggling along 'in molasses.' Listening to their reactions, bizarre thoughts, and grief confirms that I'm not *crazy* for feeling the way I do. There in the group, I don't have to explain or justify anything."

Genetic counselors can address social isolation at a variety of levels. Specific interventions that address guilt, shame, or stigmatization may reduce their impact as it affects social isolation. For some counselees, the genetic counselor's empathic acceptance of their situation and responses provides a healing experience compared to those they have encountered elsewhere. Interpretation and anticipatory guidance may be of help. Analogous to the issue of similarities and differences in coping mechanisms discussed previously in Similarities and Differences, counselees may not recognize that ineptness or defenses underlie the hurtful responses of others.

Exploration of family issues relevant to communication and direct discussion about whom to inform may promote decisions that reduce social isolation. It is sometimes useful to discuss ways of responding to the inappropriate comments, distancing, or rudeness of others. Keeping a journal of comments and possible responses, or using a tape recorder to formulate and refine responses, including ones that initially seem unacceptable, may be helpful. This approach must take into account the importance of the individual to the counselee. For anonymous "supermarket" interactions, a brief explanation or rejoinder consistent with the counselee's personality and mood will suffice. The situation is different when the individual has an important or valued relationship to the counselee, such as a family member, friend, or coworker. A comment or explanation concerning the extent of loss and pain, the desired degree of communication, or the understandable difficulty of communicating given the circumstances may substantially improve subsequent interactions. However, this places yet another responsibility on the counselee. Thus, he or she must consider how much effort, emotion, and self-exposure to expend for any given relationship (Miezio, 1983; Shapiro, 1993).

The genetic counselor also has a direct impact through referrals to social services, support groups, individuals with circumstances similar to the counselee's, and mental health professionals (Darling, 1991). The genetic counselor's knowledge of resources and her sensitivity to the counselee's needs and desires are critical. The potential value of support groups and individual contacts, which has already been discussed, is relevant here. However, counselees may also have important reasons for declining or withdrawing from such interactions. They may not (yet) wish to define themselves or their situation in the manner implied by the support group or individual contact (e.g., parent of a child with a disability). Counselees may not be ready to confront the issues or emotions that will be evoked or may wish to avoid exposure to more severe, less severe, or more advanced situations than their own. Finally, discussed later in Chapter 3 under Mental Health Referrals, a counselee's declining of a referral when it is given by no means implies that the process of making the referral is not of value.

Religion

Religious beliefs and practices are an important part of the lives of many individuals. According to a national survey conducted in the United States in 1995, the majority of respondents indicated a belief in God or a universal spirit, and a substantial minority reported that they attend church or read religious literature weekly (Gallup, 1996). Studies in the medical literature suggest that some patients would prefer that their physicians include religion in a discussion of treatment and adaptation to medical conditions (Oyama & Koenig, 1998). In investigations involving genetic counseling, Beeson and Doksum (in press), Rapp (1998), and Weil (1991) are among those who have found that, for a significant proportion of counselees, religious beliefs influence reproductive decision making and the process of coping with adverse events such as prenatal diagnosis results or the birth of an affected child.

Religion and spirituality may affect individuals in a number of ways relevant to genetic counseling. Religious beliefs may provide answers to the existential search for meaning following an untoward event. For example, counselees may believe the birth of a child with a disability represents God's will or is a test that God has set for them. Such beliefs may be interpreted in largely positive, if painful, terms. However, they may also involve divine retribution, as in the belief that the affected child is punishment for a previous elective abortion or for premarital sex (Bosk, 1993a). There are many ways in which religion can provide support and solace during difficult times. These include belief in God or a higher entity, prayer, attendance at religious services, direct religious or spiritual experiences, religious or spiritual literature, the blessing or absolution of a clergyperson, and the experience of the communal support of church and congregation. Funerals or spiritually oriented memorial services allow both mourning for and commemoration of a person who has died. More broadly, in the fracturing of hopes, expectations, and assumptions that follow a severe crisis, religious beliefs and practices may provide guidance and support for the adaptive restructuring of life in response to new circumstances (Hines, 1998; Walsh, 1998). As Pargament (1997, p. 221–222) states, "suffering may become something explainable, bearable, and even valuable."

The relationship between religion and genetic counseling is complex with respect to reproductive issues such as genetic screening, genetic testing, prenatal diagnosis, and elective abortion. Most commonly, the fundamental issue involves a religious prohibition against abortion. However, religious practices may also influence other matters such as the acceptability of adoption following the birth of an affected child or spouse selection with respect to carrier status for a recessive disorder (Greb, 1998; Rapp, 1998). For some counselees, religious beliefs support or strengthen a decision to forgo elective abortion or test procedures that could potentially lead to it. This decision may be based on adherence to religious doctrine, belief in divine or spiritual support for a healthy outcome, or a willingness to accept the child as fate or God's will (Sandelowski & Jones, 1996).

However, other counselees experience tension or conflict between the teachings of their religion and the personal values and life circumstances upon which a decision is based. For some, there is an acknowledgment that personal circumstances may prevail, such that a decision is made with the understanding that it may conflict with religious precepts. For others, the conflict is acute and involves difficult, sometimes painful weighing of personal circumstances and values against conscience and religious beliefs (Beeson & Doksum, in press; Rapp, 1988). This conflict may be particularly likely when the need to address the issues is unanticipated, as when routine obstetric ultrasound reveals fetal abnormalities or prenatal diagnosis has been undertaken without consideration of possible abnormal findings and their implications.

Genetic counselors should be prepared to address issues of religion and spirituality with counselees. In many instances, the genetic counselor must open the discussion, since the counselee may not consider these topics to be relevant, appropriate, or of interest to the counselor. Opening the topic may involve following cues given by the counselee, such as a passing mention of church or spiritual practice. Discussion may also be initiated with a general question such as, "Do you see yourself as a religious or spiritual person?" or "Do you have a religious or spiritual affiliation or community that would be helpful?" If the initial response so indicates, more directed inquiry can then follow concerning sources of support or impact on decision making. In some instances, the diagnosis of a genetic disease or birth defect may lead the counselee to a new or deeper attention to religious beliefs, and the genetic counselor can be supportive of this process (Hines, 1998; Whipperman & Perlstein, 1987).

When there is a conflict between the counselee's personal values and circumstances and the precepts of his or her religion, the genetic counselor should offer empathy and support concerning the emotional and spiritual pain or confusion this conflict produces and attempt to identify resources from which the counselee might benefit. This response does not require knowledge of the religion or an attempt to adjudicate the issue. It does draw on the counseling skills that would be used in addressing any other issue confronting the counselee. In so doing, it may be helpful to inquire how the counselee understands the relevant religious precepts (Telfair & Nash, 1996).

Referral to a clergyperson may be appropriate, either to advise during the decision-making process or to discuss a decision after it has been made. This referral may be particularly helpful when it results in acknowledgment of the moral dilemma facing the counselee and offers acceptance or reconciliation within the moral framework of the religion (Vetrano & Siegel, 1987). For this reason, it is important, if at all possible, to be familiar with the attitudes and approach of the clergy to whom referral is made. Religious staff within the medical institution or clergy liaison groups in the community may work very effectively when they have been involved in two-way consultation and sharing of experience with the genetic counseling unit (R. Tung, 1999, personal communication).

3

TECHNIQUES OF PSYCHOSOCIAL GENETIC COUNSELING

===

THE preceding chapters address the complex psychosocial context in which genetic counseling takes place. This chapter begins a discussion of methods for identifying, evoking, assessing, and addressing the relevant issues. The genetic counselor has the crucial task of presenting complicated information of great importance to counselees' lives in a manner that actively assists the counselee to understand its significance, cope with its implications, and integrate it into a set of critical decisions. Viewed alternatively, the genetic counselor is an intermediary, sometimes the only intermediary, between the vast and growing body of knowledge and techniques of clinical genetics and the individual counselees, many of whom never anticipated that they would be called on to confront these issues. Thus, the genetic counselor must take an active role in the psychosocial as well as the informational aspects of genetic counseling (Kessler, 1997b).

Unconditional Positive Regard, Empathy, and Genuineness

Carl Rogers's Client-Centered Therapy has played a central role in the development of genetic counseling (Djurdjinovic, 1998). In Rogers's therapeutic approach, the relationship between therapist and client is fundamental to the healing process and includes three critical elements: unconditional positive regard, empathy, and genuineness (Bohart, 1995).

> *Unconditional positive regard* involves respecting and accepting the counselee as a complete individual, including his or her strengths, weaknesses, and full range of feelings and behaviors. While it is unconditional with respect to the individual, it need not be so with respect to specific behaviors or aspects of personality. Thus, the counselor acknowledges to herself that the counselee has some less positive aspects, and she addresses them in an appropriate manner. This includes setting limits on unacceptable or threatening behavior.
>
> *Empathy* involves an understanding, insofar as possible, of the counselee's lived reality. This includes his or her past and present experiences, emotions, and perceptions of the world, and the role these play in shaping behavior.
>
> *Genuineness* involves the counselor's openness to her own emotional experiences in the interaction with the counselee, and a modulated but honest expression of this in her interactions with the counselee.

Unconditional positive regard, empathy, and genuineness are also important in everyday life. Knowing that one is "heard," that one is accepted despite one's current troubles and trouble-driven behaviors, and that someone else understands and cares underlie caring, helpful interactions among family members, couples, friends, and social acquaintances and are central to the relief that one obtains from such interactions. Thus, genetic counselors can draw on their personal experiences of giving and receiving such care in shaping their interactions with counselees. However, just as this approach does not always come easily in personal life, genetic counselors must draw on their knowledge, skills, and self-awareness when using this approach in a professional setting. An understanding of the individual and interpersonal dynamics discussed in the preceding chapters provides one basis for understanding and valuing the person "behind" behaviors that are difficult to accept or respond to positively. Furthermore, an awareness of one's own emotional responses and their origins is critical to empathy and genuineness in the professional situation.

Unconditional positive regard, empathy, and genuineness send a strong message concerning the genetic counselor's readiness to accept the counselee as a person and provide assistance with respect to emotional issues. These three qualities lay the groundwork for more active psychosocial interventions, and their importance cannot be overemphasized (Kessler, 1999). When any of the three is missing, a message is given that emotional issues are not relevant to the counseling process. However, the potential impact runs far deeper. When emotional issues are absent, the implicit message is that they are too scary to address or too abnormal to be tractable, or that the bearer is too needy, pathological, or unacceptable to be helped (Kessler, 1979a). And the more the counselee suffers from anxiety, guilt, shame, low self-esteem, or weakened psychological defenses, the more likely is he or she to internalize these messages, to the detriment of the counseling process and of subsequent functioning.

In some instances, unconditional positive regard, empathy, and genuineness on the part of the genetic counselor run contrary to the counselee's conscious or unconscious expectations. When this is the case, the genetic counselor's stance may provide a curative experience that leads to altered attitudes and behavior in the session and which may, like any therapeutic interaction, contribute to more long-term change. This is illustrated in the following example.

The husband of a woman referred for prenatal genetic counseling following a screen-positive expanded alphafetoprotein result was openly hostile to the genetic counselor. He expressed anger toward his wife's obstetrician, whom he felt had not discussed the potentially frightening outcome of the "test" that had been recommended. He rose from his chair as he indicated a more general distrust of the medical profession based on his own experiences as a child with severe asthma. The genetic counselor respectfully requested that he sit down, which he did. Despite her visceral response to his anger, she said she could well understand that he was angry, because of his feeling that his wife had not been adequately informed of the possible ramifications of the test. Furthermore, the counselor said, she could see that his experiences as a child made him very sensitive and protective concerning the anxiety his wife was now experiencing. She would do all she could to give them the information they needed to make an informed decision that was right for them. The husband's mood softened considerably. He was an active, if not particularly forthcoming, participant in the subsequent discussion. At the end of the session he thanked the genetic counselor for helping them understand how to reach an appropriate decision.

In this example, the counselee's initial behavior caused the genetic counselor to feel both anxious about her own physical safety and angry at his dismissal of the referring physician and then, by implication, of her own profession and professional abilities. However, drawing on her knowledge and experience, and acknowledging but controlling her emotional responses (genuineness), she treated him respectfully as an individual while setting limits to his behavior (positive regard). She attempted to understand his perceptions, emotions, and responses and responded accordingly (empathy). The result was a significant change in his behavior, indicating that he felt heard and validated as an individual.

As this example illustrates, expressing unconditional positive regard, empathy, and genuineness in the professional situation can be demanding and complex. However, as it also demonstrates, these qualities may play a major role in setting the tone of the session and facilitating further, more active interventions (Baker, 1998).

The qualities of unconditional positive regard, empathy, and genuineness are considered essential to the curative process of a wide variety of psychotherapeutic approaches, although they may be referred to by different names (Gurman & Messer, 1995). However, as indicated in later therapeutic approaches derived from Carl Rogers's work (Bohart, 1995) and in recent discussions in genetic counseling (Eunpu, 1997b; Kessler, 1997b), those qualities alone are not sufficient. More active techniques to be discussed later are also of critical importance.

Informed Observation

In any genetic counseling encounter, clues abound concerning the intrapersonal and interpersonal dynamics of the counselee(s). Virtually any aspect of the discussion or session may be relevant. The counselee's demeanor in the waiting room and during introductions, the manner in which individuals enter the counseling office and take their seats, how and by whom the conversation is initiated, all provide potentially useful information. Facial expressions may indicate anxiety, withdrawal, openness, anger, love, and a host of other emotions. Body stances such as arms and legs folded protectively, tense gripping of a chair arm, or body turned away from a partner all communicate mood and emotion (Djurdjinovic, 1998).

Within the verbal domain there are also many dimensions. Tone of voice and rate and volume of speaking may be relevant, especially if they shift when new information or topics are introduced or in response to a statement by another counselee. Questions or emotional statements early in a session may signal matters that are of particular importance to the counselee. Their early timing may indicate an intensity of need or a desire to assert some control over the agenda. When topics are avoided or deflected, it is likely that they are frightening or painful or that one counselee is attempting to protect another or to avoid conflict over the issue. When a question is asked repeatedly despite the genetic counselor's attempt to answer, it is likely that the counselee is seeking clarification or reassurance at an emotional level that has not yet been addressed (Baker, 1998). Inappropriate laughter or use of humor is often a defense against painful emotions or issues (Kelly, 1977). Metaphors or turns of phrase such as "a snake in the grass waiting to kill you" (counselee with Marfan syndrome concerning the risk of aortic aneurysm), "time bomb" (woman at risk for breast cancer), or "failure" (parent of a child with Down syndrome) can be powerful indicators of emotions and sense of self (Baker, 1998). When a couple or family is present, it is important to assess whether different members are granted or can make the opportunity to speak for themselves, whether statements made acknowledge the emotions that are being expressed, and whether one speaker's comments build upon or contradict those of the previous speaker (Eunpu, 1997b).

It is essential that the counselees' strengths as well as deficits be assessed (Kessler, 1997b). Counselees frequently indicate, even if haltingly, areas of competence and success in themselves and others. Efforts to influence the agenda of the session and to control the level of emotional intensity may demonstrate self-esteem, autonomy, and efficacy. Love, loyalty, honest communication, and effective problem solving are commonly observed among counselees.

Such observations should be treated as working hypotheses. Any particular reaction or communication may have alternate personal, social, or cultural explanations. As the session unfolds, and as interventions based on the genetic counselor's inferences provide further information relevant to assessment, the hypothesis can be further confirmed, revised, or rejected. Thus, there is an ongoing, dynamic process of hypothesis generation, testing, and revision through which the genetic counselor obtains a better understanding of the counselee and develops and refines her responses.

A nephew of the husband in a couple receiving genetic counseling for multiple miscarriages had a documented unbalanced chromosome translocation. The genetic counselor gave a clear explanation, with drawings, of the cytogenetics and its potential relevance to the counselees. The husband asked a number of questions that indicated an understanding of the explanation. Later in the session he repeated several of these questions. The genetic counselor, somewhat surprised, repeated the relevant portions of the explanation. Finally, as the session was concluding, the husband asked if the carrier of a balanced translocation is "normal." The genetic counselor inferred that this was not a request for further information but was driven by his anxiety and the need for reassurance that he was not biologically responsible for his wife's miscarriages. When she responded from this perspective, the husband visibly relaxed, providing strong support for her revised hypothesis concerning the reason for his questions.

Sensitivity to verbal and nonverbal sources of information develops with experience. It requires that the genetic counselor be sufficiently at ease with factual material and with managing the session's agenda for attention to be paid to these aspects of communication. Sensitivity is also influenced by the genetic counselor's own psychological issues and emotional responses. For example, if the genetic counselor is uncomfortable with anger between partners, she may fail to recognize subtle expressions of anger because she defensively represses or denies her perceptions. Alternatively, if her discomfort causes her to be vigilant in looking for signs of anger, she may mistakenly perceive anger in a strongly stated but non-angry exchange of views. Because of her discomfort with anger, she may unconsciously guide the session away from expressions of anger. However, as with all countertransference, the genetic counselor's issues may also be areas of particular sensitivity and understanding. Thus, for example, if the genetic counselor has explored the origins of her own discomfort with anger and can recognize the effects of this discomfort on her responses to counselees, she may be able to identify subtle expressions of anger in others and work effectively with couples around these issues.

Kelly (1977), Kessler (1979b) (Kessler et al., 1984), Minuchin & Fishman (1981), Applebaum & Firestein (1983), Guerin and colleagues (1987), and Marks and associates (1989) present vignettes that illustrate the perception and interpretation of verbal and nonverbal communication. Although presented with reference to more active interventions, they can be usefully studied with respect to the issues just discussed.

Developing Emotional Intensity

Having initiated, insofar as possible, an empathic, respectful relationship with the counselee, and drawing on her clinical observations, the genetic counselor may now weave psychosocial issues into the framework of the counseling session. It is essential to address any emotion that is strongly expressed, either directly or indirectly, in the session. Strong feelings of anxiety, confusion, withdrawal, guilt, shame, anger, grief, or despair will, if not addressed, seriously affect the counselee's ability to interact fully with the genetic counselor and other medical staff and to understand and utilize the information provided (Buckman, 1992). Furthermore, as discussed peviously, failure to acknowledge and address these emotions sends strong negative messages concerning the intensity or normality of the emotion and the ability of the genetic counselor to assist the counselee in the emotional realm.

A twenty-two-year-old man experiencing the early symptoms of limb girdle muscular dystrophy had come to believe, owing to a misunderstanding of information obtained on the Internet, that he had Duchenne muscular dystrophy (DMD). Unable to address the implications of DMD with his fiancé, he had broken off their engagement, claiming a different, spurious reason. He came to a first genetic counseling session experiencing great despair and social isolation due to the presumed impact of the disease on his life, including his relationship with his fiancé. The genetic counselor's repeated explanations and reassurances concerning the probable relatively mild course of his disease were met with disbelief and mounting anger. An empathic inquiry into the source of his anger led to an anguished expression of his despair. After this he was able, guardedly in the first session and more fully in a follow-up session, to accept the much more favorable prognosis and begin to consider how he might attempt to reconcile with his fiancé.

In the absence of strongly expressed emotions, or when such emotions have received attention, the genetic counselor faces decisions about which psychosocial issues to explore from among those implied by the emotions and interactions expressed in the session or inferred on the basis of other information. Many counselees initially express little or no emotion, even when discussing emotional topics, or they focus primarily or exclusively on factual information. It is essential to respect the counselee's individual and culturally based wishes and needs regarding the expression of emotions. For example, psychological defenses against feeling emotions may be needed to cope with the situation; the counselee may fear that the emotion, once opened in the session, will be endless or overwhelming; or cultural values may lead to a deep sense of shame about expressing emotions to someone outside the family. However, both the exploration of issues and the helpful effects of counseling are often facilitated when counselees are able to be more emotionally expressive. The following techniques are helpful in eliciting and developing emotional responses so that they can be more meaningfully addressed.

Empathic Responses

An empathic comment in response to an expressed or inferred emotion can be used to elicit further expression or elaboration (Djurdjinovic, 1998).

It's scary to be given a diagnosis when you thought everything was OK.

That must have made you very angry.

I can see how upsetting this information is to you.

The comment may refer to some aspect of the session itself:

It must have been upsetting and confusing to have so many doctors examining your child in such a short time.

Not infrequently, a statement of this sort involves some degree of inference or "playing a hunch." If the emotion is not clearly expressed, the genetic counselor must attempt to identify its nature and at least some element that contributes to it (Kessler, 1980). In addition, she must assess whether the counselee is potentially open to further addressing the emotion at that time. If her judgments are basically correct, there may be an emotional response or an acknowledgment of her statement, and this may then allow further interventions.

> *Genetic Counselor:* It's scary to be given a diagnosis when you thought everything was OK.
> *Counselee (sighing deeply):* Yes, it really was scary.
> *Genetic Counselor:* Now that you and your husband are over the initial shock, how are you taking care of yourselves? [supporting coping and defenses]
> *(The counselee begins to cry.)*
> *Genetic Counselor (after a suitable silence):* I'm sorry. [social support] *(Then, as the counselee's crying subsides):* I wonder if you ever feel like it was your fault? [management of guilt and shame]

If this approach and others discussed later are used with reasonable thoughtfulness and care, the chance that they will harm or injure the counselee by opening up material that is too painful or frightening is small. In most cases, counselees are sufficiently resilient, defended, and in control of the situation to deflect or deny emotions and thoughts that are too difficult or painful to address at the time (Mintzer et al., 1984). When this occurs, the counselee may refute the comment, act as if it had not been made, or change the topic of discussion. This behavior indicates that the genetic counselor has made one or more of several possible misjudgments: She did not correctly assess the counselee's emotional state; she assessed it correctly but erred with respect to its origins (e.g., the counselee is indeed sad, but it is because of an argument with his spouse regarding an issue unrelated to the genetic counseling); her timing was inappropriate (e.g., the counselee is anxiously focused on the forthcoming specific prenatal diagnosis results); or the counselee is sufficiently defended concerning the emotion or the factors contributing to it to block expression or acknowledgment. Thus, although the session has not deepened emotionally, the genetic counselor has obtained additional information relevant to her working hypotheses concerning the counselee.

Direct Statements

The genetic counselor may also be more direct in commenting on emotional material.

It's quite confusing.

I have the feeling that you are pretty angry about this.

For counselees who are sufficiently open and undefended, this can be effective and enabling.

A more sophisticated approach that may overcome moderate defensiveness or resistance involves relating the statement to an aspect of the genetic counselor's professional judgment and agenda.

I'm concerned about trying to explain chromosomes when you are still feeling so anxious about the amniocentesis procedure.

From my experience, I think it will be hard to focus on what this means for your daughter until we've spent some time talking about how you feel about the fact that she inherited the gene from you.

Statements of this sort combine several elements: First, the statement is a nonjudgmental recognition of the counselee's emotional state. This may be experienced as empathic and understanding. Second, it invokes the authority of the genetic counselor's professional judgment and experience concerning the counselee's emotions, the counseling agenda, and the relationship between the two. This sends the message that the genetic counselor understands and takes responsibility for where the discussion is headed. Third, it expresses the genetic counselor's own humanity, feelings, and fallibility (e.g., "I'm concerned . . ." "From my experience . . ."). This helps overcome the image of the genetic counselor as an emotionally distanced professional and presents her as a helping, emotionally involved, concerned person. The former image may be promoted by the medical setting, the counselee's expectations, the multiple ways in which the genetic counselor must assume responsibility and authority in the session, and intentional and unintentional messages to that effect from the genetic counselor.

Questions

Questions may be used in several ways to enhance the emotional content of the session. Questions that can be answered with a single word or simple comment may elicit a useful response, but they encourage an answer devoid of emotional content.

> *Genetic Counselor:* Did that make you feel upset?
> *Counselee:* Yes. *(stated in a tone that signals an end to the response)*
> *or:* No.

Open-ended questions invite a more expansive, emotionally open response and are less easily answered with an inquiry-inhibiting comment (Baker, 1998).

> *Genetic Counselor:* How did you feel when you heard that?
> *Counselee:* It was really scary. I felt like the ground was crumbling under me.

Open-ended questions are often useful when the genetic counselor infers there is a significant emotional element but is unclear what it is or was (Buckman, 1992).

Another useful type of question evokes a time or situation in which there is high emotional content.

> What do you say to yourself when you are thinking about your son's neurofibromatosis?

> When you wake up at 2 AM, what is your worst fear?

As with the example in the preceding section, this question also conveys the genetic counselor's cohumanity and empathy, either by implication ("I know to ask because I've experienced it too.") or by direct comment ("That happens to me sometimes.").

Reducing Emotional Intensity

The genetic counselor must also have techniques for reducing the emotional intensity of the session when it appears to have become too intense, prolonged, or anxiety provoking for the counselee. It may be helpful to acknowledge the situation, since this implies empathy, understanding, and a willingness to assume responsibility.

> I can see this is very difficult to talk about right now.

Emotional intensity may be reduced by intentionally shifting to a more cognitive activity such as explaining medical genetic information or taking a family or medical history. This is easiest when one is in the midst of the activity and can return to it rather naturally.

Let me tell you some more about the procedure.

One may also reduce the emotional intensity by supporting or evoking the counselee's defenses and coping mechanisms. For example, one could turn to a discussion of how a mother is effectively meeting her mentally retarded child's needs. For a counselee who uses information as a means of coping and defense, one could return to an explanation of technical material. If the counselee has used humor in a modulated, seemingly appropriate manner, one might, with care, interject a bit of humor.

It is important, however, to avoid unconsciously mirroring the counselee's defensive operations. To do so sends the message, often unconscious to both counselor and counselee, that the emotions are too intense or frightening and that counselor *and* counselee should avoid them. For example, what was intended as a humorous comment to lighten the mood evolves into an extended humorous interchange that is inappropriate to the seriousness of the situation. Or, after a counselee cries, counselee and counselor collude in becoming overly invested in discussing technical information. I am not suggesting that one should avoid taking the counselee's defenses into consideration. Rather, the fact that the interaction is unconscious places it outside the genetic counselor's direct control and thus reduces the effectiveness of the interaction (see the later discussion under Countertransference).

Presentation of Self

The manner in which the genetic counselor presents herself, the information she provides, and the basis for her questions and inquiries have a major impact on the emotional tenor of the session. There are situations in which an attitude of knowledgeable authority is critical. An example involves presenting information indicating that a parent bears no responsibility for the occurrence of his or her child's disorder. At the conscious level, it is important that this information be presented with all the authority and assurance that is consistent with scientific data and the genetic counselor's knowledge of it. At the unconscious level, this stance may also evoke the counselee's positive attitude toward internalized authority figures, thus adding to the sense of reassurance.

However, an authoritative stance also creates emotional distance between counselor and counselee, and it may activate unconscious negative responses to authority figures. Several techniques can be used to reduce this emotional distance.

The genetic counselor may include herself in statements about emotions, responses to situations, and existential dilemmas.

> It's normal to feel angry when something bad happens, even if you know that no one is to blame. That has certainly happened to me.

By including herself in this normalizing comment, the genetic counselor puts herself on the same level of human experience as the counselee, thus setting up a situation of equality and human relatedness as opposed to one of authority (Kessler et al., 1984). Her statement explicitly indicates that she is subject to the same psychological response of anger as the counselee. Implicitly, it also suggests she is vulnerable to the ensuing guilt, shame, self-recrimination, or isolation that the normalizing comment addresses in the counselee. Furthermore, her statement changes the normalizing frame of reference from an abstraction—"you and other people"—to the engaged, self-inclusive "all of us."

Questions may be stated in a manner that suggests uncertainty on the genetic counselor's part or an effort to understand the counselee (Kessler, 1997b).

> I'm trying to understand this. Your brother's experiences with hemophilia greatly affect your view of the disease, but you are beginning to realize it's not always that severe.
>
> From what you've said, I get the feeling that you would like to tell your mother that this decision is up to you and your wife.
>
> Tell me if I'm wrong, but it sounds like the higher miscarriage rate with CVS (chorionic villi sampling) makes a big difference to you.

In each case the genetic counselor may have had a clear perception of the situation (whether correct or incorrect), which could have been stated in an unequivocal manner, for example:

> Your brother's experiences with hemophilia greatly affect your view of the disease, but as we've discussed, it's not always that severe.

By suggesting her own uncertainty, the genetic counselor puts herself on a par with the counselee as someone who is struggling for understanding in a complex, emotion-laden situation. Putting the comment in this context encourages the counselee to explore the situation further, as opposed to responding, perhaps defensively, to the preceding authoritative statement.

Comments about scientific uncertainty or limits to knowledge may be presented in a similar fashion.

> Although scientists have known about the maternal age effect for a long time, they are still searching for an explanation of why older mothers are more likely to have a child with Down syndrome.

Contrast this with the more authoritative statement

> There is still no explanation for why older mothers are more likely to have a child with Down syndrome.

The latter projects the counselee into the realm of unexplained, random, existentially meaningless events. The former establishes a context of humankind's ongoing efforts to understand and eventually prevent such events.

Promoting Competence and Autonomy

Despite the multiple strengths of most counselees, the circumstances that lead to genetic counseling and the process itself may produce stress, anxiety, depression, self-doubt, and low self-esteem. According to Kessler (1999), given the genetic counseling goals of promoting autonomy in decision making and providing assistance in coping with practical and emotional issues, interventions that support and enhance counselees' sense of competence and autonomy are essential. As Kessler (1997b, p. 382) states, "[C]lients almost always crave the approval, high regard, and respect of professionals."

This can often be accomplished with direct comments that highlight, support, and praise counselees' perceptions, actions, and coping mechanisms.

> I can see that you've been able to figure out the most important issues to consider in making this decision.

Your quick follow-up on the referral for physical therapy really contributed to your son's improvement.

You've obviously learned how to use the information we gave you to help you through rough emotional periods.

Comments of this sort may also refer to couple or family issues.

I see you've been able to support each other even though your coping styles are very different.

Telling your mother how angry you felt really helped clarify things. Now you are getting the support you wanted and certainly deserve.

Supportive statements of this sort are often unexpected, which adds to their emotional impact. These comments help repair previous experiences of feeling judged, stigmatized, or treated with insufficient respect for autonomy. As with all reparative interventions, they may have a longer-term impact on self-esteem and efficacy.

Reframing

Reframing involves restating a situation in a manner that casts it in a more favorable light, broadens the counselee's perception of possible strengths and solutions, or normalizes what had been perceived as deficits or failings (Kessler, 1997b).

A classic example is to reframe a couple's different coping mechanisms, which have been a source of disagreement and anger, as a division of responsibilities.

To one partner: I see that you have been the one who has acknowledged and expressed how hard this has been for both of you.
To the other partner: And you have helped hold things together by keeping a stiff upper lip and working hard to ensure there are adequate financial resources.

For each partner, this reframes the behavior of the other in a more functional, sympathetic light. It may also alter or clarify each partner's self-image. As with any intervention, if the counselees appear reasonably receptive, one can continue.

It's been working reasonably well in terms of taking care of business, but it has caused a lot of stress between the two of you. Maybe you could help each other out and begin to share the responsibilities more evenly.

Separating the practical from the emotional allows the genetic counselor to point out that there has been a positive, functional aspect to these dynamics, despite the emotional costs. Reframing the pain, anger, and sense of abandonment as a "misunderstanding" promotes the idea that this situation is due to limitations of communication, perception, and empathy rather than to willfully hurtful behaviors. The genetic counselor then reframes the options and available competencies: With increased understanding and empathy, you can improve your relationship and help your partner.

This example illustrates another important aspect of reframing. Some reframing statements may immediately feel correct to the counselee.

Counselee (internally or verbally): Yes, I can see that he (or she) was trying too!

When this occurs, the genetic counselor can move forward fairly readily from such a statement. However, some reframing statements may be difficult for the counselee to accept.

Counselee: To call the pain and anger I've been feeling a "misunderstanding" is bullshit.

When this occurs, the initial reframing statement serves as the opening step in a more extended attempt to provide the counselee with an expanded, more positive set of perceptions and potential options.

Genetic Counselor: I don't mean to deny your pain and anger, but let's take a minute to look at how misunderstandings may have contributed to what happened. Will you give me a chance to try and explain what I meant?

Both approaches (and all those in between) are appropriate as interventions. However, one must assess the counselee's ability to accept any given reframe and respond accordingly.

Reframing can be used in many situations. The counselee's perception of the options available for addressing a problem and of the personal and social resources that can be utilized may be broadened. Problematic interpersonal relationships may be improved by reframing the emotions underlying behaviors and the possible ways of responding. Emotions that are seen as negative or inappropriate can be reframed as normal, expected, and well within the genetic counselor's experience, given the circumstances. Reframing can aid in the search for meaning and in addressing issues of guilt and shame.

Some counselees display a rigid, "black-or-white" assessment of emotions, behaviors, or self-worth. Reframing can help promote more nuanced, "shades-of-gray" perceptions.

A mother whose daughter had just been diagnosed with Sanfilippo syndrome said, "I wish I had insisted on a referral eight months ago when I *knew* something was wrong. If I had, we would already be getting the treatment and services Jane needs. I feel so bad that I didn't argue more forcefully then." In addition to clear feelings of guilt, the genetic counselor inferred from this and other statements, that the mother's self-evaluation was: "If I had insisted, I would be a good mother; since I didn't I am a bad mother."

The genetic counselor responded: "I know you felt something was wrong. But you also had to consider the doctor's reassurances, and you had good reasons from the past to trust his judgment. I know how hard you tried to figure out what to do, and I think you did the best you could under the circumstances." With this reframing of the mother's self-perceptions, the genetic counselor was in a better position to address the feelings of guilt.

Modeling and Role Play

By their very nature, anticipatory guidance and coping strategies suggested by the genetic counselor often involve changes in behavior and thought patterns on the part of the counselee. Since changes of this sort are difficult for most people, the genetic counselor can assist the counselee in enacting the changes and experiencing both the resistance and the benefits.

One approach is to elicit and model the behavior in the session. This is particularly useful with respect to communication styles (Eunpu, 1997b). For example, if one member of a couple is dominating a session, the genetic counselor may actively elicit comments and opinions from the other. In a similar manner, the genetic counselor may mediate the discussion among a larger number of individuals, ensuring that each has an opportunity to speak and that responses are directed to the content of each statement. If the discussion of an issue is highly emotional, the genetic counselor can model clear statements about the relevant information and incorporate them into a consideration of options. The individual and interpersonal dynamics discussed in Chapters 1 and 2 often contribute to the communication styles just discussed and they are not readily changed. Nevertheless, the genetic counselor can often influence the course of discussion in the session, and in some cases this will have a more long-term effect on counselee functioning.

The technique of role play allows the counselee(s) to try out or "walk through" an anticipated situation, with the genetic counselor commonly playing one of the roles (Kessler, 1997b; Tuttle, 1998). As readers who have encountered role play in their clinical training will recognize, this can be a powerful and evocative experience. The initial role play often brings out unanticipated ineptness or emotionality on the part of one or more individuals. This can be normalized as understandable under the circumstances, and the role play can be repeated. It often helps to have a role reversal, in which the genetic counselor plays the counselee and the counselee plays the other individual.

The parents of a twelve-year-old boy with moderately severe spina bifida were concerned about enforcing responsibility for appropriate household chores, which they considered to be a model for a child's developing a broader sense of responsibility. Their son had become adept at using his disability to argue his way out of the situation. The mother, a full-time homemaker, confronted the issue most of the time. The father was invited to role play how he might help his wife with this situation, by addressing his "son," played by the genetic counselor. In the initial try, the father quickly capitulated, owing in part to feelings of guilt and shame. When the roles were reversed and the genetic counselor modeled a firmer response, the father experienced how supportive and reaffirming it would be for his son to receive a clear message of paternal expectations and confidence in his ability to carry out the chores. On the third role play, the father, once again in the role of "father," made a clear statement about his expectations and followed this with a strong affirmation of confidence in his son's ability to do the tasks.

Addressing Guilt and Shame

Feelings of guilt and shame are common among counselees, and the genetic counselor has an important, sometimes unique opportunity to assist the counselee in addressing them. Furthermore, therapeutic approaches to addressing guilt and shame illustrate the interrelated use of many of the techniques that have already been presented. For these reasons, the treatment of guilt and shame is discussed in detail at this point. This section is based in large part on the excellent paper by Kessler, Kessler, and Ward (1984), which is recommended for additional reading. In addition, the section on Guilt and Shame in Chapter 1 should be reviewed in conjunction with this section.

As with most psychosocial issues, there are three interrelated components to addressing guilt and shame: assessment, expression and elaboration, and response or intervention.

Assessing Guilt and Shame

Guilt and shame are difficult to distinguish because of varying uses of the terms, differing acknowledgment and denial of each in different cultures, the fact that each may be a defense against the other, and the fact that cycles of guilt and shame may occur. However, in the short-term work of genetic counseling, the goal should be to identify and address the dominant emotion as expressed in the session.

Feelings of guilt or shame may be revealed through any of the forms of communication discussed previously. Counselees may state their feelings directly, although among members of the dominant culture of the United States, they are more likely to do so regarding guilt than shame. Demeanor, such as downcast eyes when discussing a child with a disability or unconscious protective crossing of arms and legs while describing a reproductive loss may be evidence of shame. The words used in describing a situation, oneself, or another person may be highly indicative. Terms such as "failure," "vegetable," or "condemned" suggest strong emotions that may well involve guilt or shame. Reported behaviors are also important. Avoiding public settings with a child is highly suggestive of shame. Failing to inform family members or withholding genetic information is more complex. It may indicate a sense of shame and/or guilt. Alternatively, actual or anticipated responses from family members may play a role in the counselee's sense of guilt or shame and be the reason for withholding information.

Beliefs about causality should be carefully noted, as they may provide important clues. Belief in or concern about a specific cause, such as industrial or recreational exposure, sexual or reproductive history, or use of medications may indicate a sense of guilt.

I think all those fumes when we used the motorboat are what caused it.

An emphasis on low risk figures, the unlikely nature of the event, or the absence of a contributory family history may indicate a sense of having been singled out, with underlying feelings of guilt or shame.

The doctor said this only happens once in 10,000 births.

No one else in our family, as far back as I can go, has had a child with cystic fibrosis.

Dwelling on unknown causality may have similar implications.

The doctor said that calling this a "developmental error" really just says science doesn't understand what caused it.

Each of the above statements is plausible as an item of information or a possible cause, and each can be addressed from this perspective by the genetic counselor. However, if the counselee appears to be dwelling on the issue or to have strong emotions about it, possible feelings of guilt or shame should be explored.

In general, guilt is suggested by behaviors and comments that indicate a feeling of failure as a responsible agent in the world—something wrong was done or there was an error of omission. Upon exploration, guilt often involves rather detailed thoughts, memories, or internal dialogue. For example, "I just say over and over to myself, 'If I had paid attention to those fliers about Tay-Sachs screening, we would have known we were at risk.'" In contrast, shame is indicated by statements, behaviors, and demeanor that indicate a feeling of exposure and of judgment, either by others or by one's own standards for behavior and responsibility. Upon exploration, shame is likely to lead to the silence of "shame about shame" or to a further demonstration or description of feeling states (Kaufman, 1996). For example, "Some days I just don't want to go into the office and be asked, or be met with that pregnant silence, about how Jimmy is doing."

Individuals also differ in their degree of psychological development with respect to feelings of guilt and shame. The developmental level is indicated by the extent of cognitive elaboration concerning causality and culpability and by the nature and intensity of the emotions that accompany guilt and shame. In guilt or shame that is relatively undeveloped psychologically, there is a focus on external judgment and on the threat of punishment or retribution. Self-judgment is harsh, and the possibility of forgiveness or compensatory actions seems remote or impossible. Global comments concerning self or causality suggest limited psychological development of guilt or shame.

I feel so guilty.

God is punishing me.

I wish I could just hide.

When guilt or shame are more psychologically developed, the focus tends to be internal, with a sense of personal culpability, transgression, failure, or falling short of standards. Emotions are better modulated and behavior is more appropriately goal oriented. There is greater recognition of the specific events or interactions that led to the feelings of guilt or shame and a greater sense that one may find means of penance, forgiveness, or rehabilitation in the eyes of others. In other words, there is a better articulated understanding of the psychological, interactional, and situational factors that contribute to the feelings, and thus of the possibility of their amelioration. Thus, a more elaborated statement of cause and effect and of personal responsibility indicates a higher level of psychological development.

If I hadn't been in the car accident when I was pregnant, my daughter would be okay.

I feel like I am being punished for having had an abortion when I was a teenager.

I feel so ashamed when Joey acts out while I am shopping with him.

The emotions and behaviors accompanying undeveloped guilt and shame are intense and poorly modulated. Strong emotions of hopelessness or despair suggest a poorly developed, global experience of guilt or shame. This is often accompanied by feelings of deep narcissistic injury, painful vulnerability to exposure, or loss of control. Rage is common.

Sometimes I feel so angry about what has happened I just want to smash everything.

By contrast, more modulated emotions suggest a more advanced developmental level. A more advanced level is also suggested when the counselee recognizes that feelings of guilt or shame are normal or expectable under the circumstances. This indicates that the counselee recognizes the psychosocial origins of the emotions rather than experiencing them as defining attributes of self.

Sometimes I feel really angry, and it takes a while before I can calm myself down by understanding that that's pretty normal under these circumstances.

Not infrequently, counselees will comment that their feelings of guilt or shame seem "irrational."

I know it's crazy, but I just can't shake this guilty feeling.

Statements of this sort may appear to involve the global, harsh self-evaluation indicative of a low level of development. However, they more likely indicate a relatively high developmental level, in that the counselee recognizes that the feelings are not based in external reality despite their intensity and intrusiveness.

Expression and Elaboration

The counselee's expression of emotions and beliefs during the session is a critical step in the process of addressing feelings of guilt and shame (Kessler et al., 1984). When this occurs, the counselee experiences the healing relief of confession, and the genetic counselor obtains information that is crucial to devising more specific interventions.

A common impediment to addressing issues of guilt and shame is premature reassurance, normalization, and/or closure by the genetic counselor. Such actions reduce or inhibit the process of expression and elaboration. Beyond this, they also risk increasing the feelings of guilt or shame by replicating the interpersonal interactions and internal dynamics that contributed to the origins of these emotions. To the counselee who is experiencing feelings of guilt, the message conveyed by premature reassurance, normalization, or closure is, "Your transgression is too immense or the implications too frightening for me, the genetic counselor, to be able to address them with you." Although this message is often unconscious for both counselor and counselee, it repeats the internalized parental and societal messages of moral/ethical failure and impending rejection or punishment that are the origins of guilt. To the counselee who is experiencing shame, these premature responses constitute a failure of empathy and an experience of rejection that recapitulates the formative stages of shame (Kaufman, 1996).

Thus, the most important advice concerning the management of guilt and shame is: GO SLOWLY. As with so much in psychosocial genetic counseling, this need not involve large amounts of time; two or three minutes spent exploring feelings and eliciting their expression may make a big difference. In the following example, the genetic counselor's premature normalizing statement will in all likelihood bring the exploration of guilt to an end, unless the genetic counselor subsequently makes a *corrective* intervention.

> *Counselee:* I know it's crazy, but I just can't shake this guilty feeling.
> *Genetic Counselor:* It's very normal to feel guilty with an experience like yours.

As an alternative, consider the following approach, in which the genetic counselor encourages the counselee to elaborate on the feelings of guilt:

> *Counselee:* I know it's crazy, but I just can't shake this guilty feeling.
> *Genetic Counselor:* What do you say to yourself when that feeling comes over you?
> *Counselee (crying softly):* I just wish we hadn't taken that long ride in the motorboat.
> *Genetic Counselor:* It must be very hard to carry the feeling that you are responsible for your daughter's birth defect.
> *Counselee:* Yes it is. I've been told that couldn't have caused it, but the feeling of responsibility is so strong.

In this interchange the genetic counselor has communicated her ability and willingness to address the counselee's sense of guilt and his or her beliefs concerning the presumed transgression. From the counselee's perspective, the genetic counselor is not overwhelmed. Instead, she demonstrates confidence in her ability to understand and help the counselee. The counselee has been able to express some of the deep feelings of guilt and has experienced the relief of confession. But beyond this, the unconsciously feared judgment of the counselor, who represents society and on whom the counselee projects parental voices and judgments, has not been rendered. The way is now open for the counselor to use additional interventions discussed in the next section. And this entire interaction has taken no more than 60 seconds.

Interventions Related to Guilt

Helping the counselee express feelings of guilt or shame and experience the empathic, nonjudgmental responses of the genetic counselor is the core intervention. Further interventions explore the beliefs associated with guilt or shame and build on the genetic counselor's critical, if brief, therapeutic relationship with the counselee. Kessler, Kessler, and Ward (1984) discuss four guilt-alleviating tactics that may be used.

Use of authority. The genetic counselor uses her authority to assert that there is no factual basis for the counselee's feelings of guilt.

> Those are understandable feelings, but I can assure you from everything we know, Down syndrome is determined before conception when the egg or sperm is formed. Nothing you did during your pregnancy caused your daughter to have Down syndrome.

This authority rests on the genetic counselor's knowledge and experience regarding genetics, embryology, and teratology, coupled with access to and the backing of other medical genetics professionals and the research literature. To reiterate once more the importance of allowing expression and confession, the counselee's experience of this authority also rests on the fact that the genetic counselor has a relatively clear understanding of the counselee's thoughts and feelings. Thus, the counselee is less likely to have internal responses such as,

> But she doesn't understand what I really think I did to cause it.
>
> She wouldn't be saying that if she knew how I really feel.

Counselees will often experience a continuing struggle between a cognitive understanding that there is no rational basis for guilt, on the one hand, and recurring, intrusive feelings of guilt, on the other. Thus, clear, authoritative statements by the genetic counselor, reiterated when possible in follow-up conversations and stated in the report or letter to the counselee, are important, since they can all be drawn on to support cognitive understanding and processing.

Normalization. The genetic counselor states that feelings of guilt are common and normal under the circumstances.

> In my experience, most people have feelings of guilt when they face a situation like this, and I'm sure I would too. It's normal, and we've discussed some of the reasons such feelings arise.

This intervention draws on the genetic counselor's authority and experience in the psychosocial domain. It also involves the counselor's use of self. This helps reduce both the counselee's sense of social isolation and the sense that the guilty feelings are an added burden or stigma. Furthermore, it supports the counselee's cognitive understanding that the feelings have a psychosocial origin rather than being attributes of self.

Reframing. The counselee's actions and perceptions are reframed in a more positive light.

> Your feelings demonstrate your wish that you could have had the knowledge and power to change the outcome. They show your sense of responsibility and love, even though no one could have changed this.

Limiting liability. Limiting liability involves partitioning liability into areas in which there was and was not responsibility or the possibility of control over the outcome.

> You did have a responsibility to take care of yourself and your child when you were pregnant, and as you've said, you did that. But there is no way you could have affected the chromosomes your child received.

This statement limits and makes explicit the area in which there was no possibility of controlling the outcome. It supports the counselee's positive actions and sense of responsibility and uses these in an attempt to reduce the sense of global guilt and failure of responsibility. In some respects it involves reframing, and it draws on the genetic counselor's authority, thus once again illustrating that the different interventions overlap and are interrelated in actual clinical work.

The counselee's developmental stage with respect to guilt should be considered in selecting and formulating interventions. With relatively undeveloped guilt, which is experienced more globally and as an attribute of self, interventions should focus on the counselee's feelings and sense of self. For example, using authority and normalization, the genetic counselor would subtly emphasize her professional knowledge and experience, seeking to counteract harsher, more blaming voices heard in the present or internalized from the past.

> I've worked with a lot of families whose child has a birth defect, and almost all of them have had feelings of guilt, even though there was nothing they could have done to prevent it.

With more developmentally advanced guilt, in which there is an elaboration of thoughts and some recognition of psychosocial origins, interventions should include developing and expanding cognitive understanding. Thus, in using authority and normalization, the genetic counselor would explain and clarify.

> I know, both from training and experience, that guilty feelings are normal and common in situations like yours. They are a way of saying to one's self, "I wish there had been a way I could have protected my son. I would rather feel I had tried and made a mistake than that I had no control over what happened."

Interventions Related to Shame

When responding to counselees' expressions of shame, the empathic, non-judgmental approach should be continued and extended. This helps the counselee perceive the counselor as an understanding, competent professional who will be supportive and helpful. It furthers the reparative process of acceptance and validation and avoids the feared rejection and shameful exposure. In taking this approach, the genetic counselor helps the counselee gain an improved sense of self-worth and greater potential control. Validation, reframing, and normalization may be used. Practical problem solving and anticipatory guidance serve the same ends (Kessler et al., 1984).

> It's understandable that you feel self-conscious taking your daughter shopping, and I know that people's comments can sometimes be hurtful. But the fact that you do take her shopping anyway shows your concern that she not feel socially isolated. Let's see if we can think of some other ways for you to answer people who make inappropriate comments.

This example involves the sequential use of normalization, validation, and problem solving.

As is true for relatively undeveloped guilt, undeveloped shame requires that the genetic counselor concentrate more on the emotional, alliance-building aspects of the interaction and less on cognitive aspects. In such cases, the fact that one is accepting and helpful may be more important than the specific suggestions or assistance in problem solving. However, when the counselee expresses hopelessness, despair, or especially rage, the genetic counselor's ability to be accepting and helpful may be challenged. Faced with these emotions, the counselor must recognize and handle her own reactions constructively. At the same time, she must attempt to sustain an emotional connection with the counselee and overcome the barriers to interaction that these emotions create. When the genetic counselor can remain empathic and involved under these circumstances, there is a real possibility that the emotions will subside and a warmer response will be elicited. This is primarily because the counselee's expectations of rejection and of a comparable emotion induced in the genetic counselor (projective identification, see Chapter 1 under Psychological Defenses) are not fulfilled. Thus, there is a reparative experience that, at least for the moment, moderates the counselee's emotions and defenses.

> The husband of a successful professional couple referred for prenatal diagnosis after three years of infertility treatments expressed outrage when informed there was a risk of miscarriage associated with the procedure. He accused the medical profession of repeatedly prescribing further money-making treatments and of callous disregard for the additional anxiety that this information about risk created for him and his wife. For five minutes, the genetic counselor sat with him through this tirade, making brief comments of acknowledgment when she could get a word in edgewise. When he began to calm down, she said it was understandable that this information was very upsetting, since he had had no idea that there was a risk associated with this new procedure.
>
> This explicit acknowledgment produced the first glimmer of an interactive response since the outburst had begun: He looked at her, grunted agreement, and was silent. The genetic counselor then said, "It must have been very difficult to meet over and over again with doctors and other health care professionals during the infertility treatments, when you experienced so many rounds of disappointment." At this his mouth quivered, he put his face in his hands, and perhaps for the first time, acknowledged the grief and shame he had felt throughout the three years. His wife had appeared immobilized during his outburst, and her face and posture suggested shame. At this point she looked appreciatively at the genetic counselor and relaxed visibly.

As with any single expression of emotions or behavior, the genetic counselor could not determine if this was an isolated incident brought on by the stresses of the specific situation, a type of response that had developed during the anxiety and frustration of the extended infertility treatments, or a more general way of responding to life's stresses based in all likelihood on childhood experiences. However, the wife's behavior suggests that his outbursts have occurred before and they leave her feeling isolated and helpless. The husband's potentially deeper psychological issues, the wife's shame and immobilization, and the impact of all this on their relationship cannot be addressed in genetic counseling. However, the observed behaviors and emotions could be the basis for an empathic referral for individual or couple counseling.

If the husband's shame and rage involve long-standing patterns, they probably affect his perceptions as well as his behavior. Thus, any description he gives of interactions with other health care professionals must be treated with caution. Imagine how he might have later described this interaction, had the depth of his shame and the strength of his defenses precluded the emotional breakthrough that did occur. Indeed, his memory of this session may drift, owing to ingrained thought patterns and the strength of his defenses, toward a habitual sense of being misunderstood, mistreated, and shamed.

Giving Bad News

Inevitably, and repeatedly, the genetic counselor must undertake the task of delivering bad news. However, the circumstances vary widely. In prenatal and presymptomatic testing, the counselee(s) usually recognize the potential for bad news. In the case of abnormalities detected by ultrasound during prenatal diagnosis or routine obstetric care, the bad news may be totally unanticipated. Test-positive expanded maternal alphafetoprotein (triple screen) results may be delivered to counselees who are unaware they had consented to a procedure with the potential for such an outcome. Definitive or provisional postnatal diagnosis varies from the unexpected, as in the case of a newborn with Down syndrome, to the anticipated although dreaded confirmation of a serious disorder in a child or adult who is obviously ill or developmentally delayed. Sometimes no news is bad news. This occurs when the parents of an ill or developmentally delayed child must be informed that, once again, no definitive diagnosis can be made. It also occurs when presymptomatic linkage or mutation analysis proves to be uninformative.

Bad news involves information "that drastically and negatively alters the [counselee's] view of her or his future" (Buckman, 1992, p. 15). Its impact depends on the short- and long-term medical, cognitive, and social implications. However, it is also influenced by "what the patient already knows or suspects about the future"[, and thus by] "the size of the gap between the patient's expectations (including his or her ambitions and plans) and the . . . reality of the situation" (Buckman, 1992, p. 15). The impact of bad news may be exacerbated by uncertainty about the future. This may be due to clinical variability in the diagnosed disorder or by lack of a definitive diagnosis. However, uncertainty is more generally due to anxiety and fear concerning the unknown social and emotional burdens and concerning the adequacy of internal and external resources for coping.

The process of giving bad news begins when the genetic counselor obtains the relevant genetic or medical information. Even if brief, the period between obtaining the information and informing the counselee(s) provides time for planning and emotional preparation. Planning includes a review of what is known or can be inferred about the counselee's knowledge, expectations, potential responses, and resources for coping.

The subsequent step of informing the counselee should be carried out in an empathic, concerned manner (Djurdjinovic, 1998). Insofar as possible, the counselor should provide some form of forewarning that permits the opportunity for cognitive and emotional preparation. This helps soften the blow and initiates the next, complex step of assisting the counselee in dealing with the impact of the information. Forewarning and the opportunity for preparation depend upon the genetic counselor creating a time interval, however brief, between alerting the counselee that bad news is coming and the actual act of stating the information. This involves making a statement or evoking a "cognitive step" (Kessler, 1998, p. 274) that connects the counselee's prior state of understanding and preparation to the information that is to be provided.

Genetic Counselor (to the parents of a seriously ill child who have been seeking a diagnosis): I know you have been hoping for a long time that there would be a diagnosis for Billy's condition. Based on our examination and a review of the previous test results, we are now pretty certain we can make a diagnosis. However, I have to tell you that the long-term implications are serious.

Genetic Counselor (to a woman who has undertaken BRCA1/BRCA2 mutation testing because of a family history of breast cancer): We now have the test results related to your family's history of breast cancer. As we thought they might, they provide an explanation for the fact that a number of people in your family have had breast cancer.

Genetic Counselor (to a pregnant couple who have been referred because of abnormalities detected on routine ultrasound): I know you went to Dr. Smith expecting a routine obstetric check-in, and he found some potential problems when he did the ultrasound. Tell me what you heard from him about what is happening to your baby.

Genetic Counselor (making an evening telephone call to a prenatal diagnosis client and speaking slowly, in a quiet tone): I'm calling with the results of the test on your baby. Is your husband at home too?

The last example indicates the value of discussing the possibility of bad news even when, as in the case of prenatal diagnosis counseling for low expanded maternal alphafetoprotein screen results, the counselee shows some resistance and the genetic counselor wants to be reassuring given the high rate of false positives. Such a discussion fosters preparation and mobilization of resources by the counselee, provides the genetic counselor with useful information concerning how the counselee may respond, and allows a decision about the time and manner of informing that maximize coping resources and social support.

Having informed the counselee of the bad news, the genetic counselor must now turn her attention to the counselee's responses and to the therapeutic task of assisting the counselee in the initial stages of shock and coping. This involves shifting from the relatively well planned agenda for informing the counselee to more flexible, receptive attention to the counselee's emotions and behaviors and to the counselee's emerging agenda (Buckman, 1992). There are many responses to bad news. However, an understanding of the nature and variability of the shock response, the coping process, psychological defenses, and coping mechanisms provides guidance in how to be helpful and supportive.

In the moments following the delivery of bad news, counselees often feel highly vulnerable. To varying degrees, counselees will experience a flood of emotions: feelings of helplessness, disorientation, and numbness; autonomic responses such as muscle weakness, dizziness, and shortness of breath; and feelings of isolation or abandonment—from a hopeful future, from a "normal" course of events, or from the powers that be in the universe. The genetic counselor should allow the counselee to recover from the most acute, immediate reactions, and then express her empathy and concern.

Genetic Counselor: I am so sorry it has turned out this way.

This indicates briefly but clearly, not only empathy, but a willingness and ability to remain emotionally engaged. Whatever happens subsequently, be it a flood of tears or angry lashing out at the bearer of bad news, the genetic counselor's response helps the counselee experience acceptance and support rather than rejection and further isolation.

The genetic counselor's primary tasks now become to respond with empathy and support to the counselee's emotions and defenses and to help the counselee mobilize internal and external coping resources. The relevant principles and techniques are discussed in Chapters 1 and 2 and in the preceding sections of the present chapter. Specific issues that arise when prenatal diagnosis results are communicated by telephone are addressed in Chapter 6 under Counseling Following Medically Positive Results. That discussion is also relevant to other situations in which medically positive test results are initially given by telephone.

When appropriate, the genetic counselor should give the counselee or counselees an opportunity to be alone. This may occur very early, if the counselees need privacy to cry and grieve, or later if they need time to discuss options and make a decision. A brief statement to the effect that, "It seems as if you could use some time alone," is often gratefully accepted. Under other circumstances, the genetic counselor may remain with the counselees but stay silent. Her physical presence and ability to bear witness provide support and reassurance without unduly interfering with emotional processing and interpersonal interactions (Kessler, 1998).

It is a common experience, often reported later by counselees, that little is heard following the statement of bad news. This has several implications. If technical information must be discussed, it should be presented in small amounts, with frequent check-ins regarding questions and understanding. The genetic counselor should acknowledge the difficulty of attending to technical information under the circumstances and anticipate the need to present the information again at a later time. If decisions are required, the genetic counselor should provide guidance and clarification concerning the advantages and disadvantages of the available options and help the counselees with the process of discussing the options and deciding among them. Under these circumstances, counselees' questions or requests for information often reflect a need for guidance or reassurance rather than a desire or ability to attend to the specific details. The genetic counselor should be sensitive to this need and respond accordingly (Buckman, 1992).

> *Father who has just been informed that his son has Down syndrome:* I've heard that Down syndrome is caused when the egg or sperm has an extra copy of some chromosome or other. Is that right?
> *Genetic Counselor:* That is our way of understanding what causes Down syndrome and why it occurs so unexpectedly. We'll have a chance to discuss that it in more detail when we meet again.

Instead of going into an explanation and clarification, which the father would probably not remember, the genetic counselor responds to his need to feel that there is an explanation for this unexpected blow to his hopes and expectations. Implicitly, she also acknowledges his confusion by deferring the explanation, and she reassures him that she will provide guidance and support during this difficult period when he feels confused and overwhelmed.

Giving bad news is hard, painful work. It evokes strong emotions and may activate any of the responses discussed later under Countertransference. However, certain countertransference issues are particularly relevant (Buckman, 1992; Kessler, 1998). There is pain and discomfort at "causing" pain in others. The feeling that the bearer of bad news "causes" the pain is normal, and is true in some respects. However, if the genetic counselor frequently has deeper feelings of responsibility or guilt, these should be addressed, because in reality the situation exists independent of the genetic counselor's involvement or actions. There may be anxiety about the counselee's emotional responses. This may involve discomfort with emotional intensity in general; with specific emotions and reactions such as grief, anger, or blame; or with the responsibility for providing support and comfort. The genetic counselor may worry that she does not know enough about how to handle the situation or will make hurtful mistakes. In addition, giving bad news and addressing the immediate sequelae may evoke strong feelings of one's own vulnerability or memories and images of past tragedies or losses.

Any of these countertransference responses may lead to avoidance, short-cuts, or emotional distancing involving any or all aspects of the process of giving bad news. Countertransference may intensify if there are several difficult cases in a short period of time or after a particularly difficult case. This intensification may involve one genetic counselor or several who work together. When the intensity of emotions involved in giving bad news increases, it is important to address the issues, either individually or through group consultation and processing. This helps maintain the quality of work with individual counselees and reduces genetic counselor burn-out.

Mental Health Referrals

A variety of situations may lead the genetic counselor to consider referring the counselee or counselees to a mental health professional for individual, couple, or family therapy or counseling. The decision to suggest or make such a referral involves assessment of both the counselee(s)' psychosocial situation, on the one hand, and receptiveness to a referral, on the other. By attending to both aspects of assessment, the probability of acceptance is enhanced.

Many psychosocial situations may indicate the potential value of referral to a mental health professional. At the individual level, these include what appear to be unduly intense and/or sustained experiences of guilt, shame, grief, depression, anxiety, social isolation, deterioration in work or social life, or inability to reach a critical time-limited decision (e.g., after a medically positive prenatal diagnosis result). With children and adolescents, indications of the dynamics just discussed may be expressed through behavioral acting out, deterioration in academic work, or social withdrawal. For couples, intense or protracted discord involving poor communication, differences in coping and defenses, sexual dysfunction, physical or emotional violence, or bitterness are relevant. At the family level, failures of communication, anger, violence, major changes involving either social withdrawal as a unit or structural disintegration, and missed individual or family developmental milestones are indicative (Hand-Mauser, 1989). The presumably rare but important issue of the suicidal counselee is discussed in an excellent article by Peters (1994b).

Because of the specific issues involved in reproductive decisions, reproductive losses, genetic diseases, birth defects, chronic illness, and death, referrals should be made to mental health professionals with experience in these areas. It is therefore very important for the genetic counselor to be acquainted with appropriate mental health professionals in the geographic area she serves, based if possible on personal contacts. Individuals trained and licensed under a number of professional categories including psychology; marriage and family therapy; marriage, family, and child counseling; clinical social work; and psychiatry may have relevant experience. The information obtained and personal relationships thus established help the genetic counselor choose an appropriate referral and personalize the referral process with the counselee. In addition, professionals with whom the genetic counselor has established a relationship may provide useful consultation concerning potential referrals (Hand-Mauser, 1989; Peters, 1994b).

Some counselees request or welcome a mental health referral. Others will, for a variety of reasons, overtly reject counseling or psychotherapy. If such feelings have been expressed, they should be respected or, if the need seems pressing and the rejection is not angry or adamant, addressed directly. For the majority of counselees, discussion of a mental health referral may raise substantial resistance. There is normal resistance to addressing pain and dysfunction directly and of embarking on the painful, yet potentially useful path of self-exploration and more open communication. In addition, such a referral may be experienced as an indication of failure, abnormality, mental illness, or stigmatization (Kelly, 1977).

A number of techniques may be used to address or bypass these sources of resistance. The most important is to base the discussion on an empathic, normalizing response to the counselee's pain or difficulty coping with the situation (Kelly, 1977). Two options follow.

Genetic Counselor: It's very difficult adjusting to having a child with a serious disability, and I can see how hard you have tried using your own resources.

Genetic Counselor: It is normal for two people to respond differently to a difficult situation. And even when there is a lot of love between them, misunderstandings and hurt can develop because of that.

Either statement would serve several ends: they normalize the counselee's mental functioning and efforts to cope, stress the situational component of the difficulties being experienced, and place the genetic counselor in a position of empathy and concern rather than of appearing to blame, judge, or make a clinical diagnosis. From this basis, the genetic counselor can then address the potential value of professional assistance.

In my experience, it can be helpful to work with a professional who understands these problems and has experience helping people deal with them.

Specific information concerning the mental health professional and his or her background and experience makes the referral more personal and tangible (Kelly, 1977; Peters, 1994b).

I know a counselor who has worked with many families whose child has a birth defect. I've spoken to her a number of times. She is very thoughtful and caring, and she understands the types of problems that come up for the parents of a child with disabilities.

The tenor of the referral may be further softened by suggesting a consultation rather than counseling or therapy.

I know she is willing to set up a single session, so that you could begin to get to know her and discuss how you might work with her.

There are situations in which the genetic counselor may help overcome a practical or psychological block by offering to make the initial contact for the counselee. However, in most cases this should be left to the counselee. Both the decision and the action involved in contacting the mental health professional involve autonomy and commitment that promote the successful initiation of treatment.

With some counselees, long-standing individual, couple, or family dysfunction or psychopathology will form the primary reason for suggesting a mental health referral. Unless the individual or family unit has had prior positive experiences with counseling or psychotherapy, a referral made on this basis is likely to encounter substantial resistance. This includes resistance and denial related to the psychopathology and maintenance of the dysfunctional system, as well as the fact that most counselees have no expectation of receiving such a referral during genetic counseling. Thus, if a referral is suggested, it is best to base it insofar as appropriate on the specific situation related to genetic counseling. In other cases, a couple or family may perceive that their problems are due an individual family member, often a child with mood, academic, or behavior problems, although the genetic counselor's professional assessment suggests broader, systemic dysfunction. This involves the concept of the "identified patient." In these cases, it is appropriate to use the counselees' perceptions as the primary focus of discussion regarding a referral. Both these approaches rest on a common aspect of psychotherapy or counseling: a transition from the client(s)' initial conceptualization of the problem and its origins to broader psychodynamic and systemic factors (Minuchin & Fishman, 1981; Wachtel, 1994). It is often useful for the genetic counselor to discuss these issues with the mental health professional.

The mental health referral is part of a process. Although some counselees will act relatively quickly, the majority will probably respond more slowly, if at all. This is borne out by my experience as a psychotherapist. Over the years, a number of clients have contacted me long after receiving a referral from a genetic counselor. Substantial time had been required for them to recognize that the problems they faced were more severe or difficult to resolve than they had appreciated and to accommodate to the idea of seeking professional help. Once the decision was made, they engaged fully in psychotherapy or couple counseling. Thus, the success of mental health referrals should not be judged on short-term "uptake" statistics. This aspect of genetic counseling is successful insofar as it helps counselees better understand the nature and origins of their emotional difficulties and become more open to alternative and professional sources of assistance.

It should also be noted that many of the issues and techniques discussed in this section are relevant to referrals for other forms of community and professional assistance, including physical, occupational, and speech therapy and professional and peer support groups.

Countertransference

Genetic counselors work in a highly charged emotional environment. Repeatedly, those whom they assist confront anxiety, uncertainty, difficult decisions, and, in a significant portion of cases, bad news and its consequences. The genetic counselor, by working in an empathic, engaged manner, opens herself to the reality of the counselees' situations and the emotional consequences of interacting with them. There can be no doubt that genetic counselors are affected emotionally and psychologically by their work (Djurdjinovic, 1998; Kessler, 1992c).

Freud introduced the term *countertransference* to describe unconscious psychological processes induced in the psychoanalyst by interactions with the client. Thus defined, countertransference involves a replay of perceptions, emotions, fantasies, and behaviors derived from childhood or other formative life periods, rather than from the reality of the client's personality and behavior. The comparable process in the client, called *transference*, is a critical therapeutic element in psychoanalysis and psychoanalytically based psychotherapies (Scharff & Scharff, 1991b).

The term countertransference is now often applied to a broader set of clinical situations and may be used to include conscious as well as unconscious processes. This expanded definition includes emotions, fantasies, behaviors, and perceptions, both conscious and unconscious, that are induced by the counselee, his or her circumstances, or aspects of the counseling situation. Despite the utility of this broader definition, the unconscious components of countertransference retain a particular significance. Because they are outside consciousness, they are more likely to distort or interfere with the genetic counselor's activities in ways that limit her clinical effectiveness (Djurdjinovic, 1998; Kessler, 1979d).

Countertransference can be induced by virtually any element in the counseling situation. The circumstances confronting counselees are a common source of countertransference. Informing and assisting counselees with respect to the risk or occurrence of mental retardation, physical disabilities, chronic illness, genetic disorders, infertility, or fetal loss may activate the genetic counselor's anxieties, fears, and fantasies (Buckman, 1992; Burke & Kolker, 1994a). This may occur in response to the specific aspects of individual cases or through the accumulated impact of many cases (Swinford et al., 1988). When the genetic counselor has had experiences similar to those of the counselee, specific memories and emotions may be evoked (Djurdjinovic, 1998). More generally, empathic involvement with the stresses, pain, and losses of others will activate the counselor's psychological defenses, may induce universally experienced emotions such as anxiety and fear of loss, and can weaken defenses against the sense of vulnerability or of a meaningless universe (Rolland, 1994).

The genetic counselor's goals, expectations, and fantasies concerning her professional work also play a role. The need to feel a sense of competence and success, the desire to be seen as an expert, or the fantasy of being able to handle any and all cases despite their medical and emotional complexity influence the counselor's feelings and responses. Genetic counselors inevitably address situations that are beyond the control of counselor and counselee alike and work with counselees whose decisions and actions run counter to the genetic counselor's sense of what would be appropriate and efficacious. These circumstances can lead to feelings of incompetence, shame, or hopelessness and can induce anger toward the counselee or the situation (Rolland, 1994; Whipperman & Perlstein, 1987).

Strong counselee emotions such as anger, helplessness, fear, or rage commonly elicit countertransference, which often relates to how these emotions were handled in the genetic counselor's childhood. A parent may have expressed such emotions in a manner or under circumstances that were frightening to the child, or there may have been overt and covert messages that expressing such emotions was unacceptable and would lead to negative responses from the parent or other family members. Countertransference around these issues can lead to loss of empathy, to rejection or emotional distancing from the counselee, and to reciprocal expression of the emotion by the genetic counselor.

Counselees' defenses can also readily induce countertransference (Djurdjinovic, 1998). The genetic counselor may have negative responses, as when she perceives the defense of intellectualization to be inappropriate, dysfunctional, or an impediment to her desire to feel professionally effective and competent. However, it is also common to have positive responses, particularly when the counselee's defense is similar to the genetic counselor's. For example, in the face of painful information, the counselor may collude with the counselee in intellectualizing or in using defensive laughter or humor. Counselees' decisions and aspects of personality, and couple and family dynamics may all evoke strong countertransference. Common examples include decisions to abort for conditions that seem inappropriate to the genetic counselor and couples in which the woman has or appears to have a subordinate role (Kessler, 1992c; Rolland, 1994).

It is important to recognize that situations that are independent of the counselee may induce countertransference that affects interactions with the counselee (Whipperman & Perlstein, 1987). For example, if the genetic counselor has an uncomfortable relationship with another professional who is also involved in the session, the genetic counselor may be withdrawn or angry, or feel incompetent, inhibited, or unusually assertive.

Countertransference can affect clinical work in a variety of ways. The genetic counselor's anxiety, pain, or wish to avoid specific emotions or situations can result in emotional distancing, failure to follow appropriate lines of inquiry, failure to provide empathic responses, and, more generally, premature closure, as discussed earlier in Addressing Guilt and Shame. Anger, frustration, or disapproval on the genetic counselor's part may lead to responses or actions that are not centered in the counselee's best interests. The counselor's body language may express these emotions. Or the counselor may become directive, prematurely end the session or interaction, refer or defer to other professionals, or fail to provide appropriate follow-up. Given the emphasis on empathy and positive regard in the training of genetic counselors, I suspect that emotions such as anger, frustration, or disapproval are particularly likely to be unconscious unless specific attention is given to countertransference in training and ongoing professional development.

"Boundary issues" involving the emotional and behavioral relationship between genetic counselor and counselee are a major countertransference issue (Djurdjinovic, 1998). The genetic counselor may feel a sense of understanding and identification with the counselee due to a perceived similarity in age, stage in the individual or family life cycle, life situation, circumstances involving genetic counseling, or preferred defenses and coping mechanisms. This can be therapeutically valuable. However, it may also lead the counselor to an inflated opinion of her understanding and empathy, for in reality, the circumstances of one life always differ in many important ways from those of another (Kessler, 1992c). A sense of identification, especially when unconscious, can lead the genetic counselor to project her own wishes and perceptions onto the counselee or to become more directive in her counseling. For example, if the counselor identifies with the counselee with respect to age and childlessness, the counselor might skew her counseling in favor of the course of action she would wish to take. A strong sense of identification is also another potential cause of premature closure, when the genetic counselor feels that her insight and understanding preclude the need for further inquiry and exploration.

Self-disclosure by the genetic counselor spans a broad spectrum. Brief, general self-inclusion, as discussed previously in Presentation of Self, lies at one end. Providing information about specific circumstances, such as having had a miscarriage or experiencing high anxiety while awaiting prenatal diagnosis results, lies at the other. Self-disclosure may, in selected circumstances, lead the counselee to an increased sense of trust and of being understood. However, it must be used with great care. From the counselee's perspective, there is the danger that the genetic counselor's self-disclosure will shift the focus of the session from counselee to counselor with respect to emotions, experiences, and need for care (Kessler, 1992c). Furthermore, self-disclosure may activate a variety of psychological responses in the counselee. On the one hand, conscious and unconscious desires for friendship, help, and empathy may lead to unrealistic expectations of continued or inappropriate involvement with the counselor. This can lead, for example, to repeated telephone calls to the counselor, whose purpose is less the explicitly stated reason than the desire to maintain or increase contact. On the other hand, anxiety about the counselor's needs, or fear of increased emotional involvement, may cause the counselee to withdraw emotionally.

From the genetic counselor's perspective, it is essential to attend to countertransference issues that may underlie the impetus to self-disclosure. They may involve expectations or frustration concerning the emotional engagement of the counselee, or the wish to be more helpful than is possible in the genetic counseling encounter. Alternatively, they may result from a need to share unresolved issues or pain with someone who, it is believed, will be empathic and understanding due to shared circumstances (Kessler, 1992c; Rolland, 1994).

Despite the numerous pitfalls involving countertransference, it can also have a very positive role in clinical work (Djurdjinovic, 1998). The developmental experiences and psychological processes involved in countertransference heighten the genetic counselor's perceptions and engender emotional re- sponses that can be an important source of insight, empathy, and guidance. For example, the genetic counselor whose childhood experiences have made her anxious when others express anger may be particularly sensitive in recog- nizing a counselee's repressed anger when it is expressed through body lan- guage or covert comments. The counselor's experiences have led her to be vig- ilant regarding the anger of others, and one of her clues may be a familiar anxiety she feels when others are angry. In another example, a counselor who has experienced a fetal loss may feel a special bond of empathy with a coun- selee who has faced a similar situation. The genetic counselor may have an in- nate understanding of the many, sometimes subtle ways in which social inter- actions can be hurtful, and thus she may be particularly skillful and sensitive in exploring these issues and providing support and guidance.

Furthermore, the genetic counselor's emotions concerning the counselee and the course of the session are important sources of insight. If the counselor feels a sense of transient hopelessness, it may be a signal that the counselee feels hopeless, although it has not been expressed directly. If the counselor feels an- gry, perhaps the counselee is displacing anger onto the counselor. If the coun- selor feels a sense of discomfort with how the session is going, it may be a clue that she is colluding with the counselee in defensive intellectualization or humor. However, the value of these perceptions depends greatly on the genetic counselor's having addressed her own countertransference issues, so that she has a basis for sorting out her own issues from those of the counselee.

Because of the inevitable emotional impact of genetic counseling on the ge- netic counselor and the significance of countertransference to the process of genetic counseling, it is essential that genetic counselors attend to counter- transference issues. Attention to one's own emotions before, during, and after counseling interactions is very important. Strong feelings are not in themselves problematic. However, they suggest the possibility of countertransference. If particular types of clients or counseling situations are experienced as difficult or anxiety producing, or if one makes repeated clinical mistakes or errors that appear to have a pattern, the matter should be explored. Swinford, Phelps, and Mather (1988) present a list of potential countertransference issues that it is helpful to review periodically. Rolland (1994, p. 270) provides a useful exer- cise for exploring personal and family issues related to clinical work.

Because the most significant countertransference issues are unconscious, the assistance of another, knowledgeable person is often essential to recognizing countertransference and exploring it adequately. Clinical supervision, peer con- sultation, or discussion of difficult emotions and cases with colleagues on an as-needed basis can be very helpful. However, for these interactions to be ef- fective, there must be understanding and trust among the participants con- cerning confidentiality, fears and potential consequences of self-revelation, and boundaries to discussing past experiences and current personal life. When such understanding is achieved, genetic counselors, like their counselees, may benefit not only from exploration and clarification, but from normalization and a reduced sense of isolation concerning these difficult professional issues (Djurdjinovic, 1998; Kessler, 1992c; Whipperman & Perlstein, 1987).

Psychotherapy or personal counseling can help address issues related to countertransference. They can lead to increased self-awareness of the developmental origins and contemporary precipitants of emotions and behaviors and to a reduction of repetitious, dysfunctional responses. These insights give the genetic counselor increased conscious control over potentially negative countertransference reactions. However, beyond this, these insights can also enhance the positive role of countertransference. When one can, with reasonable reliability, identify one's own countertransference issues, one's emotional responses to the counselee have greater value and trustworthiness as a guide to clinical work.

Personal or family issues of any magnitude may have an emotional impact on the genetic counselor's work. However, they may be particularly significant when they involve major losses or transitions such as infertility, fetal loss, disability, marital separation, divorce, or the death of a close family member or friend. In the early stages of coping and grieving, related counseling situations may evoke very painful emotions. Limits may need to be set concerning the types of cases with which the genetic counselor is involved. With time, the acute reactions will subside, but pain, grief, anger, and strong feelings about counselees' reactions and decisions may remain. These require careful attention, both to ease the genetic counselor's emotional burden and to address countertransference issues in her work.

A significant issue, particularly in the early stages of grieving, involves setting limits to discussion and expression of emotions in the workplace. On the one hand, genetic counselors often have warm friendships with colleagues and perceive coworkers to be empathic and supportive, so the workplace is a potential source of emotional support. On the other hand, there is the need to limit one's emotional reactions while at work so that they do not become too intrusive during interactions with counselees. Such limits may also be desirable so that work provides a defense and a respite for the stresses in one's personal life. It is important for the genetic counselor and her coworkers to recognize the need for understanding and open communication concerning when, how much, and with whom these issues will be discussed.

4

THE STRUCTURE OF PSYCHOSOCIAL GENETIC COUNSELING

═══════════════════
═══════════════════

G ENETIC counseling interactions vary greatly in length and complexity. At one extreme lies the teratogen telephone consultation in those cases which allow reassurance to be readily provided. At the other lies a family's ongoing involvement with a specialty medical service such as a hemoglobinopathies, metabolic, or cystic fibrosis clinic. This relationship includes multiple family members and spans successive stages in the individual, family, and disease life cycles. More medial is the single face-to-face session, which may also include intake and/or follow-up interactions. Despite this diversity, and the array of other differences that characterize genetic counseling with specific counselees, certain elements are common to most genetic counseling cases. These are examined in the present chapter. This chapter is not intended to promote uniformity or a formula-based approach to genetic counseling. The purpose is to discuss how the sequential, yet overlapping and interconnected elements of the genetic counseling process contribute to successfully addressing the counselee's psychosocial circumstances and concerns.

The medical-genetic components of genetic counseling are tightly interwoven in this process. They may include obtaining and evaluating medical records, evaluation of the medical history and pedigree, clinical examination, clinical laboratory tests, and referral to and report from other medical specialties. The primary genetic counselor, whatever her professional specialty, may be involved in some or all of these procedures. However, the medical-genetic components will commonly involve other professionals as well. Conversely, other professionals may play a direct role in addressing psychosocial issues. Even when they do not, their interactions with the counselee(s) and the genetic counselor play a significant role in how well the stage is set and the tenor maintained for eliciting and addressing psychosocial issues. Thus, although many of the issues are beyond the scope of this discussion, multidisciplinary teamwork and professional interactions among clinic personnel and with outside professionals are of great importance.

In what follows, reference will frequently be made to the genetic counseling "session." However, it is always recognized that multiple sessions, and contacts other than those that are face-to-face, may be involved in the situations under discussion.

Initial Contacts

The circumstances that initiate genetic counseling vary tremendously. For many counselees genetic counseling begins with a physician's referral. This may occur under relatively routine circumstances, such as the referral for prenatal diagnosis based on maternal age of a woman with a normally progressing pregnancy. It may occur with substantially higher anxiety and tension, as when family history puts a pregnancy at significant risk for an affected fetus; when a physician suspects or diagnoses a genetic disorder in an infant, child, or adult; or following test-positive results on expanded alphafetoprotein (AFP) screening. It may occur under crisis circumstances, when severe abnormalities are identified in a newborn infant or in a fetus during routine obstetric ultrasound.

Furthermore, many social factors influence the knowledge and attitudes with which counselees enter genetic counseling. These include information in the media about prenatal screening and diagnosis, carrier testing, and cancer risk screening and testing; the discussion of these procedures in the social circles of some counselees; information obtained on the Internet; and the prior experiences of the counselee, family members, colleagues, and friends. Individuals who consider genetic testing or screening to represent current standard of care, who have high anxiety concerning the relevant risks, or who feel substantial social pressure to utilize such services may request a referral from their physician or initiate contact with the genetics clinic themselves. On the other hand, counselees may have substantial resistance to genetic counseling. This can occur for many reasons, which include a lack of information about genetic counseling, anxiety about procedures or potential results, negative experiences of family or acquaintances, and personal, cultural, or religious beliefs and values. Counselees may also be resistant if they feel they must comply with a medical referral they did not desire or if they have failed to understand that a screening test such as expanded alphafetoprotein had the potential to precipitate the need for genetic counseling.

It is in the context of these multiple factors that clinic personnel respond to the counselee's first contact and, to greater or lesser extent, lay the foundation on which psychosocial genetic counseling can be developed. The essential components of the initial contact are that the counselee be treated with respect; that his or her anxieties, fears, and concerns be acknowledged; that scheduling be as expeditious as possible, with explanations for any departure from counselee request or optimal response times; and that the nature and timing of services are indicated. It is through these approaches that the nascent counselee forms initial impressions as to whether emotions, concerns, and resistance will be honored and addressed in a respectful manner and begins to learn about the ensuing process. Issues of trust, self-esteem, and openness to providing information and expressing emotions are significantly affected by the initial contacts (Kessler, 1979b).

When a genetic counselor is involved in the initial contact, or when clinic policy includes obtaining substantial medical or family history during the first phone call, subsequent stages of the genetic counseling process also begin during the initial contact.

Introductions

The introduction stage involves the initial face-to-face meeting between the genetic counselor and the counselee(s). Even when there has been prior telephone contact, the direct personal encounter, with its multiple sources of verbal and nonverbal information, plays an important role for everyone in setting the tenor of subsequent interactions. As in all such initial encounters, both the counselee and the genetic counselor engage in conscious and unconscious "sizing up" of the other person. For both, aspects of this process may include personal responses,

Do I find this person attractive, attentive, concerned, knowledgeable, respectful?

a sense of what is to be expected from oneself and the other,

What is going to be provided for me? What is going to be expected of me?

and issues of power and responsibility

> Who is the "expert"? Who will set the agenda? Will one person dominate or will there be shared responsibilities?

The counselee may have additional questions such as:

> Will the genetic counselor be kind and understanding, so that I will feel basically helped and cared for, even though what she tells me may be very hard to hear?

> Will the genetic counselor be able to explain this complicated genetics stuff in a way that I can understand (i.e., provide what I need) or will I have to ask a lot of questions to get it straight (i.e., require me to work hard, and perhaps appear stupid, to get what I need)?

> Will the genetic counselor be able to understand what I am worried about but also help me clarify it, because it is frightening and confusing?

The genetic counselor may also be asking herself questions such as:

> Will the counselee be reasonably friendly and forthcoming, so that my job will be basically pleasant, however difficult the issues that may come up?

> Will the counselee be an adequate historian with respect to family and medical history (i.e., provide what I need) or not (i.e., require me to work hard, and perhaps against resistance, to get what I need)?

> Will the counselee provide guidance as to his or her concerns and questions but still allow me to follow my agenda in providing the necessary information?
> (Baker, 1998; Kelly, 1977).

As Kessler (1979b) has discussed, the most important issue that is being assessed and established is that of trust. Trust is crucial to the genetic counselor in terms of obtaining medical and family history, assessing emotional states and coping resources, and making follow-up recommendations. It is crucial to the counselee in terms of feeling safe in expressing emotions and in answering probing questions about personal, family, behavioral, and medical matters. Trust is also an essential element in the counselee's acceptance of and belief in the information that is provided and his or her willingness to consider and follow the genetic counselor's recommendations.

The introduction stage usually involves some amount of social conversation that is either unrelated to the purpose of the session (the weather, the trip to the clinic, general questions about the family) or serves as both a social warm-up and an inquiry regarding an issue of concern (difficulty in arranging the session or in getting to the clinic) (Baker, 1998). This may be quite brief if, for example, other clinic personnel are present and pressed for time. It may be more extended if, for example, the genetic counselor is the only professional present or must walk some distance with the counselees from the meeting area to the location of the session. Introductions also provide the opportunity to establish names, pronunciations, relationships, and preferred modes of referral. When this is done in an unhurried manner, with attention to each individual, it sends the message that the genetic counselor will give time and attention to each person and provides a model of focused, clear communication (Kelly, 1977).

I know of no references that directly discuss introductions in genetic counseling with respect to the counselee's background or previous experience. I hypothesize, however, that a relatively more extended introduction, within available time constraints, would be helpful to counselees whose background or experience makes them less familiar with or less at ease with the professional and/or medical setting of the clinic. Potentially relevant to this, Bernhardt and coworkers (1997) found, concerning preferences for counseling with respect to genetic testing for breast cancer susceptibility (BRCA1 testing), that "higher SES [socioeconomic status] women would often prefer that the provider be an expert, whether or not they know the person, while lower SES women would ideally want the provider to be someone they know and trust" (p. 218). This suggests that, at least in this population, women from lower SES groups are less comfortable with a highly professionalized approach. Thus, additional time taken in introductions and personal interactions might promote a form of relationship with which these women are more comfortable and, therefore, find more trustworthy and reassuring as a source of information and support.

When more than one counselee is present in the session, it is essential to address any differences in the genetic counselor's prior contacts, which occur when the genetic counselor has had telephone contact with one member of the couple or family, but not all. It also occurs if the session begins before the arrival of one or more individuals. Acknowledging the situation, welcoming the "newcomer," and briefly describing what has been discussed help alleviate feelings of being left behind or left out with respect to factual information and alliance with the genetic counselor.

Your wife told me on the phone about your son's diagnosis and the infant stimulation program he is in. I'm very glad I will now be able to get your thoughts and observations too.

Beliefs, Understanding, and Questions

In moving from introductions into the main body of the session, it is important to inquire about the counselee's understanding of the reason for referral,
the nature, cause, and implications of the medical-genetic issue or situation to
be addressed, and the procedures and possible benefits of genetic counseling.
It is also important to ask what questions the counselee may have. The information thus obtained provides the genetic counselor with critical guidance and
insight into the counselee's expectations, areas of understanding, and areas of
misunderstanding or misconceptions. When there is more than one counselee,
the genetic counselor also obtains information about the dynamics of the couple or family in terms of similarities and differences in knowledge, beliefs, and
expectations, and how these are negotiated (Baker, 1998).

This inquiry must be made in a manner that does not induce feelings of
shame or blame due to the counselee's lack of knowledge or sense of confusion. The initial questions, in particular, must be asked with this in mind. In
this respect, a question concerning the referral process or the reason for the
genetic counseling appointment is often relatively benign (Kessler, 1979b). It
does not usually require a large amount of factual information for an answer,
and it allows the counselee to express any confusion or anger he or she may
feel.

> *Genetic Counselor:* What is your understanding of why Dr. Miller referred you
> to the genetics clinic?
> *Counselee:* He said this was a rare genetic disorder, and you are the specialists who
> could help us understand why it happened and what it means for our daughter.
> or: *Counselee:* I *don't* understand—I'm angry and confused! It seemed like he
> didn't know anything about this "rare hereditary disorder," as he called it, and he
> shunted us off to someone else as fast as he could.

Either answer provides critical information for further empathic inquiry that
does not seem judgmental or like a test.

> *Genetic Counselor:* Yes, my area of specialization is hereditary disorders, and I
> think I'll be able to answer many, but probably not all, of your questions. It would
> be helpful to me, as we get started, if you would tell me what you understood
> Dr. Miller to mean when he said it was genetic.
> or: *Genetic Counselor:* It must have been very upsetting to have the doctor you've
> worked with so closely tell you that you had to see a bunch of total strangers. I
> hope we can be helpful. It would help me get started to know what you under-
> stood when Dr. Miller called the disorder hereditary.

These responses illustrate a more general technique for reducing feelings of blame or shame. Rather than asking about specific facts or mechanisms, the questions are posed in terms of the meaning and utility of the information to the counselee. Questions concerning facts and mechanisms may cause the counselee to feel put on the spot, with a need to provide specific details. However adequate the response, the counselee may *feel* inadequate when answering an "expert." When the question addresses the meaning and utility of the information, it asks more empathically about whether the counselee has been able to put the information into a form and context that is meaningful.

Thus, for example, instead of asking

What is your understanding of how an extra copy of chromosome 21 causes Down syndrome?

the genetic counselor might say

I'm sure you have many questions. Has being told that Down syndrome is due to an extra copy of chromosome 21 helped answer any of them?

Again, different responses may lead to further lines of inquiry:

Counselee: It helped me understand that it happened before conception, and there is no way we could have prevented it.

The genetic counselor might then inquire about beliefs concerning why it did occur.

Counselee: Well, it seems like there are a lot of genes involved, so there's no way to cure it.

This suggests that the counselee initially had hoped for a cure. Thus, the genetic counselor could inquire about this and the emotional impact of learning there is no cure.

Counselee: I think I sort of get the idea, but I am confused. It doesn't help much.

The genetic counselor might then inquire what questions the counselee has.

If an empathic line of inquiry is established through these or other techniques, the counselor may then ask more detailed questions with less danger of shaming or blaming. For example,

What is your understanding of how an egg or sperm with two copies of chromosome 21 comes to be formed?

Many areas are potentially useful to explore in this manner. A choice must be made based on available time, the presenting issues and problems, and the tenor of the session as it gets started. However, by asking questions in the context of their meaning for the counselee and by using the responses as a guide to further questions, the genetic counselor increases the likelihood that she will gain useful information and that the inquiry will also help focus and guide the counselee's thinking (Kelly, 1977). It is also useful, in this part of the session, to ask what questions the counselee has. The responses will vary widely. Some counselees will have a number of specific, well-articulated questions. Others will have only one or a few questions, and these may be rather general. Yet others will have too little information or understanding to formulate questions, or the situation will be so confusing or overwhelming that organized thought about questions is impossible (Kelly, 1977; Kolker & Burke, 1993).

This part of the session involves the first substantive attention to factual and psychosocial issues; the main body of the session still lies ahead. Thus, in general, it is better not to attempt detailed answers or explanations at this time. Instead, the information obtained should be used in planning and guiding the remainder of the session (Baker, 1998). The counselee's questions and areas of confusion or misunderstanding should be noted and addressed when appropriate in the broader context of the session. In so doing, it is often helpful and reassuring to the counselee to comment that the questions have been heard and will be addressed later. There are, however, exceptions to this approach. If the counselee is highly concerned or anxious about a specific question, such that these emotions will interfere with attention and comprehension, it is often useful to provide at least a preliminary answer at this time. In addition, if the counselee has serious misunderstandings or misinformation, especially concerning the procedures or potential outcomes of the genetic counseling process, it may be necessary to address these before continuing (Kelly, 1977).

Agendas

Both the genetic counselor and the counselee(s) enter the session with ideas concerning the information to be obtained and the issues to be addressed (Baker, 1998). For both parties, the nature and complexity of the desired agenda may vary widely. The genetic counselor may have a well-defined, complex agenda that must be accomplished within a limited time, as in the case of pre-natal diagnosis counseling. Alternatively, the genetic counselor's agenda may be complex but defined only in broad terms, as in the case of a referral, with no available medical records, of a child with developmental delay of unknown etiology. Another point in this multidimensional spectrum involves the follow-up visit of a child with a metabolic disorder who is well known to the genetic counselor and medical geneticist. In this case, the genetic counselor's agenda may be relatively routine and brief.

Counselees have similarly variable agendas (Kessler, 1979b). Some arrive with well-articulated questions and concerns based on prior knowledge and under-standing. Their agendas may be well laid out in advance. Others have pressing medical, reproductive, or psychosocial concerns, but they are unable to articu-late well-defined questions or needs (Djurdjinovic, 1998; Kelly, 1977). Their agenda may include a strong desire for clarification and guidance. Yet others may have prior experiences such that the proceedings seem familiar and rela-tively routine. Coupled with these differences is the great variability in counse-lees' emotional and psychosocial circumstances. If the counselee is highly anx-ious about the implications of diagnosis or prognosis that will be presented in the session, he or she may want a quick answer to end the uncertainty and seek help in managing the anxiety. Counselees who are confused about or resistant to genetic counseling may come to the session with the intention of expressing their feelings or of confronting the genetic counselor about the need for the session. Couples or families may arrive with disagreement or discord (Kelly, 1977). When this occurs, each person may wish for validation or support from the genetic counselor but fear that this will be granted instead to the other party. Alternatively, one or more of the counselees may wish to discuss the issues in the presence of a presumably impartial referee, witness, and expert.

Negotiating and implementing the actual agenda is a complex but critical matter that is closely interconnected with the preceding stages of the session. As Kessler (1979b, p. 67) states, "As soon as the counselor and counselees meet, they begin to influence and shape each other's behavior and agendas in an at-tempt to have their respective needs met." Assessments of knowledge, trust-worthiness, willingness to assume responsibility, openness versus resistance, dominance versus passivity, and neediness, plus the specific information ob-tained, influence the evolving agendas and expectations of counselor and coun-selee alike.

Thus, the genetic counselor's role is to identify, insofar as possible, the coun-selee's agenda with respect to the nature and intensity of factual and psy-chosocial issues that he or she wishes to have addressed. This is coupled with an assessment of the intellectual, educational, motivational, and emotional re-sources the counselee brings to the task of addressing these issues. This in-ferred agenda must then be integrated, insofar as possible, with the genetic counselor's agenda (Kelly, 1977). The latter may include the need to obtain and present factual information, to assess and address psychosocial issues, to obtain informed consent, and to adhere to flexible or inflexible time constraints imposed by clinic procedures and by the counselee's needs. Clearly, the more flexible the genetic counselor can be with respect to her agenda, the more ad-equately the counselee's agenda can be accommodated.

The Pedigree as a Psychosocial Instrument

The process of obtaining or reviewing the pedigree presents an important op-portunity to assess and address psychosocial issues (Eunpu, 1997b; Schuette & Bennett, 1998). However, for many counselees, giving a family medical history or pedigree in a medical setting is unfamiliar, and for some it is unexpected. Thus, it is important that the genetic counselor explain the relevance of the pedigree to the genetic counseling process and describe in reasonably detailed form the types of information that are useful. This explanation improves the quality of the med-ical-genetic information obtained. In addition, it explains the reason for what may seem to some counselees an intrusive line of questioning, and it indicates that the genetic counselor will provide support and guidance (Bennett, 1999).

Inquiry about the family's medical history may bring up painful losses, situa-tions, or memories. The genetic counselor can respond to these as she would to any such expression of emotions to help develop a sense of empathy and accep-tance (Bennett, 1999). However, even when the inquiry does not evoke strong emotions, the process frequently induces a thoughtful frame of mind that is both inward- and outward-looking regarding family members and family dynamics. When this occurs, the genetic counselor may readily intersperse questions and comments concerning communication patterns, family interactions, sources of support, deaths and losses, and stages in personal, family, and illness cycles among questions concerning the medical history. By treating this inquiry as a normal part of the procedure, valuable psychosocial information can be obtained in parallel with medical-genetic information (Eunpu, 1997b; Schuette & Bennett, 1998).

Counselee (responding to a question concerning health and illness in her extended family): My sister's son, who is nine, has a really severe learning disability.

Genetic Counselor: I see. Have you discussed that much with her?
Counselee: When he was starting school and it was first discovered, she was very upset and we talked a lot. She tells me now that the special education he is getting is making a big difference.
Genetic Counselor: It sounds as if you gave a lot of support to your sister when she was really concerned about her son. Do you plan to tell her about your amniocentesis result?

Another example:

Wife (to husband, after pausing a moment to gather her thoughts): It seems to me that your nephew has some kind of muscular dystrophy, but *(turning to the genetic counselor)* we don't have much contact with that part of his family.
Genetic Counselor (to husband): Are there other parts of your family that you are in touch with?
Husband: I've always been closer to my other brother. I talk to him and his wife pretty often.
Genetic Counselor: Do you feel as if they will understand what the two of you are going through?

When the pedigree is completed and the genetic counselor reviews it with respect to medical-genetic implications, psychosocial issues can also be addressed in parallel.

Genetic Counselor (looking over the pedigree that has just been completed): You said your mother has been a big help in caring for your son. What does she think caused his developmental delay?

This approach allows a wide variety of issues to be addressed in a manner that conveys an interest and concern with psychosocial issues and family dynamics. It also actively promotes the point of view that medical-genetic and psychosocial information and issues are interrelated.

A number of systems have been developed for recording and analyzing family dynamics in visual, diagrammatic form. Structural family therapists use an established system for diagraming subsystems, the degree of enmeshment versus disengagement and other structural features (Hand-Mauser, 1989) (see Chapter 2 under Family Structure). The *ecomap* allows a representation of the relationship between the nuclear family and other individuals and agencies. However, the *genogram* is most easily utilized in genetic counseling, because of its congruence with the medical-genetic pedigree (Eunpu, 1997b).

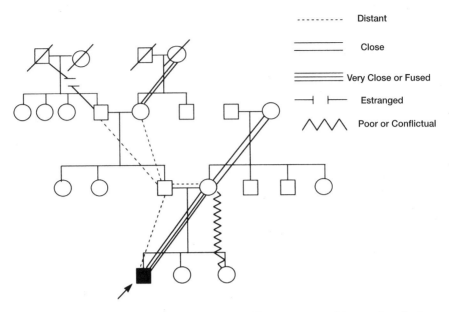

FIGURE 4.1. Mr. and Mrs. Smith have three children: a 17-year-old son John who has spina bifida and two healthy daughters, Joanne (15 years) and Julia (13 years). . . . Mr. Smith's involvement in work translates into distance from his wife, son and parents. Mr. Smith's father was out of contact with his father. Mrs. Smith maintains a close relationship with her mother (as did Mr. Smith's mother to her mother). Mrs. Smith is overly close to John. She is overprotective of him and acts as if he cannot take care of himself. Her relationship with Julia is conflicted due to Julia's unwillingness to participate in family or school responsibilities. Joanne, the middle child, does not figure in the primary family drama since she is doing well in school and ostensibly has no problems. (Adapted with permission from Eunpu, D. L. (1997). Systematically-based psychotherapeutic techniques in genetic counseling. *J Genet Counsel,* 6:1–20.)

In the genogram, genetic relationships are designated by the same conventions as in the pedigree. However, additional symbols are used to indicate the quality of psychosocial relationships with respect to variables such as closeness versus distance, conflict, and estrangement. Figure 4.1, adapted from Eunpu (1997b), illustrates a combined pedigree-genogram for a family in which a son has spina bifida. The genogram facilitates the identification and analysis of psychosocial patterns across multiple generations and among extended family members, just as the pedigree does for genetic data and processes (McGoldrick et al., 1999).

The genogram can be used in conducting and reporting psychosocial research in genetic counseling (Daly et al., 1999). In principle, it could be adopted within a genetics clinic as a standardized method of recording psychosocial data, although this would require resolution of complex practical and ethical issues involving standardization, confidentiality, and patient access to medical records. More readily, individual genetic counselors may adopt the genogram, either formally or informally, as an aid in eliciting and analyzing psychosocial information (Eunpu, 1997b). However, transcending the issue of direct utilization, the ideas embodied in the genogram help elucidate the interrelated nature of medical-genetic and psychosocial dynamics and provide conceptual guidelines for obtaining psychosocial information along with the medical-genetic pedigree.

Presenting Information

Presenting and explaining medical-genetic information lie at the heart of genetic counseling (Smith, 1998). It is at this stage of the genetic counseling process that the medical-genetic and psychosocial domains converge, because the information must be presented in a manner and context that maximizes its meaning and value for the counselee. From among the large amount of information that is pertinent to any genetic counseling situation, the genetic counselor must select both the material and a level of explanation that will meet the counselee's intellectual, educational, and emotional needs and capabilities. The information and its presentation must be accurate, and it must be balanced in its explication of uncertainties, ambiguities, the meaning of risk figures, and the positive and negative implications of prognosis and of potential impact on the family.

Clinic policy, professional guidelines (Marymee et al., 1998), the need for informed consent, and other legal and ethical considerations usually require that certain information be presented. The counselee's emotional state, education, or cognitive abilities may interfere with the ability to attend to or understand elements of this material. Presentation of the required information may take up the majority of the scheduled time, as in prenatal diagnosis clinics where a high volume of clients is seen on a schedule in which genetic counseling is followed by prenatal diagnosis procedures. Furthermore, some counselees resist or object to the presentation of this material, as in the case of those who wish to obtain prenatal diagnosis or other diagnostic tests without the requisite genetic counseling. For the above reasons, the assessment, planning, negotiation of agendas, and building of trust involved in the preceding stages of the genetic counseling process play a vital role in the successful presentation of information.

Order, Complexity, and Pacing

The order, complexity, and pacing with which information is presented have a major effect on the utility of the information for the counselee. Thus, it is at this stage that the genetic counselor's accumulated observations about the counselee's emotions, beliefs, knowledge, concerns, and agenda are brought into full play (Smith, 1998). Counselee questions that were acknowledged but deferred earlier in the session can also now be answered. Misunderstandings or incorrect information can be addressed within the broader context of presenting the relevant medical-genetic information.

Insofar as possible, the order and emphasis of information should reflect the counselee's interests and concerns. Thus, if in a given genetic counseling session, a couple whose child has been diagnosed with cystic fibrosis are primarily interested in the genetics and recurrence risk, these matters should be the first topic that is discussed. Conversely, if their principal concern is prognosis, this should be discussed first. This approach gives the couple the sense that their concerns have been understood and addressed, and it engages their full attention, which is not preoccupied by more pressing concerns or anxieties. In addition, their memory, understanding, and utilization of the information is supported, because it has high importance and meaning for them.

Based on assessments made in the earlier stages of genetic counseling and on the counselee's responses as information is provided, the genetic counselor must strive to fit the level and complexity of explanation to the counselee's needs and abilities. While it is important not to "talk down" to counselees, I believe the greater danger lies in presenting information that is too complex or detailed. The genetic counselor's ease and facility with the meaning and context of the information may make it difficult to recognize the extent to which many counselees must struggle to understand both the content and the significance of new technical information. In some instances, the counselee's cognitive, educational, or emotional circumstances may preclude an ability to understand basic concepts such as chromosomes, genes, or risk figures. When this is the case, it is essential that the counselor describe the situation in simple, meaningful lay terms that are relevant to the counselee's emotional needs and required decisions (Djurdjinovic, 1998; Finucane, 1998b). The critical issue in responding to situations such as these is the genetic counselor's ability to accept that this form of counseling, in which the relevant technical information is greatly simplified to meet the counselee's needs, represents legitimate *genetic* counseling.

Information should be presented in a stepwise fashion. Each step should involve an amount of material that can be encompassed and understood. After each such step, the genetic counselor should pause for counselee responses or ask questions to determine if the information has been understood, whether further clarification or elaboration is desired, and what the emotional impact has been. This approach promotes the counselee's sense of being understood and assisted (Smith, 1998), and provides the genetic counselor with information for ongoing adjustments in the technical complexity and pacing with which the information is presented and with the opportunity to address the emotional responses that are invoked.

Terminology

Introducing and explaining relevant medical-genetic terminology is a critical part of providing information. It is important from an educational perspective, both to facilitate the counselee's understanding during the session and to provide a basis for obtaining, understanding, and utilizing future professional services and medical or educational resources. It may also serve the counselee's coping mechanisms and psychological defenses. The counselee's understanding of relevant terminology facilitates discussion with professionals and involvement in medical decisions and treatment. It may also increase the counselee's sense of control over the situation.

However, as with any profession or area of scientific endeavor, the terminology of medical genetics is highly specialized. It serves professionals well by efficiently conveying concepts and information that are complex in terms of meaning and context. Understanding and using this terminology is an important part of professional training and socialization. For these reasons, inappropriate use of this terminology may confuse the counselee or lead to a sense of exclusion or objectification due to the counselee's lack of familiarity with the terms. These responses may also occur when familiar terms have a technical meaning that differs from lay usage. Terms such as "appreciate" (a sign or symptom), "positive family history," and "uneventful pregnancy" may have very different cognitive and emotional meanings to counselees than they do to genetic counselors and medical geneticists (Chapple et al., 1997; Rapp, 1993a).

When counselees are unfamiliar with relevant terminology, it is important to first provide an explanation in lay language and then introduce the technical terms.

Genetic Counselor (making a drawing or using a diagram): During your baby's development, one part of his spinal column failed to close completely. This left the nerves inside exposed, so some of them don't work properly below that point. The medical term for this is "spina bifida."

For the counselee who will feel helped and reassured by the use of technical terms, the last sentence is an invitation to join the professional, medical-genetic discourse. For the counselee who may feel excluded or objectified, this sentence labels the term as medical-genetic, to be used when necessary but not providing the only basis for discourse.

When the counselee has been exposed to an emotionally upsetting use of technical terminology, the genetic counselor should explain the term and the context in which it was used. It may also be appropriate to acknowledge the counselee's emotions and/or apologize for the situation.

> The father of an infant girl with Down syndrome was deeply offended when the physician, during physical examination, said that she could "appreciate a heart murmur." In the pain and anger of early grieving, he felt his daughter was being treated as an object of training and research rather than as an infant in need of medical care and treatment. The genetic counselor responded as follows: Doctors use the term "appreciate" in a special way when they are describing what they have and have not found during an examination. It means something has been detected. I'm sorry that Dr. Smith's use of the term while she was so intent on making an accurate examination was upsetting.

A different aspect of terminology is the use of alternate terms for the same condition or situation. Should the genetic counselor say "baby," or "fetus," "abortion" or "termination," "mental retardation" or "developmental delay"? At issue are the social meaning, implications, and context of the alternate terms (Finucane, 1998b). Thus, for example, the literal, grammatical meaning of "mental retardation" and "developmental delay" are nearly the same. However, the former has become more fully associated with permanent disability and stigmatization than the latter. (I recognize that there are also differences in professional usage, in that "developmental delay" is often applied to infants and young children on the basis of motor as well as cognitive assessment, or when the permanency of the delay is unknown. At issue is the use of this term when permanent cognitive deficits are known or presumed.)

Two guidelines may be used in making these decisions. First, terms that are euphemistic or are thought to be less emotionally intense should not be used as a substitute for addressing the emotional impact directly. For example, when a newborn's diagnosis clearly indicates permanent mental retardation, it is preferable to use that term, rather than "developmental delay." The emotional impact should be addressed through the timing and sensitivity with which the information is conveyed. If the counselee repeatedly uses "developmental delay," the significance of this usage and the emotions behind it should be addressed as would any other aspect of defenses and coping. Second, insofar as it is consistent with the first guideline, the genetic counselor should use the term that is preferred by the counselee. Thus, for example, if "baby" is preferred to "fetus" as less clinical and more personally and emotionally attached, it should be used (Suslak et al., 1995).

Contextual Issues in Presenting Information

The information provided by the genetic counselor is embedded in a number of different contexts, which provide the broad conceptual framework for understanding this stage of the genetic counseling process. The most general context is the impact of the genetic counseling situation on the counselee's life and on the individual and family life cycles of all those who are affected by it. These are the issues discussed in Chapters 1 and 2. They are addressed by relating the information to the counselee's previous experience and knowledge, to implications for the future, and to decisions that must be made. There is also the context of the genetic counseling session or of the sequence of contacts assumed under this term. This issue is addressed through the interconnected counseling stages discussed in the present chapter, coupled with the counseling techniques discussed in Chapter 3.

As Kessler (1979e) has stressed, there are also multiple, contextual levels of meaning and communication in any human interchange. Nonverbal communication, voice volume and quality, and the sequence of statements all convey essential information that is processed both consciously and unconsciously. In addition to the literal meaning of statements and questions, there is embedded communication concerning emotions such as anger, grief, or thankfulness and embedded requests for responses such as empathy, help, and validation.

Finally, there is the contextual organization of the explanation itself. This involves providing an overview and guidelines that help the counselee understand the significance and interrelatedness of specific facts and concepts, their relevance to the questions and concerns that have been raised, and their potential utility in decision making and problem solving (Smith, 1998).

Elements of this latter contextual approach are illustrated in the following outline of a portion of a consanguinity counseling session.

A couple who were first cousins requested consanguinity counseling. They were particularly concerned about the possibility that future children would have mental retardation. However, they also wondered about the risk for other undesirable outcomes and expressed an interest in understanding why being related increased their risks. The following outline was used in providing an explanation and risk figures, where the statements enclosed in brackets are commentary on the outline. There were frequent "check-ins" concerning the counselees' understanding, desire for more information, and emotional responses:

Mental retardation is increased among the children of first cousins.
[This is a direct, qualitative answer to the counselees' initial concern.]

However, it is just one of a number of disorders and disabilities whose frequency is increased among children of first cousins.

[This broadens the qualitative answer to include their question about other possibilities.]

Although these increases have been clearly demonstrated [The basic finding is unequivocal.] different studies have given different frequencies. [Thus, the risk figures will not be precise.]

These are very difficult data to obtain with accuracy, which is one of the reasons for the range of results.
[This is a qualitative statement that could be expanded if the counselees expressed an interest in more detail. It provides a basis for understanding, and thus perhaps for more readily accepting, the degree of uncertainty in the figures that will be given.]

Disorders with one particular pattern of inheritance are especially increased, [This part of the statement sets the stage and context for the explanation of autosomal recessive inheritance that will follow.] because consanguinity increases the chance that both parents will be carriers for a gene causing such a disorder. [This part of the statement provides a qualitative introduction to the ensuing more technical explanation.]

Autosomal recessive inheritance is explained, with the use of diagrams.
[This provides the specific explanation of the relevant inheritance pattern.]

Identity by descent and its implications for occurrence risk are presented, with the use of diagrams.
[This explains why consanguinity increases the risk.]

Approximate risk figures are given for mental retardation, including an average or consensus value and a plausible range.
[This provides the quantitative answer to the counselees' primary question. Its meaning and relevance are presumably enhanced because the counselees' request for an explanation has preceded its presentation and because the basis for the inherent uncertainty has been provided.]

Comparable figures are given for all genetic diseases and birth defects.
[This provides a quantitative answer to the counselees' broader concern.]

These figures are compared to average or consensus risk figures in the general population for mental retardation and for all birth defects and genetic diseases.
[This places the counselees' risks in the context of general population figures, the unavoidable risks with any pregnancy, and the situation they would have faced had they not been cousins.]

If the counselees indicate an interest, the derivation of the quantitative risk figures are explained based on estimates of the average number of deleterious recessive gene equivalents per human genome.

[If appropriate, the counselees' interest and coping are supported with this more detailed explanation.]

One sees in this example a weaving back and forth between contextual and specific explanations, between qualitative and quantitative answers, and between the specific questions asked and the broader or deeper questions to which, in part through the genetic counselor's sensitivity and guidance, they may lead.

With respect to presenting information, it is my firm conviction that the genetic counselor's most important area of expertise does not involve knowledge of specific facts and concepts, however complex these may be. The critical expertise involves the ability to communicate to the counselee the relationship between the various facts and the relevance of these facts and concepts to the counselee's concerns and decisions.

Meeting with Subsets of Counselees

The presence of more than one counselee may either facilitate or inhibit the expression of emotions and the willingness to acknowledge and address difficult issues. The potential value of speaking alone with one counselee is sometimes demonstrated spontaneously, as when one parent accompanies a child to be weighed in another location while the other remains with the genetic counselor, or when a follow-up telephone call involves only one of the counselees who had been present in a session. Under these circumstances, there may be a more open expression of feelings, a more complete response to questions, the airing of previously unexpressed concerns, or the presentation of previously withheld information.

When the genetic counseling session includes multiple generations, members from different branches of an extended family, or other complex groupings such as a biological mother and foster mother, serious consideration should be given to meeting with some or all of the participants individually or in smaller groups after initially meeting with all the counselees. The composition and number of such groups will depend on many factors, including the available time or number of sessions and the relationships and interactions of the counselees. However, the guiding principle is to see in appropriate subgroupings those who might be defined as the primary counselees. Thus, for example, when a couple is accompanied by parents or in-laws, the couple would be seen separately; when an affected adolescent is accompanied by one or both parents, the adolescent and the parent(s) would be seen separately.

It is best to state early in the session that one either will or might wish to meet separately with some of the counselees. It may also be stated or implied that this is a standard procedure. This statement avoids the more complex task of making the request during a subsequent stage of the session, when one or more counselees may infer that it is a response to specific statements, expressions of emotions, or interactions that have occurred. Counselees usually understand the potential value of this approach and are agreeable. Unless the genetic counselor is in a position to address interpersonal interactions in depth, nonagreement should be accepted with a brief acknowledgment of the reasons stated for declining.

The vignette presented in Chapter 2 under Couples: Triangles demonstrates the effective use of this approach.

Closing the Session

The conclusion of the session may be determined by general agreement that the relevant topics have been satisfactorily covered, by time constraints, or by an assessment that the cognitive or emotional limits of one or more counselees have been reached. If the counselor's and counselee's agendas have been adequately identified and blended and the session has gone reasonably well, the sense of completion may more or less coincide with the end of available time and allow a relatively leisurely closing stage. Under other circumstances, such as when a counselee suddenly seems to reach his or her emotional limits, or when the complexity of issues extends the session as long as possible, the time available for closing may be limited. Nevertheless, this stage involves critical issues and tasks and time must be allotted for them.

It is helpful, whenever possible, to indicate that the session is drawing to a close while sufficient time remains for the counselee(s) to bring up new or unresolved issues or questions (Kelly, 1977). Recognition that the session is ending may heighten emotions such as anxiety over unresolved issues, guilt regarding information that has been withheld, or relief that an emotionally trying situation will soon be over. For reasons such as these, counselees may disclose significant new facts or concerns during the closing stage (Baker, 1998; Tuttle, 1998). If there is time, they should be addressed. If insufficient time remains, this should be noted.

Closure involves several interrelated elements. The genetic counselor should review, summarize, and integrate the most important information that has been presented and the major issues that have been discussed. This helps consolidate the counselee's understanding and ability to remember the information and concepts. It also provides a review of how this information may be used as a basis for future action, planning, and decision making. It thus strengthens the contextual foundations on which understanding, memory, and future use are based.

Genetic Counselor (referring again to a drawing that illustrates autosomal re-cessive inheritance): As we discussed, everyone carries several recessive, disease-causing genes. While it's unfortunate that you both carried one for phenylke-tonuria, this explains why it never occurred before in either of your families, and why there is nothing you could have done ahead of time to prevent your daugh-ter being affected. As we also discussed, there is a 25% chance with each preg-nancy that it will occur again.

Related to this review is a summary distinguishing those issues that have been adequately addressed from those that require further discussion or de-cision. For example, a definitive diagnosis may have been established for the first time in the session, but decisions concerning medical treatment will be made later based on additional clinical tests and/or referral to other medical specialists.

The nature and details of genetic counseling follow-up should be reviewed and/or established. This review may involve specific information, such as the time and date of the next session. It may involve decisions, such as when and to whom the results of prenatal diagnosis should be conveyed in the event of a medically negative or medically positive outcome. It may involve further clin-ical tests or referral to other professionals. The genetic counselor's role, if any, in making arrangements, conveying reports or records, providing explanations and interpretations of results, and providing emotional support should be dis-cussed. In addition to clarifying important procedural matters, this serves to reassure the counselees, insofar as appropriate, that the genetic counselor will remain available, involved, and supportive.

Finally, closure involves personal comments and goodbyes. This is an op-portunity for the genetic counselor to say that she has enjoyed working with the counselee(s) and to comment on positive qualities she has observed. The professional techniques of unconditional positive regard, empathy, and gen-uineness play a role in this process. But these may be deepened and enriched by the working relationship, trust, and appreciation of the counselee's thought-fulness, resourcefulness, fortitude, and love that have developed during the ses-sion (Kelly, 1977).

Follow-up

Genetic counseling follow-up takes many forms. These range from those that are predominately psychosocial in nature and involve the counselee directly, such as a phone call for emotional support following a genetic abortion, to those that are predominately medical-genetic and involve a professional, such as call-ing a medical specialist to arrange an examination and evaluation. However, even at these relative extremes, elements of the alternate component may be involved. Thus, the genetic counselor may reassure the counselee that postabortion tests confirmed the diagnosis, and she may convey psychosocial information to the medical specialist.

Genetic Counselor (speaking by phone to a pediatric ophthalmologist): The parents are very concerned about the possible implications of this diagnosis for their child's vision. So even though we consider this to be a relatively routine evaluation, I would appreciate your explaining this to the parents again and giving them as much reassurance as is appropriate.

Follow-up has many modalities: transmitting medical records, sending blood or tissue samples, writing a letter to the counselee and/or physician, telephone calls, and further clinic sessions, which may involve the same or different family members and clinic team members. Follow-up may be related to a specific issue or procedure, may be part of continuing care, or may have the important role of providing case management when the number and variety of treatments, services, and specialists threaten to overwhelm the family's ability to organize and cope (Seligman, 1991). The psychosocial components of follow-up are most easily discussed in the context of a face-to-face session, where they can be pursued extensively. However, they are also relevant to telephone follow-up and other modalities.

It is important to determine the events and changes that have occurred in the time interval between contacts (Kelly, 1977). The interval may be brief, as in a telephone call a few days after a genetic abortion, or it may be long, as in an annual follow-up clinic visit. Whatever the time span, there are several potential sources of information. The genetic counselor may provide new information, such as a test result or clinical evaluation, or she may know that the counselee has received such information from other sources. The counselee may report events and changes of many sorts including emotional responses, couple or family interactions, decisions, births, deaths, and changes in social or medical status. In addition, the counselee's demeanor and emotions with the genetic counselor and the interactions between counselees provide important clues concerning how things have gone during the interval and how changes that have occurred have affected the counselee.

Sometimes a counselee will have a substantially different demeanor toward the genetic counselor on telephone follow-up than was expressed in the preceding session. There are a number of possible reasons for this. The counselor's approach in the session may have increased the counselee's trust or openness, and this is more fully expressed after the passage of time than it was during the session. The follow-up call may involve a single counselee, who expresses different or more intense emotions in the absence of other counselees who were present in the session. The counselee may have a more distant demeanor, give only curt responses to questions, or abruptly terminate the call. This may be due to the reemergence of defensive distancing that had been reduced during the session, or it may reflect a desire for closure regarding the situation or the genetic counseling process. Because of the unexpected, seemingly abrupt change and the difficulty of assessing the cause during a telephone conversation, these situations, particularly of the latter distancing type, can be a source of significant countertransference.

Follow-up also provides the opportunity to review the counselee's understanding, memory, and integration of information and concepts; to review or correct these as needed; and to further discuss how the information has been used and/or may be used in the future (Kessler, 1979b). Counselees' perceptions, understanding, or basis for decisions may have changed owing to further processing of the information, new information, changes in emotions or medical status, and input from family members or other individuals or institutions.

When relevant, the presentation and/or explanation of new results are of critical importance. When new information is provided, several stages of the genetic counseling process discussed previously may be repeated as the nature, meaning, and impact of the new information are addressed.

Finally, follow-up provides the opportunity for further evaluation, discussion, and support concerning the psychosocial impact of the situation that led to genetic counseling and of the genetic counseling process. Although busy schedules and workloads may limit the opportunities for follow-up, it is important to recognize the sense of clarification, support, and continuity that even a brief, appropriately timed telephone call can provide to many counselees.

5

NONDIRECTIVE COUNSELING, RISK PERCEPTION, AND DECISION MAKING

THE topics of nondirective counseling, risk perception, and decision making are fundamental to genetic counseling. The ethos of nondirective genetic counseling, which has a complex, still evolving history, is conceptualized in terms of the active promotion of counselee efficacy and autonomy. This conceptualization significantly influences the approach to working with counselees, including the techniques used to help each counselee reach decisions that are consistent with both the factual information and the counselee's beliefs, values, and circumstances. The psychological process of risk perception transforms the risk information provided in genetic counseling into individualized perceptions that are influenced by the counselee's life experiences and other sources of information. Cognitive and emotional factors then affect the psychological steps by which a decision is either reached or deferred, based in part on perceptions of risk. Thus, an understanding of risk perception and decision making is essential if the genetic counselor is to use the technique of nondirective counseling to facilitate counselee-based decision making.

117

Support for the eugenics movement declined during the second quarter of the twentieth century because of social and political changes that included recognition of the racist, discriminatory aspects of the resulting laws and policies; genetic advances that demonstrated that eugenicists had overestimated the role of heredity with respect to many phenotypic characteristics and assumed unduly simple patterns of inheritance and selection where heredity was involved; and the fact that the atrocities of Nazi genocide against Jews, Gypsies, homosexuals, disabled individuals, and others had been rationalized by supposed eugenic principles (Caplan, 1993).

Three successive groups of professionals contributed to the rise of nondirective genetic counseling. Beginning around the late 1930s, genetic counseling was provided by Ph.D. research geneticists located in academic settings. They provided information to individuals with a family or reproductive history involving the limited number of disorders known to have a Mendelian pattern of inheritance. Many of these geneticists endorsed some elements of eugenics. These involved the presumed effects of differential reproduction on the incidence of genetic diseases and on the human gene pool, coupled with a belief that "enlightened" individuals would use reproductive risk figures to make "wise," "socially beneficial" decisions (Sorenson, 1993). However, many of these same individuals also practiced and promoted what would now be considered nondirective counseling (Resta, 1997). They provided information while supporting the autonomy of the counselees with respect to reproductive decisions. Their nondirective approach was based on several factors. Their academic orientation and settings supported neither the social activism of the eugenics movement nor the directive ethos of the medical profession. Their intention was to provide unbiased scientific information on which decisions could be based, grounded in part on the belief just cited that this information would lead to "enlightened," "appropriate" reproductive decisions. In addition, there was the recognition that reproductive decisions were the right and the domain of the counselees. Finally, as stated by Reed (1974), there was a strategic element based on the perception that genetic counseling would be socially acceptable only if dissociated from the eugenics movement.

From the mid-1940s, genetic counseling shifted to academic medicine, where it was provided by physicians in departments of medical and clinical genetics. By training and institutional setting, and by virtue of continuing changes in social policy and genetic information, these physicians did not have a broad eugenics agenda. However, they were concerned about birth defects, and their general orientation was one of preventive medicine. Their medical training and practice were also within the prevailing medical model of providing directive medical advice. Nevertheless, several factors contributed to a nondirective orientation. Through advances in cytogenetics, population genetics, and the genetics of multifactorial disorders, it became apparent that individual reproductive decisions

Nondirective Genetic Counseling

The Evolution of Nondirective Genetic Counseling

Practices related to nondirective genetic counseling began to emerge around the second quarter of the twentieth century as genetic principles and knowledge were applied to reproductive decisions and medical diagnosis (Sorenson, 1993). These practices stood in marked contrast to the predominant orientation of the preceding half-century, which involved concepts, values, and laws based on the eugenics movement. Eugenics emphasized the maintenance and improvement of the hereditary stock of the population and nation, defined in highly normative, exclusive terms. It was based in part on what is now recognized as incorrect and inadequate science. The eugenics movement was directive in that it promoted higher reproductive rates by those judged to be most socially productive and acceptable. It was coercive when applied through laws allowing the institutionalization and involuntary sterilization of individuals deemed unfit to reproduce because of mental, physical, or social characteristics. And it was exclusive when used as a rationale for laws banning marriage between members of different "races" and for restricting immigration by individuals with nationalities or ethnicities that were considered to be hereditarily inferior (Sorenson, 1993).

The eugenics movement was social and political. As Sorenson (1976, p. 474) states, "[M]any within the movement looked to the past as an ideal and they were attempting to reconstruct an assumed lost purity of the American race, or to recapture the simplicity of an earlier form of social existence. [They also] looked to the future as an opportunity to improve men and society, through selective breeding, immigration, and social planning." However, eugenics had strong support from leading scientists of the time. It was based on "biometric" investigations initiated by Sir Francis Galton, cousin of Charles Darwin. Galton and his followers investigated the statistical correlations of physical, mental, and social characteristics among identical twins, fraternal twins and individuals with other degrees of relationship, which provided a scientific basis for investigations of heredity and evolution that preceded the rediscovery of Mendel's work at the turn of the century. Eugenic principles were also strongly supported and promoted by many of the leading geneticists in the early decades of the twentieth century (Lubinsky, 1993). By way of example, Sheldon Reed (1974), who is credited with originating the term "genetic counseling," notes that in 1916 all the members of the founding editorial board of the journal *Genetics* had been supporters or participants in the eugenics movement and that, between 1916 and 1930, all four editions of the textbook written by the prominent geneticist William Castle and published by Harvard University Press were titled *Genetics and Eugenics*.

would not lead to the prevention of genetic disease. Furthermore, in most cases the only available decision relevant to occurrence/recurrence risk remained whether or not to have (more) children, with continuing recognition of the counselee's decision-making authority in this domain (Fine, 1993). Sorenson (1993) has argued that the grounding of these early physician genetic counselors in research and scholarship rather than in clinical medicine also contributed to an ethos of providing information rather than prescribing courses of action.

Developments in the late 1950s and 1960s greatly expanded the number of actual and potential counselees. These developments included a continuing increase in the number of identified monogenic genetic diseases; the introduction of carrier screening for Tay-Sachs and sickle cell disease; the elucidation of the chromosomal basis of genetic disorders beginning with Down syndrome and Klinefelter syndrome; and the introduction of prenatal diagnosis by amniocentesis. Carrier screening and prenatal diagnosis for advanced maternal age also involved counselees whose average profile differed from those who had previously sought genetic counseling. In most cases, these counselees had no affected family member, did not define themselves as at elevated risk except based on information provided by or in support of genetic counseling, and had a much lower risk of having an affected child (Sorenson, 1993).

The growing discrepancy between the number of available genetic counselors and the projected needs, coupled with increasing understanding of the psychosocial impact of genetic diseases and prenatal diagnosis, led to the founding of the first master's degree genetic counseling training program at Sarah Lawrence College in 1969, followed by several other programs within a few years. The training programs adopted a value-neutral, nondirective approach to genetic counseling and, more specifically, adopted Carl Rogers's "nondirective," "client-centered" theory of long-term psychotherapy as a model for the psychosocial component of genetic counseling (Fine, 1993; Marks, 1993). More broadly, growing awareness of the psychosocial aspects of genetic counseling led to a more interactive form of counseling in which the counselee's beliefs and concerns were elicited and addressed (Kessler, 1980). Over the next decade and beyond, the graduates of these programs changed the makeup of those providing genetic counseling to a predominance of women, who had received training in both medical genetics and counseling with a specific emphasis on the terminology and ethos of nondirectiveness (Burke & Kolker, 1994a).

Major social-political changes also affected the development of nondirective genetic counseling. The growth of prenatal diagnosis, in which abortion or pregnancy continuation were usually the only options, coincided with the liberalization of and continued struggle over abortion rights (Caplan, 1993). This period also involved broader social change, in which the civil rights and anti-Vietnam War movements of the 1960s developed into the interrelated women's rights, patients' rights, and consumers' rights movements (Rapp, 1999; Kessler, 1997a).

I know of no extended discussion regarding the impact of these social-political changes on the practice of genetic counseling. However, it is almost certainly the case that the personal, professional, and political values of a significant number of genetic counselors, increasingly comprising master's level women professionals, supported an approach to genetic counseling that promoted the counselee's autonomy with respect to reproductive decisions and abortion (Caplan, 1993; Kenen, 1984). Conversely, there must have been a significant proportion of counselees who supported or even demanded such autonomy.

Institutional developments also promoted and reflected the ascendancy of nondirective counseling. In 1975, the American Society of Human Genetics published a definition of genetic counseling that, in part, involved helping the counselees "choose the course of action which seems appropriate to them" (Ad Hoc Committee on Genetic Counseling, 1975, p. 240). This document, by the predominant relevant professional organization of the time, is frequently cited and quoted with respect to the practice of genetic counseling. The founding of the National Society of Genetic Counselors in 1979 provided a continually growing professional organization that has promoted the professional and ethical interests and approaches of master's level genetic counselors. In the 1990s, nondirective genetic counseling was supported by the code of ethics of the National Society of Genetic Counselors (National Society of Genetic Counselors, 1992) and by several other national and international organizations representing professionals and parents and patients (Baumiller et al., 1996).

Four surveys have assessed support for a nondirective approach among those providing genetic counseling. With the exception of the earliest (Sorenson & Culbert, 1977), they have reported strong endorsement of nondirective genetic counseling by predominately M.D./Ph.D. (Sorenson et al., 1981; Wertz & Fletcher, 1988) and master's level (Bartels et al., 1997) genetic counselors in the United States and, with a few notable exceptions, by M.D./Ph.D. genetic counselors in other countries (Wertz & Fletcher, 1988).

Thus, at the beginning of the twenty-first century, nondirective genetic counseling, broadly defined, has a high level of support among those professionals who are identified as providing genetic counseling services. However, as this brief historical review indicates, historical, social, scientific, and professional developments all had significant, interrelated roles in the evolution of nondirective genetic counseling. These same factors influence current practice, theory, and critiques. They will undoubtedly also affect both the practical and theoretical application of this principle in the future.

Definitions of Nondirective Genetic Counseling

The term "nondirective" has been used generically in the preceding discussion. However, its actual use in the genetic counseling literature has not been consistent. Not infrequently, it has been used without adequate definition, and when defined, definitions have differed (White, 1997; Wolff & Jung, 1995). In addition, some of the statements cited in the preceding section that support nondirective genetic counseling have, in fact, not used the term (Baumiller et al., 1996; Ad Hoc Committee on Genetic Counseling, 1975; National Society of Genetic Counselors, 1992).

The stated and implicit definitions may be examined from two broad perspectives. In the first, nondirective genetic counseling is defined as noncoercive or nonprescriptive, in which the genetic counselor refrains from giving advice, telling counselees what to do, or making therapeutic recommendations (White, 1997). This involves far more than simply avoiding giving advice or answering specific questions about potential decisions (e.g., "What would you do?"). A wide variety of verbal and nonverbal activities may also convey the genetic counselor's attitudes, values, or beliefs concerning a decision. These include the selection and balance of information given, the tone of voice and body language with which different alternatives are presented, and the terminology used (e.g., "risk" versus "chance" or "probability"). Another aspect involves whether the counselee's questions are answered in a manner that addresses the underlying emotions and concerns, which is empowering, or in a directive or dismissive manner, which implies that the genetic counselor's agenda and perspective are the only valid basis for discussion (Kessler, 1992b).

This nonprescriptive definition is closely aligned with the principle of value-neutrality, which recognizes and validates the variety of personal, cultural, ethical, and religious beliefs and values held by different counselees. Under this principle, the values of the genetic counselor and the genetic counseling profession should not impinge on the counselee's decision-making process, and the genetic counselor should unequivocally support the counselee's decisions. This approach promotes the expression and utilization of the counselee's own values in decision making. Some authors consider value-neutrality and nondirective counseling to be related ethical principles (White, 1997). Others consider value-neutrality to be the ethical principle, with nondirective counseling serving as a technique for implementing it (Caplan, 1993). These definitions of nondirective genetic counseling are largely proscriptive, involving what not to do and what to avoid. However, they do also involve the active principles of effective communication and a balanced presentation of information and alternatives (Baumiller et al., 1996; National Society of Genetic Counselors, 1992).

The second perspective is based on the principle of counselee autonomy, which promotes the active, competent, self-confident role of the counselee in decision making. This principle has had a substantive place in genetic counseling for many years. With some authors, it is the overarching principle, with both nondirectiveness and value-neutrality considered to be means for implementing it (Gervais, 1993; White, 1997). Implicitly or explicitly, this perspective is prescriptive, in that it involves active counseling approaches and techniques to support and implement counselee autonomy (Kessler, 1997a). It thus stands in contrast to the proscriptive implications of nondirective counseling considered in the absence of an emphasis on counselee autonomy.

Both perspectives are relevant to Carl Rogers's theory of nondirective or client-centered psychotherapy. His techniques of allowing the client to set the agenda and direction of counseling are prescriptive. However, these techniques were developed and promoted to support client autonomy, in contrast to a more authoritarian medical model. Although this is of historical interest given the role of Rogers's theory in the development of genetic counseling, I fully agree with Kessler (1997a) that a more active counseling approach is required in the brief medical- and decision-oriented context of genetic counseling.

Critiques of Nondirective Genetic Counseling

Despite its central place in theory and practice and its high rate of endorsement by genetic counselors, nondirective genetic counseling has been subjected to a variety of criticisms and critiques. These range from the practicality of providing nondirective, value-free genetic counseling to the ethical sufficiency of such an approach.

As a practical and logical matter, nondirective value-free genetic counseling, when strictly defined, is at best a goal to be aspired to rather than an achievable outcome. To provide information that is useful and usable, the genetic counselor must make decisions concerning the nature, detail, balance, and timing of the information she presents. These decisions involve an assessment of the counselee's concerns, interests, education, cognitive abilities, culture, and values. And these decisions and assessments must be based on some concept of what constitutes health and illness, ability and disability, and an appropriate model of education and counseling. None of these aspects of genetic counseling is value free (Kessler, 1979a; Sorenson, 1993).

By way of example, consider a couple whose fetus has been diagnosed with trisomy 21 and who are torn between not wanting to raise a child with Down syndrome and ethical reservations about abortion. Nondirective counseling would include information about the "positive" and "negative" aspects of Down syndrome, an exploration of the meaning for the counselees of both courses of action, and implicit or explicit support for either decision. By contrast, consider a couple for whom abortion is firmly precluded for religious and cultural reasons. Nondirective counseling for them would primarily involve a discussion of practical and emotional preparation for the birth of their child, with implicit or explicit support for their unequivocal decision to continue the pregnancy. For them, the "balanced" approach used with the first couple would probably be perceived as directive, nonsupportive, and potentially coercive in its emphasis on the possibility of termination. Both the genetic counselor's values and her assessment of the counselees' values are involved in implementing "nondirective" counseling in these two situations (Brunger & Lippman, 1995).

In addition, the concepts of nondirective genetic counseling and value-neutrality are themselves highly value laden and potentially prescriptive. As discussed previously, they are the product of historical, social, scientific, and professional developments and struggles. Thus, they are neither ethically absolute nor historically immutable. Furthermore, when the counselee, for individual or cultural reasons, desires or expects direction and advice from the genetic counselor, a nondirective stance is in itself prescriptive. It places responsibility on the counselee that may be unfamiliar or undesired, and it attempts to influence the counselee's decision-making behavior (Caplan, 1993; Kessler, 1992b). As an additional consideration, in cancer risk counseling, decisions may relate more directly to medical management and thus require a reformulation of nondirective counseling along a more medical decision-making model (see Chapter 6 under Cancer Risk Counseling: Cancer Risk Counseling Techniques).

Nondirective genetic counseling has also been analyzed from broader social, historical, and ethical perspectives. It has been argued that genetic counseling cannot be nondirective, since it takes place within the context of medical-genetics, state-sponsored public health programs, clinical research, and commercial enterprises. Because these institutions promote the use of medical technology and often have an implicit or explicit commitment to reducing the frequency of genetic diseases and birth defects, the overall message to the counselee may be directive despite the genetic counselor's nondirective stance (Caplan, 1993; Clarke, 1991). Questions have also been raised as to whether value-neutrality is an adequate ethical stance for a profession that deals with many current and emerging ethical issues. Nondirectiveness and value-neutrality may in part be self-serving defenses. As such, they allow the genetic counselor and the profession to avoid taking an ethical position with respect to issues that may be considered highly significant by individual counselees and the public at large (Wolff & Jung, 1995; Burke & Kolker, 1994b; Caplan, 1993).

Between the inherent limitations to nondirective genetic counseling, on the one hand, and the broad social-ethical issues, on the other, lie questions of clinical efficacy. Strict, narrow definitions of nondirectiveness emphasize what the genetic counselor should not do. Thus, they tend to limit the role of the genetic counselor to that of information provider and to inhibit use of the full range of relevant counseling techniques (Bosk, 1993b; Kessler, 1997a). Indeed, Burke and Kolker (1994a) and Brunger and Lippman (1995) poignantly describe genetic counselors who feel torn between the realities of providing counseling to actual counselees and what they consider to be the strict nondirective ethos in which they were trained and which they feel characterizes the profession.

Broader, more forgiving definitions, backed by appropriate counseling techniques, are required to effectively assist counselees in reaching informed, autonomous decisions. Sensitivity and respect for counselees' circumstances and values are critical, as are conscientious efforts to avoid the unbalanced presentation of information and inappropriate suggestions and directions. However, I fully agree with those who argue that active, autonomy-promoting counseling is also required to provide effective, ethical genetic counseling (Eunpu, 1997b; Kessler, 1997a; White, 1997). That is the premise on which this book is based. It is also from this perspective that we now turn to the subject of decision making, addressing first the related topic of risk perception.

Risk Perception and Interpretation

The calculation, presentation, and discussion of risk figures are central to genetic counseling. Genetic counseling began with the use of Mendelian ratios to determine recurrence risks for monogenic disorders, and occurrence/recurrence risks based on Mendelian genetics remain integral to genetic counseling. Empiric risk figures have been calculated in many domains. These include occurrence and recurrence risks for chromosomal abnormalities, multifactorial disorders, and disorders of unknown etiology; the morbidity associated with prenatal diagnosis procedures; the occurrence and/or severity of specific symptoms in a multitude of disorders; lifetime and age-related risks for the onset of cancers and other adult disorders; and the increased morbidity and mortality attributable to consanguinity. Complex mathematical algorithms are applied to maximize the predictive accuracy of expanded alphafetoprotein tests. The inferential logic and sometimes complex calculations of Bayes' theorem are used to refine risk figures based on a variety of pedigree, age-of-onset, clinical, and laboratory data.

The great effort involved in developing and applying these risk figures and calculations speaks to the importance given to risk assessment and prediction in genetic counseling. Much of this effort was presumably motivated by research interests and by the need to determine the efficacy and safety of clinical procedures and public health programs. Nevertheless, each of these risk assessments is, when applicable, routinely used to provide risk figures to counselees in support of informed consent and informed decision making.

In the 1960s and 1970s, several assumptions dominated much of the discussion and research concerning reproductive risks and decision making. It was assumed, explicitly or implicitly, that the numerical recurrence risk and the medical-psychosocial "burden" associated with any given disorder represented objective facts about that disorder. It was also assumed that prospective parents would weigh the relative risks, burdens, and benefits of various courses of action to make a "rational" reproductive decision. This decision would balance the risks, burden, and benefits of having an affected child with those of having a normal child or of forgoing reproduction in a manner that would maximize the desirability of the average outcome (Palmer & Sainfort, 1993). Thus, for example, it was assumed that the relatively low probability and burden of cleft lip and palate (ca 2% recurrence risk) would lead to frequent decisions to have children, whereas the relatively high probability and burden of cystic fibrosis (25% recurrence risk) would lead to frequent decisions to forgo having children.

A number of studies during this period failed to demonstrate the clear relationship between numerical occurrence/recurrence risks and reproductive decisions (with burden adjusted for or held constant) that these assumptions predicted (Palmer & Sainfort, 1993). These results, coupled with increasing recognition of the psychological aspects of genetic counseling (Kessler, 1979c) and seminal papers concerning decision making by Lippman-Hand & Fraser (1979a-d), led to a growing recognition of the highly complex process by which risk information is perceived, processed, and incorporated into decision making. The "objective" quality of numeric risk figures and disease burden was questioned, as were the accuracy and appropriateness of fact-based, "rational" models of decision making when applied to reproductive choices in the face of genetic uncertainty.

The discussion that follows addresses multiple aspects of risk perception, processing, and decision making, including some theoretical material related to how these issues are conceptualized and studied.

"Objective" and "Subjective" Risk Figures

It is natural to use verbal descriptions such as "high," "moderate," or "low" in situations in which risk is involved. These terms describe and clarify an individual's perceptions of the chance that an event will occur and of the extent to which it will result in difficult or undesirable circumstances. However, a number of investigations have shown that individual counselees apply these terms differently to the same numerical risk figures (Palmer & Sainfort, 1993). Two examples will illustrate contrasting aspects of these findings.

Wertz and coworkers (1986) obtained responses from more than 500 counselees that included both the numeric risk figure received in genetic counseling and the verbal category they would choose to describe it. Responses from the 73 counselees who had received the Mendelian recurrence risk of 25% illustrate the diversity of subjective assessments:

very low	3%
low	19%
moderate	37%
high	27%
very high	14%

Clearly, individual circumstances and assessments affect how an individual views a given numerical risk figure.

A different aspect of risk perception is illustrated by the work of Burke and Kolker (1994a), who analyzed verbal or written responses from 36 prenatal genetic counselors. When asked for the descriptor they would apply to the risk of 1 in 200 for spontaneous abortion following CVS or amniocentesis, 73% described it as "low" or "very low." Although precise figures are not given, when the same numerical value of 1 in 200 was presented as the occurrence/recurrence risk for a genetic disorder, it "was commonly perceived as 'moderate'" (p. 42). Thus, individual genetic counselors used different descriptors for the same numerical risk depending upon the potential outcome to which it referred and the context in which it was considered.

In broad terms, these results show that the response to a given numerical risk figure may vary widely depending upon the context in which it occurs and its implications for the individual. Stated differently, verbal descriptors incorporate these contextual features, as opposed to being closely correlated with numerical value. Thus, verbal descriptions may be helpful when discussing the meaning a risk figure has for the counselee, and counselees commonly use such descriptions themselves (Shiloh & Sagi, 1989). However, these verbal descriptions are an unreliable method for communicating the numeric risk itself.

Factors Influencing the Perception of Risk Figures

Research into risk perception and choices made in the face of uncertainty has identified general principles, personality characteristics, and specific factors that influence these processes. Each has potential relevance to genetic counseling.

Tversky and Kahneman (1974) presented the following three general cognitive processes or "heuristic principles" that influence risk perception and decision making (see also Wertz et al., 1986).

Anchoring occurs when an individual has a prior belief concerning the magnitude of risk that serves as a frame of reference within which new information or risk figures are evaluated. This "anchor" limits the extent to which the new information results in an adjustment of perception or judgment. The adjustment is commonly insufficient, resulting in estimates that are biased in the direction of the initial value. For example, if a counselee initially believes that the recurrence risk is 50%, a risk figure of 25% will be judged as higher or more risky than if there had been no prior belief or if the belief had involved a value lower than 25% (Shiloh & Saxe, 1989).

Anchoring can also result from the order or the context in which risk figures are provided. This is relevant to the genetic counseling technique of giving the population-based risk figure as a basis for interpreting the counselee's specific risk. It suggests that the order in which the two risk figures are presented may influence the counselee's perception of the specific risk. Presenting the lower general risk first may create an anchor that results in a lower evaluation of the specific risk compared to the evaluation if the order of presentation were reversed.

Wertz and coworkers (1986), in the study discussed at the end of the preceding section, found that counselees' verbal descriptions of their numeric risk prior to genetic counseling were the strongest predictor of postcounseling interpretation, exceeding all other factors including the actual numerical risk. This illustrates the importance of prior beliefs on the interpretation of risk. This interpretation may be due in part to the anchoring effect itself, as suggested by the authors. However, it is based on a *qualitative* prior evaluation, which already incorporates aspects of belief that go beyond the numeric risk figure itself.

Availability refers to how easily or readily examples of the potential outcome can be brought to mind. Availability is affected by knowledge or direct experience of situations or events, by the number of such known events, and by the emotional impact they have had. Greater availability results in a higher assessment of risk. Heightened risk assessment by those who have experience or familiarity with relevant disorders has been reported in a variety of circumstances that include having an affected child (Wertz et al., 1986), knowing someone with a serious birth defect (Chase et al., 1986), and direct experience with an affected family member or close acquaintance (Bernhardt et al., 1997). Conversely, Lippman-Hand and Fraser (1979d) found that having an unaffected child in addition to an affected child reduced risk perception. It increased the availability of the outcome of having an unaffected child. Kessler (1992a) also suggests that availability explains the finding that, on average, genetic counselors rate genetic risks more highly than counselees (Abromovsky et al., 1980; Wertz et al., 1986), because genetic counselors can more readily bring to mind multiple examples of genetic disorders than can counselees.

Representativeness refers to a variety of circumstances in which individuals inappropriately use the characteristics of a small sample with which they are familiar as a basis for predicting the outcome related to a larger population.

Relevant examples would appear to be common in genetic counseling. One is the effect of having a first child or more than one child who is affected with a disorder. Either situation may lead to a higher evaluation of the recurrence risk than would occur under other circumstances (Lippman-Hand & Fraser, 1979c; Pearn, 1973). Another example is the effect on risk perception of the degree of severity of a disorder, either having a child who is more or less severely affected than average, or who is so perceived. A severely affected child may increase risk perception whereas a child with few or minor symptoms may decrease it (Sagi et al., 1992; Wertz et al., 1986).

Risks and outcomes also tend to be assessed against a reference point that is considered to be neutral, acceptable, or unavoidable (Tversky & Kahneman, 1981). Thus, knowledge of the general background risk for genetic diseases and birth defects may reduce perception of a specific risk figure, especially when the specific figure is also on the order of a few percent (Pearn, 1973).

The cognitive "bias" of "conservatism," which is "a reluctance to formulate either very high or very low subjective interpretations of objective risks" (Pearn, 1973, p. 130), was observed by Wertz and coworkers (1986). Counselees were asked to choose a verbal descriptor of their own recurrence risk ranging from "very low" to "very high." Among counselees with a 4%–5% recurrence risk, the most frequently selected (i.e., modal) descriptor was "low." Only among counselees whose risk was 3% or less was "very low" the most common choice, and even among them, more than half chose a higher descriptor. Wertz and associates attribute this effect to the desire for absolute certainty, such that even small numeric risks represent a significant departure from the wished for reassurance that a negative outcome will not occur.

Counselees differ with respect to emotional and cognitive processes affecting risk perception (Tversky & Kahneman, 1981). One variable is the extent to which individuals have an optimistic or pessimistic view of themselves, their families, and events that befall them. A pessimistic outlook may increase the apparent significance of a risk figure ("It will be just my luck"), while optimism may decrease it ("It won't happen to me"). Differences in attitude toward risk taking versus risk avoidance undoubtedly also play a role (Parsons & Atkinson, 1993).

Kessler and Levine (1987) identified individual differences in the cognitive processing of risk figures. In an experiment designed to assess the effect of presenting the same numerical risk in different ways (e.g., "one out of four" compared to "25%"), college students were asked to "imagine themselves as prospective parents at risk for a child affected with a serious genetic disorder" (p. 363). In comparing the different forms of presentation, some subjects worked directly with the numbers, which was called "numerical reasoning." In general, they perceived percentages as more risky than odds because percentages involved larger actual numbers (e.g., "25" as compared to "4"). The remaining subjects used a "person reasoning" strategy that "involved the construction of mental images of groups of faces, bodies, or people, especially infants or children which were scanned or consulted when magnitude judgments were made" (p.368). Individuals who used person reasoning commonly perceived odds as more risky than percentages, because they were more conducive to constructing a serviceable mental image (e.g., four children, one of whom is affected). However, person reasoning did not lead to differential perceptions when the ratio in question had a denominator greater than 10, such as 1/25, 1/100, etc. Consistent with other research data, images of more than ten entities apparently could not be imagined or utilized effectively.

The individual differences just discussed may involve relatively stable aspects of personality (Denayer et al., 1997). However, specific experiences can also contribute. For example, having one's first child affected by a genetic disorder or having two or more consecutive affected children may lead to pessimism concerning the ability to conceive unaffected children (Lippman-Hand & Fraser, 1979d; Pearn, 1973). In another example, family dynamics that "preselect" one individual as a presumed carrier of Huntington disease, cystic fibrosis, or other disorders may also lead to a pessimistic perception of risk (Fanos & Johnson, 1995; Kessler & Bloch, 1989). Some of these examples are similar to those previously cited in the discussion of anchoring, availability, and representativeness. Thus, there is no definitive logical or practical boundary between the individual differences just discussed and the general "heuristic principles" of Tversky and Kahneman (1974; 1982). Each addresses a different but interrelated aspect of the complex process of risk assessment.

Other factors have been identified that can affect understanding or perception of risks provided in genetic counseling. Multiple or complex risk figures may cause confusion. For example, following genetic counseling for Duchenne muscular dystrophy, some counselees confused their risk of being a carrier with their reproductive risk if they were a carrier (Parsons & Clarke, 1993). In cancer risk counseling, similar confusion can arise between the risk of carrying a predisposing mutation and the risk of cancer if one is a carrier (Richards et al., 1995). Empiric risk figures for disorders with unknown diagnosis or etiology often represent a composite of the risk for several different potential etiologies, such as autosomal recessive, X-linked, and multifactorial or sporadic. An explanation of this complexity appropriately indicates the uncertainty of the risk figure and the potential for widely differing actual recurrence risks. However, the consequence may be that the counselee perceives the risk figure as relatively nonspecific, providing little guidance for decision making (Bloch et al., 1979). Risk figures for conditions such as neurofibromatosis type I that are highly variable in severity may be difficult to assess because they do not provide the most relevant information: the probability of an outcome whose severity exceeds that which is acceptable to the counselee (Ponder et al., 1998).

Counselees may have difficulty handling numerical values or may make logical or conceptual errors in interpreting risk figures. Chase and associates (1986) found that 28% of pregnant women interviewed by telephone were unable to translate a 1/1000 risk of neural tube defects into a correct percentage figure. This included four of the 41 respondents who were college graduates. In addition, counselees may fail to understand that the outcome of each pregnancy is statistically independent, so that having one (or more) affected or unaffected child or sibling is thought to alter the risk for subsequent children or for one's own genotype (Parsons & Clarke, 1993). Counselees may believe that if the probability of having an affected child is 1 in n, n children must be born before one will be affected (Ponder et al., 1998).

Counselees may also feel that their experience or that of their families invalidates the risk figures provided in genetic counseling. Describing a woman at risk for being a carrier for Duchenne muscular dystrophy, Parsons and Clarke (1993, p. 565) state, "The doctor was defining her carrier risks of 7% as 'moderate' and yet her sister, who had been given a risk of 0.7%, had given birth to an affected boy. Mathematical probability seemed meaningless in the light of her personal experience." It is noteworthy that Fanos and Johnson (1995, p.88) also use the term "meaningless" in describing comparable situations for siblings of individuals who have cystic fibrosis.

Complexities Underlying the Concept of "Risk"

The discussion thus far has used the single term "risk" to describe the situation faced by counselees. However, risk involves two underlying concepts: *uncertainty* as to what the outcome will be and *undesirability* of the consequences (Palmer & Sainfort, 1993). A discussion of each will further elucidate the meaning of risk and its components.

In genetic counseling, uncertainty is commonly addressed by providing a numerical figure that ranges from 0, certainty of nonoccurrence, to 1, certainty of occurrence. This value may be presented in a variety of forms, such as a percentage, a ratio, or odds. The number may refer to a possible future outcome, such as the chance that a woman who is heterozygous for Duchenne muscular dystrophy (DMD) will have an affected son or that a woman aged 38 will conceive a child who has Down syndrome. Alternatively, the number may refer to a current situation or to an event that has already occurred. Examples include the chance that a counselee is heterozygous for DMD or that the karyotype of a counselee's fetus is trisomy 21.

Despite the similarity in their numerical representation, the two are logically quite different. A numerical value concerning a possible future event is a probability, calculated as the frequency with which the outcome would occur among many individuals whose circumstances are comparable to those of the counselee. A probability figure may be based on theory and experimentation (e.g., Mendelian ratios) or on empiric observations (e.g., the frequency of Down syndrome as a function of maternal age). A numerical value concerning a current situation involves an inference about the present state of affairs. It is exemplified by the use of Bayes' theorem, which combines "prior" information concerning the chance of each possible state of affairs having occurred with "conditional" information related to the likelihood that each possible state of affairs is the actual case (Hodge, 1998).

Many "risk" figures given in genetic counseling are actually likelihoods or inferences about the present, not probabilities concerning future events. These risks include figures given in prenatal diagnosis counseling concerning the likelihood that a fetus is affected based on maternal age, expanded alphafetoprotein test results, ultrasound findings, or any other type or combination of data. The risks also include figures concerning the likelihood that a counselee is a carrier for an autosomal recessive or X-linked disorder and concerning possible mutant gene status in presymptomatic/pretesting counseling for cancer risk and Huntington disease.

The other component of risk involves the impact or consequences of a given outcome. Although the outcome may be identifiable by a single term, such as "Down syndrome" or "neurofibromatosis-1," the range of potential consequences is exceedingly complex (Palmer & Sainfort, 1993). For example, the consequences of having a child with Down syndrome include the effects of trisomy 21 on cognitive, social, and emotional development and on health and medical problems at every age. Each of these has an impact on the rewards and responsibilities that are involved in raising any child. Thus, the implications for the parents and other family members depend in large part on their values, beliefs, motivations, coping mechanisms, and social circumstances. Furthermore, any attempt to evaluate these factors beforehand is limited by very substantial uncertainty about many outcomes including cognitive ability, temperament, and medical problems.

In addition, knowledge that one is at increased risk for having a child with Down syndrome introduces its own set of consequences involving responsibility for a series of potential decisions that involve fundamental personal, social, and ethical considerations. These include the desire to have children, the consequences of having an affected child, the use of prenatal diagnosis with its attendant risks, the acceptability or unacceptability of abortion and the possibility of having to decide on its use, and the responses of others to the decision-making process and the decision made (Lippman-Hand & Fraser, 1979c).

The significance and complexity of potential consequences help explain why the numerical value of the probability or likelihood figure may not be the major determinant in risk perception and decision making. Viewed alternatively, the complexity of potential consequences helps explain the diversity of responses that can occur for the same "objective" risk information. Attention to the impact of both uncertainty and consequences is essential in evaluating research involving risk perception. Furthermore, both aspects must be kept in mind when presenting and explaining risk information to counselees.

Binarization and Other Transformations of Risk Figures

Faced with the responsibility for making critical decisions about uncertain but complex outcomes, counselees commonly transform numerical risk figures into a dichotomous or binary form. Lippman-Hand and Fraser (1979b; 1979c) identified this process through observation of genetic counseling sessions involving increased reproductive risk and in-depth postcounseling interviews. "[P]arents overwhelmingly perceived their chances in binary form. That is, when they focused on the outcome of a potential pregnancy, all spoke in terms of two alternatives: either the child would be normal or affected. . . . Regardless of the probability numbers assigned by the counselors, and despite their knowledge of their rates, in the parents' view it was an either-or event. It was not so much that the chance became '50–50,' . . . but that the two alternatives exhausted the possibilities and were given equal consideration in one's thinking" (Lippman-Hand & Fraser, 1979c, p. 57). The process of binarization began during the genetic counseling session. It was identified in all 60 follow-up interviews independent of numerical recurrence risk, subjective interpretation of risk, medical condition, or sex of the parent. Beeson and Golbus (1985) also reported binarization among all counselees they interviewed who were actively considering reproductive options for an increased risk of hemophilia A or Duchenne muscular dystrophy. Green (1992) describes the same process in a narrative of her own responses following an abortion for Down syndrome.

Binarization involves a cognitive simplification in response to being at risk, with the emotional burden and responsibility for critical decisions this involves. It reflects the fact that the numerical risk figures provided in genetic counseling do not eliminate uncertainty and that the information provided concerning consequences is often ambiguous with respect to potential severity and occurrence of specific symptoms. Binarization facilitates decision making by focusing attention on the most salient definable issue: the possibility of an outcome with undesirable consequences (Lippman-Hand & Fraser, 1979b).

Binarization simplifies the content of the information provided in genetic counseling by eliminating numerical risk values and reintegrating probability with outcome. In this sense, it appears to involve the discounting of a significant proportion of the information provided. However, it meets the emotional and cognitive needs of the counselee, who must make decisions in the face of uncertainty (Lippman-Hand & Fraser, 1979c). Furthermore, in a fundamental sense, binarization reflects the statistical reality confronting the counselee. When it involves potential future events, binarization addresses the fact that, while probabilities refer to the frequency of outcomes among many "trials" or "rolls of the dice," parents must make a decision that involves a single outcome or "trial": With each reproductive decision, parents get only one "roll of the dice," whose consequences are of great significance (Shiloh, 1994). When binarization involves a current situation whose nature is unknown (e.g., mutation status, carrier status, or fetal genotype), it has a clear relationship to the inferential assumptions underlying Bayesian analysis and the calculation of numerical likelihoods: There are two possible "states of nature," which exhaust the possibilities, and one of which must in fact be the case (Murphy & Chase, 1975, p. 74).

For some counselees, the long-term emotional consequences of being at risk lead to a process of simplification more complete than binarization: an assumption of certainty that involves the complete absence or full presence of risk. Parsons and Clarke (1993) observed this among women at risk for being Duchenne muscular dystrophy carriers, with the attendant risk of having affected sons. "This tendency for women, particularly those with risks at the polarities, to resolve it into either certain carrier or non-carrier status was often accompanied by the use of descriptive 'one liners.' Jean Moffoot (CR [carrier risk] 80%) had been told by her mother that any boy she had would be affected and made no attempt to explore carrier risk or its significance. She had passed this message on to her husband before they got married. . . . Mathematical percentages and ratios had been translated into meaningful everyday statements which became potential recipes for reproductive behavior. This meant that these women were not constantly living with risk and uncertainty" (p. 565).

Wexler (1979, p. 218) describes a similar but fluctuating situation among individuals at risk for Huntington disease. "The ambiguous condition of 50% risk is extremely difficult to maintain in one's mind, if not impossible. In practice, a 50–50 risk translates to a 100% certainty that one will or will not develop the disease, but the certainty changes from one to the other from moment to moment, day to day, month to month."

Both binarization and the assumption of certainty involve a process of risk assessment that is driven by the cognitive need to encompass complex, uncertain information and the emotional desire to reduce anxiety, uncertainty, and the burden of decision making. As such, they form a bridge to the more complex process of decision making. However, before considering that topic, it is useful to review the implications for presenting and discussing risk information that arise from the discussion to this point.

Techniques for Presenting Risk Information

Several approaches to risk presentation can be used to support nondirective genetic counseling: Numerical figures should initially be presented in a simple format without the use of verbal descriptors such as "low," "very low," "high," etc. (Lippman-Hand & Fraser, 1979b). This allows the counselee to begin processing the information without value-laden, potentially directive interpretations by the genetic counselor. In addition, whereas the term "risk" implies that the outcome is undesirable, terms such as "chance" or "probability" are more neutral. Thus, use of the latter terms avoids an implicit prejudgment by the genetic counselor concerning the desirability or undesirability of the outcome. It is useful to present the probabilities for nonoccurrence as well as occurrence. This focuses attention on both possible outcomes and establishes their relative probabilities or likelihoods. It is also useful to present the figures in more than one form, for example, as a ratio and a percentage. This provides options for cognitive processing and more than one frame of reference in terms of the cognitive and emotional impact (Smith, 1998). After presenting these figures and allowing time for initial processing, an inquiry as to how they are perceived may initiate a discussion of their meaning for the counselee (Kessler, 1979b).

> *Genetic Counselor:* The chances of your having another child with phenylketonuria is one in four, or 25%. That also means there is a three in four, or 75% chance that your next child will be unaffected. *(after a pause)* How does that sound to you?

If the counselee's response indicates an understanding of the figures and begins to address their implications, little further consideration of the numerical values may be needed. However, if at this or a later point there is an indication of confusion or lack of understanding, this should be addressed. Difficulty in converting from one form to another (e.g., ratios and percentages) may indicate problems understanding the meaning of the numbers (Chase et al., 1986). What is important is that one form be identified with which the counselee is reasonably conversant and comfortable. It is critical that counselees understand the statistical independence of each conception, thus avoiding the errors of thinking that previous outcomes affect future outcomes or that some specific number of children are required before the outcome will occur. An example or analogy from other aspects of life may be helpful in explaining this concept (Kelly, 1977).

> *Genetic Counselor:* It's like tossing a coin. You might, by chance, get four heads in a row, that's not so unlikely. But the next toss still has a 50–50 chance for heads or tails; each toss is a separate chance event.

Errors or misunderstanding may, however, have a more psychodynamic origin. Examples discussed in the preceding section include the occurrence of an event that had been given a very low probability and family preselection of a presumed carrier of Huntington disease or cystic fibrosis (Fanos & Johnson, 1995; Kessler & Bloch, 1989). In such situations, the psychodynamic origins must be addressed.

The cognitive processes involved in risk assessment function unconsciously much of the time. Bringing them to the counselee's attention may reduce their influence under circumstances where they appear to limit or bias consideration.

> *Genetic Counselor (to a couple who were informed the preceding day that they had test-positive, low expanded alphafetoprotein results—i.e., below normal range, indicating an increased risk for Down syndrome):* The fact that you were told that your pregnancy is at somewhat increased risk must affect how that number looks to you. That's entirely natural. But it is important to step back and try to look at the actual figures. Even though it is scary to be informed this way, the chance that your baby has Down syndrome is one in 160, and the chance that it is normal is 159 in 160.

This may be a more appropriate, nondirective approach than to be overly reassuring, including the use of descriptors such as "low" or "very low." Excessive reassurance may have countertransference elements and may leave the counselee who subsequently receives medically positive results less well prepared to cope with the emotional and practical consequences.

Special attention must be given to situations that involve multiple or complex risk figures. These include, for example, cancer risk counseling in which both lifetime and age-interval risk figures may be given, composite risks (e.g., "Our calculations indicate there is a 32% chance that you have inherited the gene, in which case there would be a 50% chance of passing it on to each child"), and risk figures that are ambiguous with respect to the probability of specific medical or cognitive outcomes. Care must be taken that the counselee understands the complexity and that questions or sources of confusion have been addressed. These situations may also evoke emotions such as anxiety concerning the complexity of the information or anger and disappointment that more definite information cannot be provided (Kessler, 1979b).

The fact that people differ in their cognitive approaches to risk assessment is very important: There is no single, "correct" approach to presenting risk figures. Instead, as in other aspects of genetic counseling, the counselor must be alert and sensitive to the counselee's verbal and nonverbal communication in order to identify areas of confusion or misunderstanding, emotional impediments to understanding, and preferred methods of processing the information (Shiloh & Sagi, 1989). In some instances it might be useful to ask how the counselee handles the information.

Genetic Counselor: Different people think about figures like this in different ways. Some work directly with the numbers. Others think in terms of a room full of people or a number of children. I wonder what method you are using?
Counselee: I was thinking about four babies, one of whom had sickle cell disease.
Genetic Counselor: Then it might be helpful to talk first about what it would be like if you had the baby with sickle cell disease. And then we can talk about having one of the babies that doesn't have it.

All of the preceding suggestions have some support in the literature and many are undoubtedly commonly used by genetic counselors. However, almost none have been extensively evaluated with respect to their impact on risk perceptions and decision making with a variety of counselees under various circumstances. Our understanding of these approaches would benefit from systematic research and from trials, observation, and reporting by genetic counselors.

Decision Making

From the factual information of numerical risk figures and their subjective assessment, we now turn to the even more complex psychological process of decision making. Several studies have shown statistically significant correlations between numerical risk figures and subjective risk assessments, and between numerical risk or subjective risk assessments and intended or actual reproductive decisions (Parsons & Atkinson, 1993; Sagi et al., 1992). Thus, risk figures and their interpretation play a role in reproductive decision making. However, the correlations are far from complete, and a variety of quantitative and qualitative investigations have shown that decision making is often a complex process occurring over a substantial period of time, in which risk figures do not play the predominant role. Counselees bring values, beliefs, experience, previous decisions, and information, both correct and incorrect, to the process of decision making. Furthermore, these various factors often have deep personal, family, social, and cultural roots and significance (Beeson & Golbus, 1985). In order for the information provided in genetic counseling to be useful, it must be integrated into the counselee's broader values and life experiences in a manner that is personally meaningful (Kessler, 1989; Shiloh & Saxe, 1989).

Underlying Beliefs and Values

A multitude of beliefs and values underlie how the information provided in genetic counseling is perceived and processed and the decisions that are made based upon it. One of these is the desire for children. Reproductive intentions prior to genetic counseling are a major determinant of reproductive decisions made after counseling (Kessler, 1989). These include directly expressed intentions such as planning another pregnancy, a desire to have children, and perceiving one's family as not complete (Frets et al., 1990b; Parsons & Atkinson, 1993). As an example, among counselees at elevated risk for disorders not detectable by prenatal diagnosis, Sorenson and coworkers (1987, p. 349) found that "the most powerful independent correlate of clients' intending or initiating a pregnancy at the 6-month follow-up was the client's reproductive plans before counseling. The odds of intending or initiating a pregnancy was 28.8 times greater for clients who had intended, before counseling, to have a child than it was for those who had not intended a pregnancy or who had been uncertain of their plans." The relationship between prior reproductive intentions and reproductive decisions following genetic counseling may also be inferred from associations between postcounseling reproduction and factors such as the presence or absence of a living child and the number of children born before the first affected child (Evers-Kiebooms, 1987; Frets et al., 1990a).

   Direct experience of a disorder in oneself, a child, or another affected relative also has a significant influence on reproductive decisions. The lived experience provides intimate, detailed knowledge of the impact of the disorder on the affected individual and other family members. Most reports indicate that direct experience and the perceived severity of problems associated with it lead to increased acceptance of prenatal diagnosis and selective abortion and to reduced reproduction in the absence of prenatal diagnosis (Frets et al., 1990a; Ponder et al., 1998; Wertz et al., 1992)

   However, the situation is complex, as might be expected with experiences that so directly and intimately affect the counselee and his or her family. Thus, in in-depth interviews with family members of individuals with cystic fibrosis or sickle cell disease, Beeson and Doksum (in press) identified what they call "experiential resistance" to the use of prenatal diagnosis and selective abortion. This attitude was based on the rich, direct experience of living with an affected individual, with its complex mixture of love and recognition of what the individual contributed to the family, in addition to the difficulties, pain, and loss. For these family members, using genetic testing to avoid the birth of another person with the same disorder implicitly devalued the life of the affected individual and his or her relationship to the family. (See Chapter 8: Resistance to Genetic Screening, Testing, and Counseling, for Reproductive Issues.)

   Attitudes toward abortion influence the utilization or nonutilization of prenatal diagnosis as well as the decision whether to continue a pregnancy when a fetus is found to be affected. For some counselees, the unacceptability of abortion precludes using prenatal diagnosis. Others who find abortion unacceptable or undesirable nevertheless choose prenatal diagnosis. Some would continue a pregnancy following medically positive results, using the information for medical and emotional preparation. Others would terminate despite their disapproval of abortion or await the test results before making a decision (Evers-Kiebooms et al., 1990). The conflict between opposition to abortion and the desire to avoid having an affected child can be intense and may be a major element in decision making. Attitudes concerning abortion may have personal, family, social, and/or religious bases and may be intensely felt in terms of personal beliefs and values as well as social precepts and expectations (Parsons & Atkinson, 1993; Wertz et al., 1992).

Many beliefs and values in addition to those just discussed influence reproductive decisions. Very broadly, they may be grouped into four categories: those that lead to the desire for children; those, such as career commitments that conflict with or reduce the desire for children (Humphreys & Berkeley, 1987); those that influence reproduction itself, such as the acceptability and utilization of contraceptive techniques, prenatal diagnosis, and abortion, and beliefs concerning the etiology of the disorder in question; and those that involve objective and perceived coping mechanisms and sources of support, both personal and interpersonal.

For many counselees, the fundamental decision or decisions have been made by the time they begin genetic counseling (Kessler, 1989; Parsons & Atkinson, 1993). Some counselees will be explicit that they have reached a decision, while with others it can be inferred in the course of the counseling (Kessler, 1980). Sometimes the decision will have been made through active consideration of the available alternatives, with an assessment of the perceived advantages and disadvantages of each. However, as Beeson and Golbus (1985, p. 108) point out, some counselees "do not perceive themselves as engaged in a decision making process at all because only one course of action appears tenable from their perspective." This occurs when the unacceptability of abortion blocks any further consideration of prenatal diagnosis. However, it occurs in the converse situation as well, when a strong desire for a child is coupled with a strong desire to avoid having a child with disabilities and there is acceptance of technological methods for so doing. For these counselees, the intention to use prenatal diagnosis precludes further consideration of both the risks of the procedure and emotional, ethical, or moral considerations concerning abortion. In both situations, the counselee's beliefs and values provide clear guidance with respect to a course of action.

For counselees whose decision is made, genetic counseling may provide support for their decision-making process as well as social and professional legitimization of the conclusion reached. Frequently, genetic counseling provides information regarding implementation of the decision, as in a discussion of the procedures available for prenatal diagnosis. Some counselees whose decision is made welcome these services. However, others perceive genetic counseling primarily as a requirement imposed by social expectations, the referring physician, or the policies of the genetics clinic (Beeson & Golbus, 1985; Kessler, 1989).

There are situations in which new information provided in genetic counseling leads to a reassessment of what had appeared to be a firm decision. This can occur when a counselee was unaware of the availability of prenatal diagnosis for the disorder involved (Frets et al., 1990a), or when the counselee learns for the first time that there are risks associated with prenatal diagnosis procedures. The latter situation is a primary reason for requiring preprocedural genetic counseling.

It is with counselees who have not yet reached a decision, and with those for whom a previously made decision is reopened, that decision making becomes an integral aspect of genetic counseling. For these counselees, the information provided and the manner in which it is processed has a potentially significant role in the decision that is made. However, for this to occur, the information must be comprehended and used in ways that are personally meaningful in terms of the counselee's beliefs, values, experiences, and expectations.

Scenarios

The binarization of risk figures discussed previously initiates an important process by which risk information is transformed so as to be more personally meaningful. By focusing on the possibility that each potential outcome might in fact happen, the counselee begins to assess the implications of each outcome for his or her life and for the lives of other family members. This analysis takes place through what Lippman-Hand and Fraser (1979c) call the use of "scenarios": imagining or visualizing the potential outcome with its consequences. "Just as a woman reduced the problem of having an abnormal child to a simpler binary form, she also reduced the consequences to a single basic structure, a scenario, in which a sequence of outcomes imagined to result from her choice was incorporated and around which her deliberations were organized. . . . [T]he diagnosis or birth of an (other) affected child—the event—became the starting point for an imagined series of outcomes in which the dimensions most important to the woman were highlighted and her emotional responses to them surveyed" (p. 63).

The elaboration of a scenario depends upon the counselee's knowledge, prior experience, and life circumstances. These influence the consequences envisaged, the extent to which they are elaborated, and the cognitive and emotional responses to them. For example, one individual might envisage the birth of a child with Down syndrome in terms of the effects of mental retardation on education, social relationships, and achievement, visualizing the child's and family's life at various ages (Wertz, 1992). For another, the scenario might focus on the possibility of severe medical problems involving hospitalization, surgery, pain to the child, and possible death, with images of a fragile, suffering infant and fearful or grieving parents. A counselee with personal knowledge may develop a detailed scenario, while one for whom the information is new and learned through the haze of shock and grief might have only a vague idea of potential consequences. The imagined impact upon the family and its members will also vary. Thus, a counselee with sufficient financial resources might think through either of the preceding scenarios primarily in terms of the emotional consequences for all involved. However, for a counselee with resources that are already strained, concerns about the demands and limitations that would be imposed on each family member may have a prominent place in these considerations.

In Lippman-Hand and Fraser's (1979c) study, the crucial role for scenarios involved assessing the worst case outcome, to determine whether the consequences were ones with which the counselee could cope. This involved the counselee's perceptions of the genetic disorder and its potential impact. However, it was also influenced by the burden of uncertainty resulting from variability in or lack of information about severity and symptoms, by concern for social and professional judgments about the decision made, and by the potential for guilt and remorse should the outcome be unfavorable. These assessments were active processes involving review of previous experiences, evaluation of coping skills and resources, emotional preparation, and the operation of psychological defenses. For example, the previous birth of a normal child as well as an affected child led to a more positive assessment. It was proof that a normal child could be produced. It thus reduced the perception of risk, strengthened the sense of biological and social normality, and may have contributed to an illusion of control over the situation. These factors, in turn, increased the sense of internal and external resources available to cope with the possible birth of another affected child.

According to Lippman-Hand and Fraser (1979c, p. 66), "trying out the worst provided an element of control for the parents. . . . [T]hey could prepare for the worst and, by this very process of preparation, explore how manageable the problem was and attempt to come to terms with it." An affirmative assessment of the ability to cope facilitated a decision to have further children. In the absence of an affirmative assessment, reproductive decisions were commonly deferred or diffused.

Despite their value, scenarios are limited by the counselee's sources of information and experience. For example, the first scenario described earlier, involving the effects of mental retardation on a child with Down syndrome, is uninformed by knowledge or experience of the love, joy, and sense of achievement that occurs in many families who have a child with Down syndrome. The counselee's direct experience greatly influences scenarios, both in the specifics envisioned and in the degree of detail, the immediacy, and the emotional impact. However, to the extent that personal experience is not representative of the actual range of possibilities, the scenario may have a skewed perception of the range of possible outcomes. For example, the counselee's experience may involve an individual for whom the severity of a disorder lies near one end or the other of the spectrum, or it may be based on a young child for whom the major symptoms of the disorder are not yet expressed (Wertz, 1992). At a more general level, the ability to elaborate a scenario may be diminished by lack of relevant experiences, cognitive deficits, restricted imagination, anxiety, or the press of time. All these limitations point to the importance that both the information and the guidance given in genetic counseling may have in the elaboration and utilization of scenarios.

Diffusion of Responsibility

The state of being at increased reproductive risk carries with it implied responsibility for decision making. This places a burden on counselees that may, in itself, be perceived as one of the negative consequences of a disorder (Lippman-Hand & Fraser, 1979c). The required decisions may raise moral, ethical, and religious issues and involve weighing conflicting personal desires and fears. There may be concern about the judgments of others, including those such as partners who will be intimately affected. There is the need to anticipate one's own emotional responses should the choice lead to an undesired outcome. Furthermore, considerations of contraception or technological interventions such as prenatal diagnosis impinge upon some of the most intimate, emotionally profound human experiences.

A number of behaviors, beliefs, and psychological defenses can reduce this burden by diffusing responsibility for the decision itself or the actions implied by the decision. One approach is to seek advice from others, thus giving them some direct or implicit responsibility for the decision that is made. This may be conscious and overt when a counselee consults with a partner, family member, friend, clergy, or other individual who will be directly affected or has an established role in the interpretation of family, social, ethical, or religious values. It may be more indirect or unconscious when the genetic counselor or other professional is asked for her advice or when questions are asked as to how other counselees have made comparable decisions. Counselees may also diffuse responsibility by construing that circumstances require or support a given decision. For example, a single child may be seen as needing a sibling for companionship, thus supporting a decision, based on the counselee's own desire, to have another child (Lippman-Hand & Fraser, 1979d; Shiloh, 1996).

Another behavior that involves diffusing or diluting responsibility is the inefficient, sporadic, or non-use of contraception. Termed "reproductive roulette" by Lippman-Hand and Fraser (1979d, p. 80–81), "it is a choice not to decide, a choice of 'fatalism' made when one does not want to exert control." Reproductive roulette may occur when a definitive reproductive decision has not been made. It may also be used when uncertainty, ambiguity, or disagreement remain despite a stated decision to forgo reproduction or use prenatal diagnosis with the option of abortion (Evers-Kiebooms et al., 1990).

The behaviors, beliefs, and psychological defenses just described are common elements in decision making in many aspects of life. Indeed, some counselees who engaged in reproductive roulette after genetic counseling reported having used similar reproductive practices before knowing they were at increased risk. However, an understanding of the dynamics of these processes and their potential effects on making and implementing decisions is essential for effective counseling. While they can reduce the burden of and barriers to decision making, they also have the potential to lead to less than optimal decisions and outcomes. Lippman-Hand and Fraser (1979d) report that some counselees who had unaffected children following lax contraceptive practices expressed relief that they achieved pregnancy in this way. They might have been unable to take the risk had they needed to make an explicit decision. The authors conjecture that, if these counselees had had affected children, feelings of responsibility and blame might have been reduced, since it was an "accident." However, such an outcome might also result in remorse and blame. Data concerning such cases would broaden and balance our understanding of the potential impact of reproductive roulette and other processes that diffuse responsibility for decision making.

Further Complexities in Decision Making

Decision making occurs at multiple psychological and social levels. It frequently involves both conscious and unconscious conflicts between contradictory wishes, expectations, and values (Kessler, 1980). It is a dynamic process that is influenced by evolving emotions and outlook, social pressures, new information, and altered circumstances. For example, an individual's acceptance of prenatal diagnosis and abortion may decline dramatically once quickening occurs or during a pregnancy in which the possibility or reality of abortion for genetic causes is experienced. Conversely, the emotions evoked by the birth of an affected or an unaffected child in a pregnancy that did not involve prenatal diagnosis may lead to the use of prenatal diagnosis in subsequent pregnancies (Parsons & Atkinson, 1993; Wertz, 1992).

The period of time during which active decision making takes place varies greatly. At one end of the spectrum are counselees who receive medically positive results that were unanticipated, as in expanded alphafetoprotein screening or ultrasound during routine obstetric care. These individuals must make decisions on very short notice, with respect to issues that may not have been previously considered. At the other end of the spectrum, some counselees are aware from adolescence or earlier that they are at increased reproductive risk, due, for example, to known or possible carrier status. For these individuals, issues involving risk, consequences, and reproductive choices will have been considered at many times and been influenced in a variety of ways. These include how information was or was not communicated in the family of origin, the beliefs and values expressed with respect to affected individuals and reproductive choices, self-image with regard to carrier status, and the consequences of informing or not informing prospective partners. Parsons and Atkinson (1993) document how reproductive decisions and self-perception of carrier status wax and wane in importance and change in nature depending on developmental life stage, involvement in courting and family building, and the nature of the relationship in which a pregnancy occurs. Between these extremes, most counselees have some extended time period during which consideration can be given to reproductive or other relevant decisions and during which influences of the sort just discussed are operative.

Counselees may face an evolving sequence of decisions. This occurs, for example, when a decision to use prenatal diagnosis leads to medically positive results that require a decision between termination and continuation of the pregnancy, either of which then entails further decisions. A longer sequence is initiated when a decision to use expanded alphafetoprotein screening is followed by test positive and then medically positive results. A similarly complex sequence may occur in cancer risk counseling followed by DNA testing. In these and comparable situations, the sequence of decisions is paralleled by evolving information, emotions, and risk figures.

Finally, more than one person is frequently involved in the decision-making process, and those who may differ in their beliefs, perceptions, and values (Evers-Kiebooms, 1987; Van Spijker, 1992). While such differences may be a source of disagreement or conflict, they may also provide alternative viewpoints that facilitate decision making (Kolker & Burke, 1994). The conflicts and compromises involved obviously occur at both the individual and interpersonal levels. Women, in particular, may experience a need to weigh the impact a decision will have on their own lives, whose primacy is supported by their role in bearing the child and providing primary care, against the desire or need to sustain their marriage or relationship, which appears to require acceding to their partner's wishes (Rapp, 1999; Wertz, 1992). Members of the extended family may express expectations and advice in a manner intended, consciously or unconsciously, to influence decisions. These may be at variance with the beliefs, values, and decisions of the counselees. Among the many possible causes are different experiences with affected individuals, often at a time when genetic information, medical treatments, and reproductive choices were more limited (Ponder et al., 1998).

Techniques for Facilitating Decision Making

The preceding discussion leads to a number of guidelines concerning the genetic counselor's role with respect to decision making. There are several goals for this process: First, that the decision be based on an adequate assessment of available options and their potential consequences and that it be consistent with the counselee's or counselees' beliefs, values, wishes, and life circumstances. Second, that the counselee arrive at the decision through a process that provides a sense of resolution and, should the outcome be undesirable, minimizes feelings of guilt, blame, and regret, because it is seen as having been based on the relevant considerations and as the best decision that could have been made under the circumstances. Third, that the process also support and facilitate implementation of the decision.

It is important to assess the counselee's situation and needs with respect to decision making. If the principal decision has been made prior to genetic counseling, the focus should be on support and implementation, always recognizing that new information may reopen one or more aspects of the decision-making process (Kessler, 1989). If the counselee is in the process of reaching a decision, the relevant issues should be explored. If the counselee is in an acute quandary, has a sense of high anxiety or crisis concerning making a decision, or is faced with the need to make an immediate decision, issues related to making a decision should be given high priority.

Many factors may impede the process of decision making. These include shock, anxiety, stress, ambivalence, concern about judgment by others, disagreements with a partner, confusion regarding options, and misinformation or lack of information,. It is essential to assess sources of difficulty and address any that contribute substantially, using the concepts and techniques discussed throughout this book. Here, the focus is on those elements most related to the preceding sections of the present chapter.

It is essential that the presentation and discussion of numerical risk figures be treated as the beginning, not the end, of a process. After presenting such figures, the counselor should address the meanings for the counselee *of being at risk,* and discuss the available options. As with other psychosocial issues, this does not require large amounts of time in most cases. What is critical is that an opening be created to discuss these issues, and that the genetic counselor be responsive to messages and cues, both direct and indirect, provided by the counselee.

Genetic Counselor: The chance of a miscarriage occurring due to amniocentesis is about one-half of one percent, or one in 200. That means roughly 199 out of 200 times, the procedure will not result in miscarriage. *(after a pause)* How does that sound to you?

Counselee: Well, the number is small. But it's really upsetting to think that it might cause a miscarriage, after we have waited so long to get pregnant.
Genetic Counselor: So even though you would like to have the test, the fact that it might cause a miscarriage has to be thought about carefully.

With this comment the genetic counselor notes the importance of the possibility that a miscarriage might occur (binarization) and defines the immediate dilemma: the test is desired but it carries a risk. This provides an opening for further discussion. It does not preclude additional consideration of the 0.5% risk figure. However, that is likely to be more meaningful if it is returned to after the significance of a possible miscarriage has been discussed. It can then be considered in light of the scenario that has been developed concerning a miscarriage. In addition, considering the topics in this order may be perceived as more empathic by the counselee, since it moves quickly to the counselee's emotions—anxiety about a procedure-induced miscarriage—rather than staying with a discussion of numbers.

As the discussion continues, information, clarification, and guidance can be provided by further explaining the decision or decisions that need to be made and systematically reviewing the available options (Kessler, 1997b). When counselees are confused, lack information, or are misinformed about one or more options, correction and clarification are essential. Even when the counselee apparently understands all options, a brief review may reveal gaps or misinformation or provide a more balanced consideration of the choices that might be made.

The concept of scenarios suggests several important approaches. The counselee should be assisted in developing an accurate, sufficiently detailed understanding of each possible choice and the associated outcomes and consequences. No such description can ever include all possible consequences and details. Thus, the discussion should focus on those aspects most salient to the counselee, augmented by those the genetic counselor adds for completeness. By way of example, the genetic counselor could initiate discussion by asking, "When you think about neurofibromatosis, what comes to mind?" If the counselee's initial response relates to cosmetic aspects, her understanding of the relevant symptoms and her sense of their impact should be explored. If other important features such as neurological problems or cancer risk are not included in her response, these must be introduced by the genetic counselor.

With neurofibromatosis, as with many disorders, the potential variability must be discussed. Again, if it is not included in the counselee's description, it should be raised by the genetic counselor (Kessler, 1979b). The counselee may be unaware of the potential variability, or she may have an image of the disorder based on a family member or an example from the media, often involving very severe symptoms. The burden of uncertainty the variability creates with respect to decision making must be addressed. One way to do this is to develop a secondary worst case scenario involving a severe manifestation of the disorder. This can be explored and then compared to less severe outcomes, including a discussion of their relative probabilities of occurrence.

In developing and using scenarios, the critical comparison is between outcomes and their consequences, on the one hand, and the resources for coping with them, on the other. Thus, if the crux of decision making is to be addressed, it must include a discussion of the internal and external, objective and subjective resources available to the counselee (Lippman-Hand & Fraser, 1979c; Vlek, 1987) (see Chapter 1 under Coping Strategies). Once again, the counselee's description and elaboration are central, but the genetic counselor may be able to identify alternative resources, correct misconceptions, and provide guidance as these matters are discussed.

> *Genetic Counselor:* When you think about the possibility that your child might have a severe form of neurofibromatosis, what resources do you think you would have to help you?

If the counselee responds in terms of external resources, such as family support or a trusted physician, the genetic counselor could address emotional resources and coping skills.

> *Genetic Counselor:* Those sound very important. But this is not the first difficult situation you and your husband have faced. How have you taken care of yourselves and each other during other difficult times?

The goal here is not to inflate the estimation of resources. Rather, it is to develop a more complete and well-articulated sense of what resources are available. If the conclusion is that resources are too limited, that contributes to a more well grounded decision.

> *Counselee:* Well, after his father was killed in the car accident, we did get through it, and after some struggle we were able to support each other. But it was *very* hard. I don't know that I want to set us up for something so difficult that might go on for years.

These are difficult issues to think about and discuss, especially under conditions of stress, anxiety, ambiguity, or time constraints. Counselees may attempt to avoid issues and reduce anxiety by minimizing the risk or consequences, putting off decisions, diffusing responsibility, or rationalizing poorly considered decisions. Alternatively, they may engage in a rather frantic attempt to reach a decision under circumstances in which anxiety is high, memory and cognitive abilities are impaired, and there is vacillation with respect to choices and/or an impulsive ultimate decision that is poorly considered (Shiloh, 1996). Attention to the counselee's emotional state may help reduce these responses. More specific to the present discussion, the guidance, clarification, and attention to detail provided by the genetic counselor may reduce the sense of anxiety or panic and facilitate a more adequate consideration of the options and their potential consequences (Kessler, 1979b).

The values and expectations of others have several possible roles in this process. They may be perceived as sources of pressure with respect to decisions, which may contribute to ambivalence, vacillation, and postdecision regret (Parsons & Atkinson, 1993; Ponder et al., 1998). They may be perceived as sources of information, guidance, and support (Bartels et al., 1997). They may serve to diffuse responsibility for decisions. Finally, other individuals may be seen as having a direct, appropriate role in the decision-making process. These dynamics should be assessed and addressed as appropriate. These roles are not mutually exclusive, and they may shift with exploration. For example, a counselee's mother may have strong opinions about the risk of her daughter having an affected child, based on the mother's experience with the counselee's seriously affected sibling. Initially, this may be perceived as pressure and an impediment to independent decision making. However, when explored, the value of the mother's experience with a severely affected individual may emerge as a useful point of view that can be incorporated into the counselee's decision making. Furthermore, it may also become apparent that the mother's concerns are due to love and support of her daughter. Conversely, a position or decision that is initially felt to be one's own may, with exploration, be found to originate with others. This recognition may allow more independent decision making (Parsons & Atkinson, 1993).

It may be useful to open a potentially broad discussion of these various roles by asking a general question.

> *Genetic Counselor:* Who else do you feel might play some role in this decision, either as someone who could be of help and support, or as someone whose opinion of your decision is important to you?

This approach allows salient relationships to arise and implies that there are a diversity of possible dynamics involved. It might, for example, equally well evoke concern about a sibling's attitude toward abortion or the potential value of speaking to a clergyperson or spiritual advisor.

Interpersonal issues arise most directly among spouses or partners. Relevant dynamics and techniques are discussed in Chapter 2 under Couples: Similarities and Differences. However, the approaches discussed here are also applicable. Exploration and discussion of values, wishes, options, and consequences can provide guidance for couples who are unfamiliar with or unskilled in mutual decision making. Identifying areas of agreement and disagreement may increase the sense of mutual support and understanding and reduce global feelings of disagreement or anger to more manageable, specific issues (Humphreys & Berkeley, 1987).

"What Would You Do?"

The approach to decision making just presented clearly exemplifies those definitions of nondirective genetic counseling that support and implement counselee autonomy through the use of active counseling techniques. The implications of this approach can be further developed by considering the frequently discussed counselee question, "What would you do?" This question may be posed directly, in a variant of the form just indicated, or it may be posed more indirectly, as in a question concerning what other counselees do in similar circumstances (Kessler, 1979b). In either form the question creates a critical situation: Despite the genetic counselor's attempt to develop a nondirective dialogue, the counselee has made a direct request for an opinion regarding the decision that he or she faces. This situation is most fruitfully and appropriately viewed, not as an impediment or hazard to narrowly defined nondirective counseling, but as an opportunity to identify and address a key issue that confronts the counselee and/or the genetic counseling process. From this perspective, the essential response is to attempt to identify the nature of the issue or impasse, which can then be elaborated, discussed, and, potentially, reduced or resolved (Djurdjinovic, 1998; Kessler, 1997a).

A request for the genetic counselor's opinion may arise for many different reasons. The following list is expansive but not exhaustive. For each, a potential rephrasing of the question in terms of the underlying issue is presented. The question "What would you do?" may represent any of the following:

- a request for guidance due to uncertainty or confusion concerning the process by which a decision might be reached (Kessler, 1997a)

  Help me think about this in a constructive way that gets beyond my anxiety and confusion.

- a need to know how serious the situation is, often based on high anxiety (R. Tung, 1999, personal communication)

    Please tell me how serious this is.

- a desire for information and guidance based on the genetic counselor's experience with the choices and outcomes of others in similar situations (Geller et al., 1997)

    You have worked with others in my situation. What guidance can you give me from their experiences?

- an attempt to determine if and how others in a similar situation have been able to muster the necessary coping resources

    If you tell me that others have done it, then they must have felt they would be able to manage, and maybe I can too.

- concern about the social acceptability of a decision, which may include the approval or disapproval of the genetic counselor

    If you would tell me what you would do, or what others have done, then I would know that it has a degree of social acceptability.

- a desire to diffuse responsibility for the decision (Lippman-Hand & Fraser, 1979c)

    This is too big a decision for me to make alone. I have no one else to turn to for help besides you.

- the expression of tendencies toward passivity that have been unaddressed or even inadvertently promoted by the genetic counselor (Kessler, 1979b)

I felt overwhelmed before I came to this session and I still do. Tell me what I should do.

- a desire for a more empathic, personally involved approach by the genetic counselor (Kessler, 1997a)

  Please stop giving me information and posing questions and show me that you understand how scary and hard this is for me.

- a need or desire to move from consideration of numerical risk figures to a broader discussion of the meaning the potential outcomes would have in the counselee's life (Beeson & Golbus, 1985)

  I understand the numbers, but I don't understand what it would mean to me if it actually happened.

- a feeling that the genetic counselor and/or the situation presses for a premature decision (Kessler, 1979b)

  Since you seem to think I should make the decision before I feel ready, why don't you make it for me.

- an inability or unwillingness to take responsibility for a decision that, it is felt, the medical professional should make (Djurdjinovic, 1998) (see Chapter 7 under Cross-cultural Genetic Counseling Techniques: Ethnocultural Expectations, Decision Making, and Nondirective Genetic Counseling)

  I can't understand why you, the medical professional, expect me to make this medical decision.

- in the face of a disagreement between counselees, a desire for the genetic counselor to support the position of the counselee who makes the request (Kessler, 1979b)

I hope your answer will agree with my position so that he (she) will see that it is valid and I have someone who supports me.

- or to mediate the disagreement (Kessler, 1979b)

We are at an impasse. We need a referee.

These examples span the range of psychological, interpersonal, and social issues addressed throughout this book, and the potential responses to them draw on the diversity of techniques that are discussed. However, the unifying principle is this: By actively applying the full range of counseling approaches to the opportunity afforded by the question, the genetic counselor does far more than meet the minimal criteria of providing an answer that avoids direct advice. She supports and promotes the counselee's autonomy and capabilities by addressing an issue that, whether of momentary importance in the session or long-standing concern to the counselee, has been an impediment to the process of informed decision making.

6

SPECIFIC COUNSELING
SITUATIONS AND
COUNSELEES

THE previous chapters present a general approach to the theory and practice of genetic counseling. This chapter discusses specific counseling situations and categories of counselees.

Prenatal Diagnosis Counseling

Prenatal diagnosis counseling represents a substantial proportion of the total
reported genetic counseling caseload, and it is the primary professional focus
of many genetic counselors (Schneider & Kalkbrenner, 1998). It is characterized by a reasonably well defined sequence of steps and decision points. These,
rather than previously discussed principles, are the primary focus of this
section.

Preprocedure Counseling

The purpose of preprocedure counseling is to provide both the information
and the psychosocial support upon which an informed decision can be made
concerning whether or not to have prenatal diagnosis. This decision depends
upon personal, cultural, ethical, and religious beliefs and values related to re-

production, parental responsibility, disability, and abortion. It is essential that the counselee or counselees be assisted in reaching a decision that is consistent with these beliefs and values.

The primary informational and cognitive steps involved in preprocedure counseling are these:

- to present relevant occurrence/recurrence probability figures and discuss the nature and impact of the genetic disorder or birth defects involved
- to explain the relevant diagnostic procedure or procedures including the associated risks of miscarriage and other morbidity
- to explain the degree of uncertainty and/or ambiguity associated with potential test results
- to assist the counselee in reaching a decision concerning whether to have a prenatal diagnostic procedure and, when appropriate, to choose among available procedures
- to obtain informed consent based on an adequate understanding of the procedures, risks, and potential outcomes of the alternative that is chosen
- and, when prenatal diagnosis is chosen, to make arrangements concerning to whom the test results will be given and the timing and method for so doing.

Preprocedure counseling is often conducted under significant time constraints. In many clinics, limited time is scheduled for each case, with varying degrees of flexibility and opportunity for the genetic counselor to exercise her judgment concerning the need to extend the session. If the procedure is scheduled to immediately follow counseling, there may be pressure to reach a decision within time limits that do not delay or inconvenience the professionals who are responsible for the procedure.

Time constraints do not reduce the importance and necessity of addressing psychosocial issues. Anxiety, fear, anger, confusion, resistance, ambivalence concerning the pregnancy, beliefs and values concerning technological instrumentality and abortion, couple issues, and beliefs based on incorrect risk figures can all seriously compromise the counselee's ability to understand and utilize the complex information that is presented. As Grobstein (1979, p. 113) states, "Consenting to the procedure without understanding its psychosocial as well as its technical implications is not true informed consent." Thus, time constraints require the efficient, informed application of the elements of assessment, analysis, and intervention that have been presented in the preceding chapters, with attention focused on those issues most relevant to prenatal diagnosis.

The following line of inquiry provides one approach to assessing the most pertinent issues:

The reason for referral, including self-referral. This provides information concerning the basis from which the counselee approaches the process of prenatal diagnosis: physician referral, information in the media or social milieu, known risk factor, suspected risk factor, or test result such as expanded alphafetoprotein testing (Grobstein, 1979).

Understanding or beliefs concerning the nature and magnitude of the risk. This helps identify correct information, incorrect information, uncertainty, confusion, personal and cultural beliefs, and, with attention to contextual cues and nonverbal communication, the level of anxiety concerning the risk.

Was the pregnancy planned? This provides insight into the commitment to the pregnancy, ranging from the deep longing related to infertility treatment to the ambiguity of an unplanned or unwanted pregnancy.

Have there been previous pregnancy losses? This may affect anxiety about the outcome of the pregnancy as well as about the risk of spontaneous abortion due to prenatal diagnosis procedures.

The nature and degree of the father's involvement. When the husband or partner is present, this may be assessed through his participation and responses. When he is not present, direct inquiry should be made. This provides information concerning both the psychosocial circumstances of the pregnancy and the individuals who will be involved in making decisions.

Knowledge of amniocentesis, chorionic villus sampling (CVS), or other relevant procedures, including the associated risk factors. This provides essential information for planning the explanation of procedure(s) and risks.

Thoughts, questions, and current decisions concerning whether to have the procedure. This identifies the framework within which the decision-making process will take place.

This inquiry directly supports the psychosocial elements of genetic counseling. In addition, it may reduce the time required for presenting medical-genetic information by defining the counselee's knowledge and understanding and identifying psychosocial issues that might interfere with comprehension or utilization of the information. When time is restricted, these questions can be posed briefly and pursued only when the answers indicate significant relevance to prenatal diagnosis counseling. Tact and sensitivity are important, especially with respect to pregnancy planning and the father's involvement. However, the questions can be presented as routine and integral to the counseling process.

Many factors influence the degree of anxiety with which counselees enter prenatal diagnosis counseling. For some, prenatal diagnosis is an accepted aspect of modern medicine, which combines personal and social responsibility, the probability of reassurance, and the option of abortion if the fetus is seriously affected. When this is coupled with a lack of anxiety about the procedure itself, anxiety may be low (Robinson et al., 1975). For other counselees, fear or anxiety concerning the procedure may lead to tension and distraction in the session and may influence or inhibit a decision to have prenatal diagnosis. While it is important to address this anxiety, the genetic counselor must ensure that her overall approach remains nondirective and does not give the appearance of favoring a choice to have the procedure. There are several techniques for attempting to alleviate this anxiety: providing information about the procedure, including the fact that the majority of women report it is a relatively painless experience; exploring how other stressful or frightening situations have been dealt with in the past; providing emotional support or eliciting it from the partner; and offering to accompany the counselee to the procedure.

For most counselees, the fundamental anxiety relates to the possibility of a medically positive result—the fear that their baby will be identified as having a known genetic disorder or a detectable birth defect. For counselees whose medical and family history indicate no increased risk, this may be a distant concern, held at bay by its relatively low probability and by psychological defenses. Known risk factors such as teratogen exposure, parental genotype, the previous birth of an affected child, an affected family member, or other experiences that have sensitized the counselee to the occurrence and impact of birth defects or genetic disorders may greatly enhance anxiety (Blumberg, 1984; Shapiro, 1993). Perhaps most distressing, at least initially, is to be unexpectedly informed of a potential heightened risk. This occurs with test-positive results from expanded alphafetoprotein testing or when abnormalities are detected by ultrasound during prenatal diagnosis or routine obstetric care (Fonda Allen & Mulhauser, 1995).

This anxiety concerning the possibility of a medically positive result must also be addressed (Pryde et al., 1993). Its origin and intensity should be acknowledged and reassurance given consistent with the realities of the situation. However, the counselee may remain anxious throughout the stages of counseling in which information is presented and decisions must be made. Under these circumstances, it is particularly important to present information in a stepwise manner that includes frequent assessment of the counselee's understanding and emotional responses and provides guidance concerning the relevance of the information to the required decisions. This approach is critical in the crisis atmosphere that frequently surrounds the unexpected finding of abnormalities during routine ultrasound, when the counselee or counselees are likely to be in a state of shock.

The issue of providing reassurance is complex. For many counselees the objective occurrence/recurrence probability is low (e.g., 0.1%–1%) although the subjective experience is anxiety producing. Thus, there may be a legitimate basis for providing reassurance about the probable outcome. However, care must be taken that this does not lead to avoidance or underemphasis of issues related to the possibility of a medically positive result (see later under Counseling Following Medically Positive Results). Such avoidance or underemphasis leaves those counselees who ultimately receive bad news inadequately prepared. Finding the appropriate balance between reassurance and preparation requires clinical judgment based on experience with counselees who have received both medically positive and medically negative results.

Countertransference issues, unless addressed, may affect this clinical judgment. The genetic counselor may feel discomfort with the counselee's anxiety and emotional distress, which may lead to the avoidance of issues or to collusion with the counselee's defenses against the frightening possibility of a medically positive result. In my experience, countertransference is particularly common when counselees have been referred because of low expanded alphafetoprotein test results. The high frequency of false positive results and the anxiety they produce (Marteau & Slack, 1992) may lead to feelings of guilt or anger, and these must be addressed to avoid countertransference influenced responses.

Central to preprocedure counseling is the decision whether to have prenatal diagnosis, including the choice of procedure if relevant. The desired counseling objective is that both the process and the outcome be consistent with the counselee's values and beliefs and minimize the likelihood of guilt, blame, or regret should an undesirable outcome occur. Although the decision may be made prior to, during, or after the session, a discussion of the issues is essential. A meaningful decision must rest on an understanding of the potential implications, both practical and emotional, of each course of action, with particular attention to the possible undesirable outcomes (Pryde et al., 1993). If prenatal diagnosis is chosen, the implications include the possibility of miscarriage due to the procedure and of a medically positive test result with the necessity of deciding whether to continue or terminate the pregnancy. If prenatal diagnosis is not chosen, there is the possible birth of an affected child with the multiple implications of that outcome. In addition, the limitations of each choice must be understood. Medically negative test results do not ensure a normal outcome, and test results may be obtained that are ambiguous with respect to diagnosis and/or prognosis.

The counselee's attitude toward abortion is also critical and should be discussed (Grobstein, 1979). If the counselee has personal, cultural, ethical, or religious attitudes opposing the use of abortion, this discussion may help determine the limited circumstances under which abortion would be acceptable. These may include severe untreatable disorders or those that result in death either pre- or postnatally. This discussion may also help define the relevant degree of severity. For example, some counselees would abort for trisomy 21, whereas others would not. For some counselees, mental retardation represents the most serious type of abnormality, for others, physical abnormalities are the most serious, and for some, specific experiences or beliefs determine particular disorders for which the pregnancy would be terminated (Rapp, 1993a). When abortion is not an acceptable option under any circumstances, the genetic counselor should discuss the remaining options and their potential value. A medically negative result may provide reassurance, especially when there is relatively high risk for a specific disorder such as an autosomal recessive disease or when anxiety is high irrespective of the objective magnitude of the risk. A medically positive result may allow emotional and practical preparation, which for some disorders includes prenatal or perinatal medical intervention (Zuskar, 1987).

When a couple is involved, it is important that the process include both individuals in a manner that allows each to feel that her or his position has been considered and that the process as well as the outcome are mutually supportive and agreeable. Overt couple issues may interfere with this goal. In addition, the emotional intensity of the matters discussed may evoke latent couple issues. Relevant individual, couple, and family dynamics are discussed in Chapters 1 and 2. However, one couple issue that is relatively unique to prenatal diagnosis counseling will be discussed here. This is the statement by the man, in one form or another, that "It is her body, she should make the decision." While superficially supportive of the woman's rights and autonomy, I believe this is often experienced by women as a failure of responsibility and empathic support. Unless it is a truly mutual position, it may lead to anger and blame if the outcome is not favorable. The man may blame the woman for her decision, the woman may blame the man for avoiding his responsibility in a critical decision that has turned out poorly (Grobstein, 1979; Kolker & Burke, 1994). Thus, a statement of this sort should be addressed in a manner that elicits the man's involvement without criticizing his stated position.

> *Genetic Counselor (to father, after mother has stated that she wishes to have amniocentesis):* What is your feeling about whether to have amniocentesis?
> *Father:* Well, it's her body, I think she should make the decision.
> *Genetic Counselor (to mother):* That acknowledges your role in the pregnancy, but it seems as if it also puts a lot of responsibility on you. *(turning to father)* And the outcome is certainly going to have a big impact on your life as well. *(addressing both)* Are the two of you agreed that it is your decision *(indicates mother)*, or might it be better if both of you were involved?

When the decision is made to have prenatal diagnosis, it is important for the genetic counselor to lay the emotional and cognitive groundwork for the minority of counselees who will receive medically positive results. For counselees who have not ruled out abortion, this will involve the critical question of whether or not to have an abortion, which in turn rests on an understanding of the probable implications of either course of action. Given the anxiety and fear associated with this outcome, there can be substantial resistance to addressing these issues (Grobstein, 1979). Counselees may avoid discussing the possibility of medically positive results. When asked if they have considered how they would respond, they may say they have not thought about it, will deal with it if the need arises, or would rather not discuss it at the present time.

Although the genetic counselor should recognize and support appropriate coping and defenses, it is important to address these issues to the extent appropriate for the counselee. This will provide guidance and support for those who will receive bad news (Magyari et al., 1987). Furthermore, as has been discussed in other contexts, failure to address these issues sends the message that they are so difficult and anxiety provoking that the genetic counselor chooses to avoid them. This may adversely affect the counselee's ability to cope with the situation should it arise. It may also raise unconscious doubt concerning the genetic counselor's support and assistance under those circumstances.

The issue may be introduced with a straightforward question:

Genetic Counselor: Have you thought about what you would do if the test result says your baby has Down syndrome?

If the response is a statement about thoughts or plans, or if it initiates a discussion, the matter may be pursued. If the response is deflecting or defensive, the genetic counselor may either carefully pursue the matter or acknowledge the anxiety and desire to avoid the subject. This decision is based on an assessment of the counselee's level of anxiety, strength of defenses, and emotional vulnerability. Two possible conversations follow:

Counselee (thoughtfully, but without undue anxiety): We haven't thought about it much. It's pretty scary.
Genetic Counselor: Yes it is. But in my experience, it's very helpful to have given it some thought, should one have to deal with it. Perhaps we could begin to discuss it here, and then you might be able to talk about it some more later.

Counselee (anxiously, and with defensive firmness): We don't want to think about that unless we have to.
Genetic Counselor: It is difficult to think about, and I can see you've decided for now how you want to handle it.

In the latter case the genetic counselor's statement acknowledges the issue and its emotional impact while also supporting the counselee's defenses and coping mechanisms. If it seems appropriate, the issue may be highlighted again during closing statements by noting that it is potentially important, but that the counselee has chosen not to discuss it at the present time.

Anticipatory guidance should be given concerning the probable anxiety that will be experienced while waiting for the test results (Rapp, 1999; Phipps & Zinn, 1986). It may be helpful to discuss how other periods of anxious waiting have been handled, who is available for emotional support, and, if the father is involved, how the couple can support each other. Decisions should also be made concerning to whom, when, and at what location either good news or bad news will be given. With medically positive results, the counselee may wish to be called at home rather than at work and at a time when the partner or other supportive individuals are available. Agreement should also be reached concerning test results that are received by the genetic counselor shortly before the beginning of a weekend or holiday. Some counselees wish to be informed immediately, despite the unavoidable delay in scheduling a follow-up session. Others prefer to receive the news after a holiday or when the session can follow closely. These arrangements are important in their own right. However, they also serve other purposes. They demonstrate the genetic counselor's assumption of responsibility for the notification process and her commitment to inform the counselee as soon as possible consistent with the agreement. This may help reduce the frequency with which anxious counselees call to inquire about results. In addition, for counselees who have avoided discussing the possibility of medically positive results, this more limited, practical issue may provide the impetus for some consideration of that possible outcome.

When they occur, anxious phone calls from counselees must be treated in a balanced manner. This involves empathic acknowledgment of the anxiety and difficulty in waiting; guidance, if appropriate, concerning anxiety management and social support; and reassurance that the results will be conveyed as soon as possible. At the same time, limits must be set, implicitly or explicitly, concerning the genetic counselor's availability, in order to limit the number and emotional intensity of calls that must be managed.

This stage of the counseling process ends when the genetic counselor, or another professional, informs the counselee(s) of the test outcome. For those who receive medically negative, good news, this information is usually conveyed by telephone. It is a time of relief and often joy for the counselee. For the genetic counselor, it provides professional satisfaction and positive countertransference that is an important counterbalance to the difficult tasks of counseling for medically positive results. With the majority of counselees, this is the genetic counselor's last professional contact, although some counselees call to inform the counselor of a successful pregnancy outcome. However, a minority of counselees continue to experience significant anxiety based on fears and concerns that have been raised about the possibility of a genetic disease, birth defect, or procedure-induced spontaneous abortion (Blumberg, 1984). Such sustained fears may result from more fundamental anxieties or from ambivalence concerning the pregnancy. Thus, the genetic counselor should indicate her continued availability and be prepared to address such issues should the counselee call at a later date.

Counseling Following Medically Positive Results

When the test results are medically positive, the counselee's fears concerning the pregnancy and prenatal diagnosis have been borne out. The counselee is faced with the potentially lifelong implications of the information that has been conveyed and the need to make rapid yet profound decisions (Costello, 1987).

Grief and mourning are normal responses, with the early stages unfolding during the time when information must be assimilated and a decision made about continuation or termination of the pregnancy. In the early period after receiving the results, and if the pregnancy is continued, grief and mourning will involve the loss of the normal pregnancy and the wished for perfect child. If termination is chosen or if fetal or neonatal death occurs, grief and mourning will turn to the actual loss of the pregnancy and death of the child. Psychological defenses will be strongly activated and coping mechanisms must be accessed and strengthened. Guilt, shame, narcissistic injury, loss of belief in an orderly, meaningful universe, and a search for meaning are commonly experienced. Couple and family relationships may be tested by the strain of circumstances and emotions, and the dynamics of these relationships may have a major influence on the manner in which decisions are made and on the process of adaptation and coping.

The elements of counseling discussed in the preceding section have even greater applicability when counseling for medically positive results. Empathic responsiveness to the counselee's emotional pain and turmoil is essential. Information must be presented in a stepwise manner using clear language and frequent check-ins. The timing and detail with which information is presented must be adjusted for the effects of shock and other emotions on the counselee's ability to understand and process it. The range of possible decisions should be stated clearly along with the factors that are relevant to each.

This counseling process requires time. It is usually initiated with a phone call, in which a balance must be reached between providing basic information about the situation that the counselee confronts and avoiding extended counseling during the initial moments of shock and with the limitations of the telephone. Some counselees readily accept a brief telephone conversation, and a statement of empathy and sorrow by the genetic counselor suffices. Others will attempt to control their pain and anxiety by asking multiple questions. The genetic counselor should acknowledge the difficulty of waiting for an extended discussion while gently yet firmly limiting the extent of the conversation.

During the ensuing counseling session, the counselee or counselees may need time alone. This provides the opportunity to think, to organize questions, to discuss options, and to express emotions in private. This is important in its own right, and it may provide some sense of control over a situation that, in most respects, feels as if it is out of control. More than one session may be needed. The interval between sessions provides additional time to process thoughts and emotions; talk with family members, clergy, and other supportive individuals; or meet with professionals or parents of an affected child to whom the counselees have been referred (Costello, 1987).

For counselees who have not decided whether to continue or terminate the pregnancy, it is essential that the genetic counselor provide balanced, accurate information concerning the medical, physical, cognitive, and social implications of the diagnosis. This involves a number of clinical assessments and decisions. The amount and complexity of the information must be tailored to the counselee's ability to understand, retain, and process it. Thus, a balance must be struck between inclusiveness and utility. The potential positive and negative implications of the diagnosis must be addressed. The opportunities for love, joy, personal growth, and adaptation must be presented along with the physical, cognitive, and social limitations and problems that may occur.

The counselee's knowledge and experience concerning the disorder must be assessed. This knowledge and experience can be a valuable source of information, provide motivation to consider the relevant issues, and represent a starting point for discussion. However, counselees may also be misinformed, and in many cases knowledge is based on a limited range of experience. The genetic counselor should attempt to correct misinformation, while respecting individual, family, and cultural beliefs. Furthermore, the counseling should expand the counselee's understanding of the range and variability of possible clinical symptoms, social outcomes, and emotional responses beyond the limitations of his or her particular experiences.

Genetic Counselor (to a woman whose brother has hemophilia and whose fetus is affected): Hemophilia is quite variable in its severity. Your brother appears to have been mildly affected. That's very fortunate. But as you think about what to do, it's important to remember that the disease can be a lot more serious. Have you known or heard of anyone else with hemophilia?

Counselee: No. He's the only one.

Genetic Counselor: If you would like, I can give you more information. Or I could, if you wish, put you in touch with a family whose son is more severely affected. That might be hard for you at this time, but it could help you reach a decision that's right for you and your family.

The information that can be provided inevitably involves uncertainty and ambiguity. First, even well-defined diseases and syndromes for which highly accurate prenatal diagnosis is available are clinically variable. Thus, for example, the cognitive and temperamental outcomes in Down syndrome vary widely, and there may or may not be major medical complications. Second, the prognostic implications of the test results may be ambiguous, as in the case of a *de novo* balanced translocation or a mosaic karyotype. Furthermore, as Fonda Allen and Mulhauser (1995, p. 257) point out, "Increasingly, families are faced with ultrasound findings which carry a numerical risk for poor outcome rather than a specific diagnosis with a definable prognosis." Some of these findings are resolved diagnostically with prenatal diagnosis, but some are not.

In such situations, the genetic counselor must present the full range of possible outcomes, with relative probabilities to the extent they are available. In addition to providing this factual information, the genetic counselor must help the counselee address the emotional burden that the ambiguity creates. This involves empathic acknowledgment of the burden, reframing to reduce the counselee's sense of responsibility and failure, and careful consideration of the potential impact of the various possibilities. Ambiguous information increases both the complexity of the decision-making process and the possibility that an emotionally unanticipated outcome will occur. Under these circumstances, it is all the more important that the process of decision making occurs in a manner that reduces the likelihood of subsequent guilt and blame. Thus, relevant couple issues and disagreements should be addressed. Furthermore, as discussed in the previous section, it is particularly important that the man's deferral of the decision to the woman, based on the position that "it is her body," be addressed (Grobstein, 1979). These aspects of decision making and ambiguity were discussed in more detail in Chapter 5.

Counseling Those Who Choose to Terminate

When a decision is made to terminate the pregnancy, the counselee(s) face a new set of psychosocial issues. The decision finalizes the process of weighing the desire for a child against the anticipated impact of the expected disabilities, under circumstances in which either course of action has painful, undesired consequences (Rapp, 1999; Shapiro, 1993; Rothman, 1986). Immediate concerns commonly involve the pain and grief of losing the pregnancy and the wished for child; anxiety concerning the procedure, including physical pain and risk for the mother; and the desire for the process to be completed as quickly as possible, since reminders of the continuing pregnancy bring home the emotional pain of the decision that has been made (Magyari et al., 1987).

However, long-term psychosocial processes are also set in motion. These include the ongoing process of grief and mourning; the potential for feelings of guilt, inadequacy, and depression concerning both the loss and the decision to terminate; and the search for a sense of resolution concerning the decision and the process by which it was reached (Rapp, 1999; Suslak et al., 1995). Thus, as the genetic counselor assists the counselee with immediate issues, the groundwork is simultaneously laid with respect to the long term. The genetic counselor's empathic, nonjudgmental involvement throughout the process of termination can be an important source of emotional support and an indication of social acceptance of the decision (Grobstein, 1979). If it is possible and the counselee desires it, the genetic counselor may briefly meet the counselee at the hospital or abortion clinic. This act can be helpful to the counselee; and if the husband or partner is present, the genetic counselor can also offer support to him under circumstances where the partner is frequently overlooked or excluded by clinic staff.

To prepare the counselee(s) emotionally and cognitively for the process of abortion and the decisions that must be made, the details of the procedure must be explained (Blumenthal et al., 1990). If both induction of labor and dilation and evacuation are options, the practical and emotional advantages and disadvantages of each should be described. Although induction of labor is physically and emotionally more difficult, it is seen as beneficial by some counselees. The opportunity to exercise a choice of methods provides some sense of control over events. More significant in the long run, the opportunity to view or physically hold the baby following induction of labor may facilitate the grieving process, by promoting emotional attachment and a sense of reality concerning the loss (Suslak et al., 1995). Acknowledging the reality of the loss may be particularly important given social tendencies to underplay the emotional significance of fetal loss. The opportunity to see the baby's normal features may further enhance attachment and reduce unrealistic fantasies or mental images of the degree of visual abnormality. At the same time, observing the diagnostic features or abnormalities may help consolidate the reality of the diagnosis and thus the appropriateness of the decision to terminate. However, the genetic counselor must be prepared to address the fact that, at this stage of fetal development, certain abnormalities may not be visible and this may lead to guilt-based fears that the baby was in fact normal.

Given the work load and time constraints of the clinic, the genetic counselor may be unable to provide the multiple aspects of counseling before, during, and after the abortion that will be discussed later in this section. However, an understanding of the issues is essential in order to help counselees make relevant decisions and cope with the psychosocial consequences of the situation they face.

Insofar as possible, the genetic counselor should assist in arranging for the termination to take place under medically and socially suitable circumstances and should help the counselee understand the relevant issues in making a choice and arrangements. A positive emotional outcome is supported when clinic personnel understand and respect the emotional impact of an abortion following prenatal diagnosis; the mother is shielded from women undergoing normal labor and birth or women undergoing abortions for social reasons; the father can be present if that is wished; the genetic counselor may be present; and arrangements can be made for viewing, holding, or rituals, following induction of labor, if the counselee(s) so desire. Conversely, interactions with staff who are unaware of the circumstances or downplay the emotional significance of the loss, proximity to women who have given birth to a normal child, or exposure to the physical and emotional isolation and hurried routine of an abortion clinic can cause great emotional distress (Magyari et al., 1987; Suslak et al., 1995). When the baby is to be viewed or held, the professionals involved must understand the complex psychosocial context in which this occurs and use great sensitivity in presenting the baby and facilitating the process.

The potential value of activities or rituals that will acknowledge the baby's life and death and facilitate the grieving process should be discussed. These may include a verbal description, photographs, naming, a "Certificate of Delivery," a memorial or remembrance service, and burial or cremation (Magyari et al., 1987).

Counselees also need anticipatory guidance regarding the physical and emotional sequelae of genetic abortion (Blumenthal et al., 1990). Such guidance involves the beginning of mental and social preparation and it is also an essential element in addressing the potential feelings of guilt, inadequacy or depression discussed earlier in this section. While the genetic counselor must be sensitive to the counselee's beliefs, values, and wishes, a discussion of the grief and mourning process may help enlarge the options that counselees consider with respect to the type of abortion process, the difficult task of viewing or holding the baby, and possible memorial activities and rituals.

In the early postabortion period, the genetic counselor can support and normalize the common feelings of loss, grief, anger, and depression, and provide guidance for the process of mourning. Counselees may also need guidance on how to inform others, explain the circumstances, and set appropriate boundaries with respect to social interactions (Costello, 1987). Couples may need assistance in dealing with the differences in their ways of experiencing, expressing, and coping with the grief and anger (Black, 1991). These normal differences may be enhanced because of the woman's biological role in the pregnancy and the abortion, which may lead to feelings that she is responsible for both the reason for and decision of termination (Grobstein, 1979). The pregnancy due date may be a time of particular emotional difficulty. Counselees can be assisted in finding an appropriate remembrance, ritual, or memorial to mark the day and facilitate the grieving process (Suslak et al., 1995).

Support groups may help some counselees by providing emotional support, suggestions for ways of coping, and an opportunity to express and normalize emotions among others who have had similar experiences. However, it is important that counselees be given full support in assessing the advantages and disadvantages of support groups and of declining or withdrawing if that seems appropriate (Costello, 1987; Suslak et al., 1995). When grief reactions, depression, or couple issues appear particularly intense or protracted, a mental health referral may be appropriate.

The results of clinical tests, karyotype, and autopsy if authorized, must be communicated to the counselee. This often allows confirmation of the diagnosis or set of abnormalities on which the decision to terminate was based. This is an important, often final step in providing factual information in support of the decision. The implications with respect to etiology may be reviewed with respect to issues of guilt and blame. This is also the time at which recurrence risk and prenatal diagnosis options for a future pregnancy may be discussed based on all available information. Because of the emotional stress experienced during prenatal diagnosis and abortion, the counselee may remember little of what was discussed previously. Counselees may also experience strong emotions returning to the clinic, discussing test and autopsy results, and facing the decision and the emotional implications of whether to have another pregnancy. Thus, it is essential that the emotional issues be addressed and that the information be provided in a careful, stepwise manner (Costello, 1987; Magyari et al., 1987).

Although issues concerning another pregnancy may be discussed at this time, counselees should be encouraged to delay a permanent decision until they have adequately processed the grief of the lost pregnancy and child. It is particularly important for the well-being of a subsequent child that any tendency to conceive again as a replacement for the lost child be avoided. As Shapiro (1993, p. 141) states with respect to stillbirth,

> The professional may be especially supportive by helping the couple examine whether their readiness to conceive again is based on the wish to replace the child who has died or whether it is an outgrowth of their resolution of their baby's death. The pregnancy should not represent an effort to erase the loss of the stillborn baby but, rather, to acknowledge the couple's desire to build a family, incorporating their loss as integral to the fabric of that family.

The issues and processes just discussed take substantial time to reach adequate resolution and accommodation. Thus, follow-up should be provided on an ongoing basis, as needed and to the extent possible. For some counselees, this will ultimately involve genetic counseling for a subsequent pregnancy.

Counseling Those Who Continue the Pregnancy

Counselees who decide to continue the pregnancy also require support and assistance throughout the pregnancy and following the birth of the child. The variety of individual, social, cultural, and medical circumstances that contribute to such a decision affect the issues that will confront the counselees and thus the role(s) of the genetic counselor. The personal, ethical, moral, cultural, and religious values that lead to a decision to continue the pregnancy may also be important sources of individual and social support (Rapp, 1999). The genetic counselor can assist the counselee in identifying, developing, and mobilizing these resources (Fonda Allen & Mulhauser, 1995; Benkendorf, 1987).

When there is a definitive diagnosis of a serious disease or syndrome, the parents experience grief and mourning for the lost, normal pregnancy and child. At the same time, they must make emotional and practical preparations related to the pregnancy and to the birth and life of the child. These are similar to the tasks confronting the parents of a child diagnosed at or following birth, with additional complexities related to the continuation of the pregnancy. Ongoing obstetric testing or interventions, or a shift of care and/or delivery to a tertiary, high-risk facility introduce physical and emotional stress. They also isolate the counselee from the expected, normal primary care provider and setting. The genetic counselor has important roles in explaining and answering questions concerning obstetric tests and interventions; assisting with planning, coordination, and transitions involving providers and facilities; maintaining as much continuity as possible with the primary care provider; and helping the counselee focus on normal aspects of the pregnancy, which is difficult for some when they cannot yet hold and nurture the baby. Fluctuations in mood, the periodic breakthrough of strong emotions, and the cyclic aspects of grieving and coping may be experienced throughout the pregnancy. As in other circumstances in which this occurs, the genetic counselor can provide empathy, emotional support, normalization, and assistance in mobilizing individual and social resources.

When a decision to continue the pregnancy is made based on ambiguous test results, the cyclical aspects of the grieving and adaptation process may be increased. The uncertainty itself may contribute to fluctuations in optimism/pessimism, anxiety, and despair. Furthermore, monitoring or testing over the course of the pregnancy may result in changes in the diagnosis and prognosis or in the degree of certainty associated with each. This changing medical information can lead to additional shifts in mood and in the counselee's sense of ability to cope and adapt (Fonda Allen & Mulhauser, 1995).

If a medically positive diagnosis is confirmed at birth, or if severe abnormalities are identified, the counselee then faces the issues related to having an affected child. If all indications at birth are normal, there may be substantial relief. However, continued medical monitoring may be indicated, thus sustaining the anxiety. Even when evaluations are normal and the child's development is on course in the parents' eyes, fear and anxiety engendered by the initial circumstances may continue for years. Counselees can be assisted in dealing with these continuing uncertainties by appropriate authoritative reassurance from the genetic counselor and other medical providers and by empathic normalization of these persistent anxieties.

If the decision to continue the pregnancy is based on a perception that the abnormalities and prognosis are relatively benign, emotional and practical preparations must still be made. In these situations, uncertainty as to outcome may also persist for an extended period, as in the case of sex chromosome abnormalities.

Counselees facing any of the above situations may benefit from referral to a support group or to another family facing a similar situation. However, the same caveats discussed in the preceding section are relevant here.

Cancer Risk Counseling

Cancer risk counseling has grown rapidly in recent years to become a major area of specialization within genetic counseling. Its development has been due to several converging factors. These include the isolation and cloning of BRCA1, BRCA2, and other cancer susceptibility genes; intense public concern about cancer and familial contributions to cancer susceptibility; media publicity concerning cancer risks and the development of genetic tests; and the establishment and marketing of commercial testing services. While cancer risk counseling builds upon the general principles of genetic counseling, it also involves new types of information, concepts, and professional interactions. Furthermore, cancer risk counseling often requires sustained attention to psychosocial issues, in part because of the intensity of personal and family issues that are involved. However, other factors contribute as well. These include the complexity of risk figures and concepts that must be explained, the time period required to obtain medical records after initial counselee contacts, and the uncertainty surrounding the efficacy of potential preventive measures (Schneider & Marnane, 1997).

Given the current state of cancer risk counseling, much of the discussion that follows is based on breast/ovarian cancer. However, the field is evolving rapidly in many respects, including the identification of susceptibility genes for other forms of cancer, information concerning the effectiveness of medical management techniques, and understanding of the relevant psychosocial issues. In addition, any consideration of cancer and cancer risk counseling must take into account the fact that cancer is a generic term referring to a broad range of specific disorders. These differ significantly with respect to medical and psychosocial impact, the contribution of inherited mutations, the levels of risk that result from genetic factors, and the efficacy of surveillance and prophylactic measures.

In addition to its direct importance, cancer risk counseling is of interest with respect to the evolution of genetic counseling. Prenatal diagnosis counseling was the first major specialty area to develop (Kolker & Burke, 1994); cancer risk counseling is the second. Furthermore, cancer risk counseling is the first to cover common adult-onset disorders. Other specialty areas include sickle cell disease/hemoglobinopathy counseling and presymptomatic testing for Huntington disease. When looked at broadly, these specialty areas help define the types of issues that genetic counselors encounter when they enter and help develop new areas of practice (Walker, 1998). These issues include new information, concepts, techniques, methods of risk assessment, medical practice, interactions with professional colleagues, mix of emotional and psychosocial issues, and need to address counselee anxieties and expectations generated in part by the popular media and commercial interests. Thus, a discussion of the emerging field of cancer risk counseling also serves to anticipate the types of challenges that genetic counselors will confront as additional specialty services arise in areas such as cardiovascular risk counseling and presymptomatic testing for common neurogenetic disorders such as Alzheimer disease.

Counselee Beliefs and Concerns

At present the majority of counselees request cancer risk assessment or genetic testing because one or more family member has had cancer (Hopwood, 1997). Thus, many counselees begin the counseling process with strong emotions born out of experiences within their own families. Their experiences may include the fear that arises when cancer is diagnosed, the temporary disabling and disfiguring consequences of radiation or chemotherapy, the physical and emotional consequences of surgery, and the illness and death of a parent or other family members. Counselees may have specific fears concerning their own possible illness, disfigurement, or death as well as the possibility of further illness and loss for their children and families. They may be experiencing anger, isolation, loss of control, grief over past and possible future deaths within the family, and guilt due to a sense of having failed to do enough for family members with cancer. Intense concern about their children's chance of developing cancer is also common (Kelly, 1991; Schneider, 1994).

Given these emotions and concerns, counselees often experience substantial anxiety. It may be general, free floating, and preoccupying. It may be cyclical, decreasing after good news from a periodic cancer screen and then rising over time. It may be triggered by specific events or time periods, such as nearing the age at which a relative, especially the counselee's mother, was diagnosed with or died from cancer. It may be alleviated in part by passing the age at which diagnosis or death occurred. Counselees' anxiety must be addressed, both to alleviate the emotional pain it produces and because anxiety can interfere with the ability to understand and utilize the information provided during counseling. In addition, fear and high anxiety may lead to a defensive avoidance of thoughts and actions related to the issue of concern. As a counselee of Kelly's (1991, p. 3) stated, "It's a tug between the hysterical part of you that doesn't want to know, and the rational part that wants to do more than worry." Furthermore, the effects of unaddressed anxiety can extend beyond the counseling process. Several studies have found that high anxiety among women at risk for breast cancer adversely affects preventive care. On the one hand, it may inhibit breast self-examination and the utilization of medical examinations and mammography; on the other hand, it may lead to excessive self-examination and screening (Lerman et al., 1995).

High anxiety may lead to an approach-avoidance cycle toward cancer risk counseling. In the approach phase, with anxiety-driven desire to obtain information and assistance, counselees may contact the clinic, request information, attend education sessions, or obtain family records. However, as anxiety rises further or defenses weaken, counselees may cancel, postpone, or miss appointments, or withdraw from active involvement in obtaining records. Attention to the counselee's emotional issues may reduce the number or intensity of these cycles, help alleviate the emotional distress involved, and reduce the time required to reach a satisfactory decision concerning whether to undertake risk counseling or genetic testing. Since an avoidant phase may be activated following an early clinic contact or an education session, it is useful to address emotional issues in the early stages of the counseling process and to avoid a strict partition between the "education" and "counseling" phases (B. Crawford, 1999, personal communication).

Counselees frequently feel that the risk of developing cancer is exceedingly high, or that cancer is inevitable. In part, these perceptions result from misunderstandings about the complex risk figures relevant to cancer, coupled with publicity about the high incidence of cancer in general and breast cancer in particular. However, these perceptions may also involve beliefs that are unrelated to specific risk figures or cancer genetics. Counselees may believe they are at high risk because cancer has occurred in their family. They may feel particularly vulnerable because they share physical characteristics, or aspects of personality, life-style, or age, with an affected family member, especially a parent. Counselees also interpret their own life experiences, including age, child bearing, age in relation to menopause, and experience with breast lumps or other physical characteristics, in terms of public information and private beliefs about the relationship of these factors to cancer (Bernhardt et al., 1997; Kelly, 1991).

Owing to these psychological factors, counselees' beliefs about the risk of developing cancer may be resistant to change (Lynch et al., 1997). Information alone, even when it involves substantially lower objective risk figures than the counselee has anticipated, may not lead to more accurate risk perception or a reduction of anxiety. When this is the case, the underlying issues must be explored, in order to help the counselee process the information and incorporate it into perceptions and beliefs.

Not uncommonly, counselees use graphic metaphors with violent imagery to describe their sense of vulnerability. For example, Kelly (1991, p. 29) quotes a counselee who said of herself, "I'm a walking time bomb that could go off at any minute." Similarly, after having had oophorectomy explained, a counselee of Crawford's (1999, personal communication) said, "Oh. That means, if I have a basket full of hand grenades and I take some out, I have reduced my chances of being killed by cancer." Metaphors such as these speak to the counselee's underlying experiences. Thus, they provide an important key to addressing perceptions and concerns. The genetic counselor should note them and incorporate them into the exploration of life experiences, beliefs, fears, and misperceptions.

> *Genetic Counselor:* You said earlier you feel as if you have a hand grenade in your pocket, and someone is about to pull the pin.
> *Counselee:* Yes. I feel that way a lot, and it's terrifying.
> *Genetic Counselor (drawing on previously elicited information):* You were in your early teens when your mother was so sick and then died. You must have felt that the world was falling apart. And people were so concerned about your mother that no one could hear your grief and your anger.
> *Counselee:* Yes. I felt like I was just a chance survivor. Some days I thought I would die of sorrow, and others I thought I would explode with rage.
> *Genetic Counselor:* You still have those feelings, like many women whose mothers died of cancer. But the numbers say there's a good chance you won't get cancer, and there are ways to reduce your risk further. Even more important, there are people now who can hear your fear and anger.
> *Counselee:* Maybe so. Some of it is old stuff that isn't as true any more.
> *Genetic Counselor:* Maybe the pin on that hand grenade is more secure than you think.

By using the metaphor in this way, the genetic counselor does not deny the risk, but instead addresses the issue of perceived control or lack thereof.

Family Dynamics

As the preceding section indicates, the occurrence of cancer in one or more members of a family can have a deep impact on other members. The nature of the family's interactions in many areas, including coping skills, communication, and openness to outside assistance, influences how each member responds emotionally and behaviorally. These issues are potentially present in every counseling interaction. Furthermore, they may be significantly influenced by the process of cancer risk counseling itself, through the attention to family medical history, the review of medical records, and the identification of family members who are at increased risk (Schneider, 1994).

The illness or death of a parent from cancer can profoundly affect the children, and the consequences may be manifest many years later. In general terms, the impact appears to be greater if the child is young at the time of his or her parent's illness and/or death, and it may be greatest if the child is an adolescent. However, many other factors are also important. These include the family's ability to communicate about the disease and the parent's death if it occurred, the quality of relationships if the surviving parent remarries or forms another partnership, and the family's acknowledgment and support of the child's grief. Thus, it is essential to obtain such information when working with counselees (Baty et al., 1997; Schneider, 1994).

These issues have been explored as they affect women whose mothers have had cancer. At the time of her mother's illness, the daughter, regardless of age, may experience fear, confusion, denial, grief, and a sense of lost maternal attention and guidance. If the family withholds information about the nature or severity of the disease, the daughter may be unprepared for her mother's illness, treatment, or death, and is thus left with intense feelings of guilt because of the limited attention or sympathy she gave to her mother. In later life, the impact of these events may lead to lowered self-esteem, feelings of guilt, difficulty establishing close relationships, heightened fears of developing cancer, and an implicit belief that cancer will lead to the same outcomes as the mother experienced, be it disfigurement, death, or leaving her children motherless (Lewis, 1996; Matloff, 1997).

Memories and emotions about the mother's illness may emerge with high, often unexpected intensity during cancer risk counseling. Not uncommonly, the counselee will have had little or no previous opportunity to discuss her experiences and feelings. Thus, if these issues are adequately addressed, there is the possibility of significant emotional release and healing. For example, Matloff (1997), Eunpu (1997a), and Djurdjinovic (1997) discuss a poignant case involving two adult sisters, themselves parents, who were nine and ten years old when their mother died after several years' illness with breast cancer. Supported by an empathic genetic counselor, they reviewed their mother's medical records, including their own births and her course of cancer treatment. From this review came a healing sense of reconnection with a mother they felt they had hardly known. This included aspects of their own births and childhoods they had been unable to ask her about, a recognition of her deep desire to live for them, and an understanding of her illness and pain that had been unexplained when they were children.

The emotions, fears, and responses to risk counseling just discussed may also arise from other cancer-related experiences and losses. These include the illness or death of a father, other family members, nonfamily members of importance to the counselee, or acquaintances. The impact may be heightened if death has occurred to an individual with dependent children or if the counselee has experienced the illness or death of multiple family members. The death of a parent or of many family members may leave the counselee feeling that the family's continuity through the generations has been broken, with a loss of personal relationships as well as the memories and family knowledge of the affected generation(s). Matloff (1997) refers to this as "generations lost," and Crawford (1999, personal communication) speaks of "truncated families." These losses and truncations affect the counselee's sense of self. However, they may also interfere with the process of obtaining family information and medical records, because of both lack of information and loss of family cohesion (Green et al., 1993; Schneider, 1994).

Many aspects of cancer risk counseling may evoke family issues for the counselee as well as for other family members, such as constructing the pedigree, determining the family's medical history, locating and obtaining medical records, and contacting family members regarding medical history, at-risk status, or genetic testing. All the elements of family interactions, including communication styles, coping mechanisms, and adaptability to change, both in general and with respect to the family's experience with cancer, influence the process. Individual family members may accept or reject requests for information or involvement. Their responses depend, in part, on the quality of their relationships with the counselee, the patterns of communication within the family, and their degree of openness to or avoidance of the issues surrounding cancer within the family. As discussed previously, an individual's responses often reflect ambivalence or fluctuation between a desire to help or a wish to act on the fear of cancer, on the one hand, and denial or avoidance of anxiety and emotional pain, on the other (Schneider, 1994; Smith et al., 1999).

DudokdeWit and coworkers (1997) characterize two roles that individuals may have within a family relevant to cancer risk assessment and testing. The first involves the individual who initiates the investigation of a potential genetic etiology and contacts family members requesting information and informing them of counseling or testing options. If family members reject the contacts or are angry, resentful, or emotionally hurt, this person may feel socially isolated or guilty for having revived painful emotions and memories. For some, the process stops at this point because of the anger and rejection that are anticipated or encountered. Exploration of these issues by the genetic counselor and discussion of methods for contacting family members may allow the process to move forward again. Other individuals, for whom the motivation to pursue information and/or testing is high, may persist in their efforts despite resistance within the family. When counselees demonstrate such persistence, it is important that the genetic counselor not underestimate the emotional costs involved, overestimate the psychological strengths the individual brings to the situation, or overlook the ambivalence concerning pursuit of these issues that he or she may also be experiencing. Support and assistance may be very helpful, despite the appearance of strong motivation and resolve.

The second role described by DudokdeWit and associates (1997) involves the first family member to utilize genetic testing or other interventions. Again, the response of family members may be receptive and supportive, rejecting and avoidant, or mixed and ambivalent. This individual may feel pressure to demonstrate the value of his or her actions, in part to counterbalance the increased anxiety and emotional pain that family members may experience as the family becomes involved in cancer risk counseling and/or testing. He or she may also feel the burden of being "first and strongest" (p. 68), and thus desire emotional support from other members and the genetic counselor.

Given the potential for complex, intense interactions among family members, it is critical to explore family dynamics with counselees. While the counselee's concerns must be the primary focus, the genetic counselor must also protect the privacy of other family members and avoid supporting or colluding in coercive efforts to obtain their involvement in counseling or testing (Baty et al., 1997).

The Complexity of Cancer Risk Figures

Counselees face a dauntingly complex set of likelihood and probability figures relevant to cancer risk. For example, risk assessment and testing, if it occurs, commonly generate the following sequential set of risk figures (Hallowell et al., 1998):

- the likelihood that the cancers in the counselee's family are due to a mutation in a cancer susceptibility gene
- if so, the likelihood that the counselee or other family members carry the mutation
- then, depending on the outcome of risk assessment and/or genetic testing, the probability that the counselee or other family members will develop specific types of cancer, for example, breast, ovarian, uterine, colon, etc.

When the probability of developing cancer is discussed, figures may be given in terms of cumulative lifetime risk or the risk pertaining to a given age interval. The figure given may represent absolute risk, relative risk compared to the general population or other reference group, or percentage increase in risk. Counselees may also encounter risks of which they were unaware, such as the risk of ovarian cancer when there is familial breast cancer, the risk of breast cancer in men, or the risk of multiple forms of cancer in Li-Fraumeni syndrome. Furthermore, they may encounter new risk-related concepts, such as the risk of transmission of breast/ovarian cancer susceptibility through males or the possibility that multiple cases of cancer within the family are due to chance rather than a gene mutation (Baty et al., 1997; Schneider, 1994).

Even if the genetic counselor uses a limited, carefully selected set of risk figures, counselees may have information in other forms from other sources, and these may lead to misperceptions or confusion. In addition, individual and family dynamics may contribute to the difficulties in understanding risk or in adjusting beliefs and perceptions in response to new information. It is thus very important that the counselee's understanding and sources of information be explored, and that careful attention be given to the manner in which risk information is provided. Furthermore, when multiple forms of risk figures are presented or discussed, the genetic counselor's ability to provide a conceptual framework for understanding the information and guidance concerning the relationship between different types of data is critical.

For example, before discussing specific cumulative lifetime risk figures and age-specific risk figures, the genetic counselor could provide an overview of the two types of calculations, indicate their differences, and place them in the context of the anxiety that occurs when one is confused for the other (Kelly, 1991):

Genetic Counselor: There are two ways that the risk of developing cancer can be calculated. One way is to figure out the chance that a woman will develop cancer at any time in her life. This is usually done by calculating the risk if a woman lives to age 80 or 100, since that covers most people's life span. The other way is to calculate the chance of developing cancer during some particular period of life. For example, since you are 40, a relevant calculation would be the chance of getting cancer between ages 41 and 50. You can see that the two approaches give very different risk figures, since one is for an entire lifetime and the other is just for a limited period. Often, this isn't explained very well, and people confuse the two. It can be very scary if you read or hear a lifetime risk figure and think it is the risk over the next few years.

Cancer Gene Testing

The ability to test for mutations in cancer susceptibility genes raises complex issues that must be addressed at a number of times during cancer risk counseling. As counselees receive information, their understanding of genetic testing may change substantially and new emotional issues and responses may emerge. Counselees may initially believe that genetic testing is a relatively straightforward matter that will resolve uncertainty, relieve anxiety, explain the occurrence of cancer in the family, and provide guidance with respect to medical surveillance, life-style changes, or prophylactic measures. However, depending on the family history, the adequacy of medical records, and the type of cancer(s) involved, any or all of these expectations may require revision, with emotional consequences (Bernhardt et al., 1997; Schneider et al., 1997). For example, when a review of the family medical history does not support an inherited etiology for the cancers that have occurred, counselees may experience relief due to a perceived reduction in the risk of cancer and of having passed a susceptibility mutation on to their children. However, this outcome, or a failure to meet the criteria for genetic testing, may also give rise to renewed anxiety, anger, or disappointment that the hoped for resolution of genetic testing is unavailable.

The advantages and limitations of genetic testing must be carefully explained and the counselee's reactions explored. The known or possible limitations in test outcome and prognostic value should be discussed. In addition, it is important to address what is known about the efficacy of surveillance, life-style, or prophylactic measures that might be instituted on the basis of test results. The possibility of insurance discrimination and of discrimination or stigmatization in the workplace and in social interactions must also be addressed (Baty et al., 1997).

The potential emotional consequences of test results must be thoroughly discussed. A negative result can lead to relief, joy, decreased anxiety and fear, and the avoidance of costly, uncomfortable surveillance procedures (e.g., colonoscopy) or prophylactic surgery. However, it may also lead to sadness or survivor guilt regarding affected or mutation-bearing relatives and, in some cases, to a disorienting loss of a concern and preoccupation with cancer that was a central feature of the counselee's life. A positive result may lead to welcome relief from uncertainty and to high risk surveillance, prophylactic measures, and a health care regimen that reduce the risk of cancer. However, positive results may also lead to sadness, hopelessness, depression, fear, greater uncertainty, lessened life expectations, or heightened anxiety. In addition, positive results may involve the counselee in complex, emotionally difficult health care decisions such as whether to have prophylactic surgery. An uninformative test result may lead to sadness, anger, or depression over the lost hoped for resolution of a test result. In discussing these potential outcomes, it is essential that the counselee's reasons for undertaking testing, including hopes, expectations, and beliefs about possible outcomes, be very carefully explored. This helps identify incorrect information or assumptions and unrealistic expectations. Moreover, in broader terms, it assists the counselee in assessing the advantages and disadvantages of testing in the light of more fully articulated values and expectations (Baty et al., 1997; Schneider et al., 1997).

The potential effects on interactions and relationships within the family should also be discussed. As indicated previously, these effects often begin with the family interactions involved in obtaining medical information and records.

When there are living affected family members, genetic testing often begins with one or more of them in order to identify the specific gene mutation that is involved. The potential effects of this order of testing should be addressed. Differences in the opinions of family members concerning the desirability and value of testing are important, as is the potential impact of test results on family members and their relationships to one another. A given family member may participate in testing to benefit other family members who desire risk information, without realizing that information will also be obtained relevant to his or her own risk of developing cancer. When there are differences of opinion or desires concerning participation in testing, the rights of individual family members must be respected and supported with regard to privacy, confidentiality, and the right to not participate or not be informed of test results.

The presentation of test results initiates a new stage in the counseling process. The counselee's emotional responses must be carefully assessed. In addition, the options and limitations of available surveillance methods, life-style changes, and prophylactic surgery must be discussed. Both the emotional and medical aspects require long-term, integrated assessment and follow-up by the genetic counselor. The counselee's coping mechanisms, family and social supports, and current or previous counseling or psychotherapy must be assessed and the counselee assisted in utilizing them. The availability of support groups and mental health professionals should be discussed and referrals made if requested. In addition to addressing these issues at the time test results are given, the genetic counselor should also schedule telephone follow-ups or check-ins during the following few months (Baty et al., 1997; Peters, 1994a; Schneider et al., 1997).

For some counselees at increased risk for breast cancer, the decision concerning prophylactic mastectomy is particularly difficult. On the one hand, it reduces but does not eliminate the probability of developing breast cancer; on the other hand, the effects on body image, sense of sexuality, erogenous responses, and sexual relationships can be great. Fear of cancer, often based on the experiences of other family members, can have a major impact on the decision-making process. Tamoxifen treatment and oophorectomy also have significant sexual and physiological effects, of which counselees may be unaware. Thus, it is critical to address the emotional as well as factual aspects of these procedures in an ongoing process of exploration and explanation, with the inclusion of the counselee's partner if at all possible (Karp et al., 1999; Schneider et al., 1997).

Cancer Risk Counseling Techniques

The counseling techniques discussed throughout this book are applicable to cancer risk counseling. However, certain specific approaches are particularly useful and relevant.

Given the intensity and complexity of individual and family issues, the importance of exploring issues thoroughly can hardly be overstated. In broad terms this involves discussing the counselee's beliefs concerning the causes and risk of cancer, the meanings of cancer in his or her life and in the experiences of the family, and the fears, expectations, and other emotions that influence the perception of the disease and the decisions that are to be made (Djurdjinovic, 1997; Schneider, 1994).

This exploration serves several purposes. It helps the client express emotions and thus experience the relief that this can produce. Having the support of a counselor who is able to accept, normalize, and help contain the emotions can also be beneficial. Sometimes, emotions that feel frighteningly intense or infinite in depth appear less overwhelming once they are expressed. The counselee may discover that the crying, trembling, or outburst of anger begins to subside within minutes, rather than continuing endlessly as had been feared. This is particularly likely to occur if the counselee has had little or no opportunity to express the emotion, or if it is based on childhood experiences that have not been adequately processed. In some instances, a more extensive process of healing can occur, as counselees explore and process events from the past. The case of the two sisters who reviewed their deceased mother's medical records, discussed earlier in Family Dynamics, is an excellent example. The reduction in anxiety, fear, or other emotions that may result from such exploration reduces the impact of these emotions on decision making, on avoidance or denial of issues and procedures, and on the approach/avoidance cycle. In addition, exploration helps identify the beliefs and perceptions the counselee brings to the counseling process. It may clarify issues for the counselee, and it helps the counselor identify issues that require further discussion.

Insofar as time allows, and with attention to the counselee's level of comfort and resilience, asking small detailed questions is an effective way to evoke emotions and elicit a finely textured recounting of experiences and their meanings.

Genetic Counselor (exploring the counselee's responses to her sister's cancer): What was it like for you when you first learned that Sue had ovarian cancer?
Counselee: Well, at first I just felt numb. The whole family seemed numb. We were all very emotional, but we could hardly talk about it.
Genetic Counselor: How long would you say that lasted?
Counselee: Maybe a week.
Genetic Counselor: That must have been a very hard time. Do you remember what happened when things began to change?
Counselee: I began to be able to think a little more straight, and we all began talking more.
Genetic Counselor: And what were you thinking?
Counselee: I was thinking how sad it was for Sue, with her two children. And then I thought, with Mom having had breast cancer, maybe we're all at risk.

When the circumstances being discussed have occurred in the past, it is useful to inquire about the feelings experienced then as well as in the present. It can be helpful and enlightening for the counselee to perceive how much her emotions have changed over time, especially if the events occurred during childhood (Kelly, 1991).

In the face of difficult decisions, counselors can help counselees find options of which they were not initially aware.

> A woman with several cases of breast cancer in her family came to counseling in great anxiety. She felt emotionally unprepared to deal with the results of gene testing. However, she felt that not being tested was irresponsible toward herself and her daughters, who were in their twenties. In addition, she felt guilty that she was unable to resolve this quandary and "just grit my teeth and take the test." The genetic counselor suggested that the counselee, and her daughters if they wished, undertake breast self-examinations and medical surveillance "as if" they carried the mutation. This was presented as "responsible health care under the circumstances," which would give the counselee time to deal with the emotional issues surrounding testing. The counselee found this suggestion helpful and her acute anxiety subsided. In the more settled emotional state that resulted, and with the confidence she had gained in the counselor's ability to be helpful, she reached a decision seven months later to have testing.

By suggesting alternative options, counselors may also help counselees overcome a sense of the inevitable repetition of family experiences. Eunpu (1997a) provides examples of this in the case involving the two adult sisters discussed previously (see Family Dynamics). Eunpu suggests that they might find new ways to support each other and their children, if either developed breast cancer. Possibilities included each sister being available to the other's children for information, mothering, and support; finding ways of interacting with their children that differed from those they had experienced as children; and writing a life book or journal that could be shared with their children. Thus, should the need arise, they would have ways of reducing the children's sense of being cut off from their mother and, by so doing, avoid the sense of another "generation lost" that they so feared.

It may be helpful to discuss with the counselee issues involved in communicating with other family members, such as requests for information, for authorization to obtain medical records, or to consider genetic testing. Another issue may involve communicating the results of risk analysis or DNA testing to other family members including adult or minor children. An exploration of family communication patterns, coping mechanisms, and what has worked or not worked under other circumstances can help clarify these issues for the counselee and provide useful information for the genetic counselor. Various possible circumstances and means of communication should be considered: in person, either one-on-one or with other family members present; by phone; or by mail. It is useful to discuss ways of presenting information or requests that respect the autonomy of the other person, the types of responses the counselee expects, the pace at which different family members are likely to process the communication and respond, and whether other family members might help with the communication process (Bennett, 1999). When minor children are involved, the counselor can discuss age-appropriate ways of talking about difficult issues with children, and the counselor may offer to play an active role if the counselee so wishes (Baty et al., 1997) (see this chapter, Genetic Counseling with Children)

Genetic Counselor: So you haven't talked to your mother's younger sister in several years?

Counselee: No. And the last few times I did, she was pretty distant. I think she felt left out when my mother got so much attention from the family during her illness.

Genetic Counselor: Is there anyone else who might help in communicating with her about this?

Counselee: Well, her other sister, who is the oldest, was always the peacemaker when there was a squabble. And I do talk to her more often.

Genetic Counselor: Do you think she might help break the ice?

Counselee: That's a good idea. I can at least talk to her and see what she thinks.

Cancer risk counseling raises new issues concerning the appropriateness and effectiveness of nondirective counseling. On the one hand, the decisions that arise in cancer risk counseling do not involve reproduction, which was the primary area of concern during the historical development of nondirective genetic counseling. On the other hand, some decisions relate more directly to medical management. For example, for an individual at risk for hereditary nonpolyposis colon cancer or familial adenomatous polyposis, gene testing, if positive, can lead to life-saving colonoscopies and prophylactic surgery. If the test result is negative, the expense and discomfort of colonoscopy can be avoided. Thus, while the decision remains the counselee's, a counseling model based on a medical recommendation that also recognizes the patient's role in the decision-making process may, under some circumstances, be appropriate (Peters & Stopfer, 1996).

The situation is less clear when, as at present in the case of breast cancer, the efficacy of the available methods of medical management is unknown. However, in this regard, Bernhardt and coworkers (1997) found that the majority of women who participated in focus groups concerning BRCA1 testing preferred a medical recommendation that left the final decision to the counselee over a nondirective approach. The issue of nondirectiveness in cancer risk counseling requires further analysis, discussion, and clarification in clinical practice. However, it is important to recognize that the circumstances are variable, a strict application of nondirectiveness may not always be appropriate, and responsibility for a medically based recommendation may sometimes fall to the counselor or other members of the clinical staff.

Cancer risk counseling can evoke powerful countertransference issues. In part, this relates to the intensity of counselees' experiences and emotions, to the family issues that arise, and to the length of time and depth of involvement required by this type of counseling. However, countertransference is also evoked by the genetic counselor's concerns, fears, and experiences, both with cancer in general and with specific forms such as breast cancer. Moreover, given the high frequency of cancer, genetic counselors engaged in cancer risk counseling confront a sense of vulnerability for themselves and their families much greater than that encountered in most other forms of genetic counseling (Matloff, 1997). Given the significance of these issues in cancer risk counseling, some form of peer discussion and support, consultation or personal counseling or therapy, can be of great value.

Genetic Counseling with Children

Children are frequently present in genetic counseling sessions and, even more frequently, are affected by the circumstances that lead to and follow from genetic counseling. Yet despite this obvious situation, there is very little literature or commonly shared body of experience related to genetic counseling with children. In my opinion, genetic counselors have an opportunity and an obligation to extend their practice to include children. As with adults, genetic counseling can assist children in better understanding the situations they face and can provide an opportunity for expressing, validating, and addressing their emotions. This has the potential to enhance the lives of both affected and unaffected children and to improve the interactions and functioning of their families (Benkendorf, 1987).

In broad terms the situation is comparable to that of genetic counseling with adults two or three decades ago: There is a very substantial body of relevant theory and practice that can be drawn upon. However, it must be adapted to the context of genetic counseling, assessed through clinical practice and research, and discussed and reported within the profession. In addition, many genetic counselors can draw on their own experience as children, parents, and family members, and on prior experience in related professions, as they expand their practice to include genetic counseling with children.

The following three sections discuss the effects of genetic diseases and birth defects on children, the family context of children's lives, and child psychosocial development and functioning. The treatment of these highly complex subjects is of necessity very brief. The purpose is to provide a basic framework from which to then discuss techniques for genetic counseling with children.

The Impact of Genetic Diseases and Birth Defects on Children

Genetic diseases, syndromes, and birth defects affect children in a multitude of ways, depending in substantial part on the nature and severity of the disorder (Hobbs et al., 1985; Thompson, 1985). Affected children must adapt to the direct physical, cognitive, and social effects of their disorder. With visible physical abnormalities or impairments in cognitive or behavioral functioning, the child faces issues of self-image, self-esteem, and stigmatization. By the school age years, limitations in the ability to participate in peer group activities or to advance through the normal school regimen may significantly affect these aspects of development as well as the child's social competence and sphere of social experience. The parents' interactions with the child and responses to the disorder play a central role in how the child adapts to his or her situation. Emotional support; empathic assistance in dealing with physical, cognitive, or social limitations; normalization coupled with realism; and an appropriate balance between support and protection, on the one hand, and opportunities for trial-and-error and learning by experience, on the other hand, all contribute to the child's development. Overprotection, social isolation, or a sense of shame or stigmatization on the parent's part that is imparted to the child, all present impediments to development.

Some affected children are subject to painful, frightening medical procedures, which may include brief or extended hospitalizations. Children who have severe, progressive, or fatal disorders face the impact of disability and/or impending death far earlier than most individuals. Finally, the genetic counseling process itself may create anxiety or fear related to clinical or medical procedures; exposure to seemingly invasive professionals, sometimes in substantial numbers or in a confusingly shifting sequence; and sensitization to the hospital or clinic environment (Hobbs et al., 1985).

Siblings of children with genetic diseases, syndromes, or birth defects are also affected in many ways. As discussed in Chapter 2, the presence of an affected child influences family interactions and development in many domains and inevitably influences the lives of the other children. The effects on their psychosocial functioning, sense of self, and view of the world may extend into adulthood as powerful psychosocial dynamics that have both positive and negative effects on adult functioning. Siblings may be affected by their parents' sadness, depression, grief, fear, anger, or sense of shame and stigmatization. The needs of the affected child as well as psychodynamically driven parental overinvolvement or overprotection may leave other children feeling deficient in parental attention and support or competing among themselves for these resources. Lack of communication within the family concerning the disorder and its emotional consequences or the requirement to maintain confidentiality with respect to the outside world may lead to confusion, social isolation, distrust, and the sense of carrying a "family secret" (Fanos, 1996; Hobbs et al., 1985).

Unaffected siblings may have responsibilities toward the family or the affected child that set them apart from peers and involve parental roles for which they are developmentally unprepared. They may experience strong feelings of protectiveness toward their affected sibling or be expected by their parents to perform such a role, and these emotions and demands may conflict with the need for independent and peer-oriented interactions and development. Medical tests, hospitalizations, disease progression, and impending death may all lead to deep fears about the well-being and fate of the affected child as well as the vulnerability and fate of the self and the family unit (Seligman & Darling, 1989).

Unaffected siblings may also have fears and misunderstandings about their own vulnerability and their risk of developing the disorder. They may believe that the disorder is contagious or can have delayed onset; they may be confused about carrier status or the meaning and significance of tests to which the sibling is subjected. Some of this fear and misunderstanding is due to misinformation or lack of information. However, some is also the result of deeper psychodynamic responses including a generalized sense of personal and family vulnerability, a high level of identification with the affected sibling, and the assuming of symptoms as a means for competing with the affected child for parental attention (Fanos, 1996). Thus, there are a host of cognitive and psychosocial issues of relevance to siblings of affected children.

As an example, in the course of my psychotherapeutic work with siblings of children who have Down syndrome, a dynamic of surprising uniformity has emerged. On the one hand, the sibling feels intense love and protectiveness toward the affected brother or sister. This extends to the attitudes and behaviors of friends and peers toward the affected child, including teasing and stigmatization. On the other hand, the sibling has an intense desire and need to define his or her life and peer relationships independent of the affected child. This often includes an occasional desire to participate in the teasing or stigmatization of the affected child by peers. Much of the emotional distress experienced by the sibling with respect to this dynamic is due to the conflicting pull of these two sets of feelings and behaviors and to the confusion and guilt this engenders.

Although my understanding of this dynamic developed in the course of long-term child therapy, I now find that a brief, age-appropriate statement of the dynamic creates an almost instantaneous sense of being understood and accepted on the part of the child. This is true of school age children and of adolescents, and it includes situations in which the child is initially resistant to interacting with me.

> *Therapist (to eight-year-old sister of a ten-year-old girl with Down syndrome):* I knew another girl whose sister had Down syndrome. She told me that she really loves her sister and that sometimes she really wants to protect her. But other times she wants to play with her friends, even if they tease her sister. I bet you feel that way sometimes too.
> *Child (visibly relaxing and moving slightly away from her mother):* Yes.
> *Therapist:* And what I've found out is, that's okay. Everybody feels that way sometimes.

An understanding of this dynamic, which has also been reported in more general terms by others (Fanos, 1996; Seligman & Darling, 1989), is useful in its own right. However, it serves the broader purpose of demonstrating the intense emotional conflicts that siblings may experience and the potential effectiveness of a concise, age-appropriate empathic comment for engaging a child, whether in ongoing therapy or in the short-term interactions of genetic counseling.

Children are also affected when a parent experiences a genetic disease or birth defect (Rolland, 1994). As discussed in Chapter 2 under The Family in a Temporal and Social Context a parent's chronic disease or disability influences all aspects of family structure and of its development over time. Children face the loss in capabilities and functioning of the affected parent. In addition, the physical and emotional availability of the unaffected parent may be greatly reduced owing to increased responsibilities and the impact of anxiety, grief, or depression. Even when sufficient physical, financial and emotional resources are available, major changes in family interactions and responsibilities may occur. The child may be called upon to assume duties and responsibilities that would otherwise have remained those of the parents. Increased responsibilities, financial restrictions, reduced family mobility, and the nature of the parent's disorder may lead to limitations in social opportunities for the child and may involve stigmatization or the need to bear family secrets. The child may have deep anxieties or fears concerning the parent's well-being and survival, and family communication patterns may or may not allow these concerns to be addressed. When the parent has a dominant disorder, guilt over known or possible transmission to the child may lead to parental overprotection. Conversely, the child may harbor realistic or unrealistic fears of contracting the adult's disorder.

A seven-year-old boy was treated in child therapy for behavioral and school performance problems including difficulty reading. His mother was blind as a consequence of prophylactic surgery for bilateral retinoblastoma. In the early sessions the child frequently rubbed his eyes and complained that they hurt, and his mother reported that this also occurred at home and at school. Through the process of talking and play therapy, the therapist inferred that the boy had an unconscious fear of blindness, and this was then confirmed and brought to his consciousness through play and talking. After consulting with me, the therapist explained to the child in age-appropriate but authoritatively confident terms that his mother had had cancer in her eyes, that her eyes had been removed to save her life, and that once a child reached the age of six without getting the cancer there was no chance it would happen. The child was also offered the opportunity, which he declined, to talk to a genetic counselor, who was described as "someone who knows a lot about that kind of cancer and how it affects families."

Following the therapist's explanation, there was a dramatic cessation of eye rubbing and an improvement in school performance that included an end to statements that his eyes hurt and that he couldn't read. In therapy the boy demonstrated greatly reduced anxiety concerning himself. However, he remained concerned about his three-year-old sister who, he recognized, was still within the age range for onset of retinoblastoma.

As with the previous example of siblings of children with Down syndrome, this unconscious dynamic emerged in the course of ongoing child therapy. However, the connection between a mother who was blind as a result of retinoblastoma and a child's compulsive eye rubbing and complaints of hurting eyes and inability to read might reasonably have been inferred and explored in the course of genetic counseling. Alternatively, had the relevant factual issues been discussed in genetic counseling with the child at an earlier time, his anxiety, fear, and misunderstanding might have been reduced or avoided. This example also illustrates that, as with adults, a straightforward, authoritative explanation may provide a child with substantial and immediate relief.

Finally, fetal loss may also affect children through grief and sadness over the death of an anticipated sibling and through the emotional impact on the parents (Green, 1992).

The Family Context

For the child even more than the adult, the family provides the context of life and is thus essential to understanding and addressing the child's situation and needs (Chethik, 1989). The infant and young child's physical, emotional, and developmental needs are almost entirely met by the immediate family and any other immediate caretakers. Social interactions and resources for fulfilling needs broaden as the child grows. However, for most children the family remains central at least into adolescence. Furthermore, as the child moves from the family into widening social circles, the interactions among family members must meet the competing demands of holding on versus letting go and of stabilizing continuity versus flexible adaptation. Thus, the family is also intensely and immediately involved in the child's movements out of and away from it.

For the child who confronts issues related to genetic counseling, the manner in which the parents and other family members respond to the situation has a profound impact on how the child is affected. Furthermore, the child's ability to understand the situation and handle the emotional consequences will be greatly affected by the family's strengths and weaknesses in this regard. Familial behaviors include the ways in which emotional issues and stressors are processed within the family and the extent to which the child is included in age-appropriate discussions of what is taking place (Hobbs et al., 1985; Rolland, 1994). Thus, in working with children, the counselor should draw as much as possible on the family's strengths, coping mechanisms, ways of dealing with emotional issues, and beliefs and values, and parents or other central family members should be included in the work.

Psychosocial Development and Functioning

The child's life course from infancy to adolescence involves dramatic growth and development in all areas, therefore an understanding of the processes by which this growth occurs is as important as knowledge of specific stages and capabilities. At any given time the child will have certain capabilities for cognitive understanding; control of emotions and behavior; ability to maintain a sense of integrated self in the face of physical, emotional, and social stressors; and ability to interact in functional and socially acceptable ways with others (Bukatko & Daehler, 1992; Greenspan, 1991).

However, the situation is highly dynamic. The toddler who one minute courageously explores the outer reaches of the room and the next minute returns to the comfort and reassurance of being next to mother, and the child who on one day meets the challenges of school with eager anticipation and the next day pleads to stay home both illustrate normal fluctuations in capabilities, functioning, and sense of self. Serious stressors such as illness, major medical interventions, hospitalization, parental disability, anxiety, or depression may lead to more sustained "regression" in functioning (Kaslow, 1986). The extent to which the developmental challenges of previous stages of psychosocial development have been successfully achieved and psychosocial conflicts resolved has much to do with the strengths and weaknesses the child brings to subsequent stages, and these processes can be very significantly affected by illness or disability (Garrison & McQuiston, 1989; O'Dougherty, 1983). Thus, the effectiveness of parents, family, and the larger social environment in providing a stable structure that also supports growth through trial and error will affect both the child's current level of functioning and his or her potential for further growth. Finally, as with family development, the changes involved do not occur in a uniform, quantitative manner. Instead, periods of relative stability and consolidation are interspersed with periods of relatively rapid development in which there are qualitative changes in capabilities.

Three aspects of the young child's cognitive process are particularly relevant to genetic counseling. First, the child's view is egocentric. It is difficult for the child to perceive the world other than from the perspective of his or her own perceptions, beliefs, and experiences. Thus, alternate points of view involving either the perceptions of others or alternative explanations for situations are relatively difficult for the child to understand or perceive. In addition, the child sees itself as a central figure in the workings of the universe. This can result in unrealistic beliefs concerning the effect of the child's thoughts or actions on subsequent events. Second, the child's thinking is relatively concrete. Attempts to understand situations and apply reasoning depend in substantial part on having the objects or circumstances immediately available, either physically or in the form of specific mental images. Abstract thinking is difficult. Thus words, explanations, and causal relationships may be understood in terms of their surface or literal meanings or relationships (Bukatko & Daehler, 1992). Third, the child has a limited ability to distinguish internal psychological states and processes such as thoughts, wishes, and emotions from the external world and "reality" as perceived by others (Chethik, 1989). Thus, wishes, beliefs, and fantasies may be experienced as objective reality or as having the power to influence events in the external world.

These cognitive limitations play a significant role in children's misunderstanding of causal relationships and in their tendency to feel a sense of responsibility and guilt for adverse events (O'Dougherty, 1983). For example, an affected boy may believe that a hospitalization is punishment for angry feelings toward a healthy sister. Conversely, the sister may feel guilt and remorse due to a belief that her angry thoughts toward her brother caused the medical setback or emergency. To expand on the latter example, her egocentricity leads her to believe that the medical crisis is her fault. Her inability to adequately distinguish internal from external processes leads to a belief that her thoughts had a direct effect on the child's health. And her concrete thinking precludes understanding more complex explanations when these are offered.

These cognitive limitations are not absolute. Even young children have some capabilities in these respects, and they increase greatly with cognitive development. However, these limitations are significant into adolescence (Bukatko & Daehler, 1992) and, indeed, into adulthood (see Chapter 1 under Psychological Defenses and Guilt and Shame). Thus, it is important not to underestimate their significance when working with children. The assessment of these cognitive limitations can be a particular problem with children who have well-developed verbal or social abilities, since these abilities may suggest a level of cognitive functioning higher than is actually the case. Therefore, when working with children, it is important to use language and explanations that are clear and appropriate to the child's level of understanding; to check frequently on what the child has understood; and, insofar as possible, to determine the child's beliefs and perceptions so these may be addressed.

The child's understanding of the concept of death provides a pertinent example of cognitive development. A broad outline of children's concepts of death, with approximate ages, follows (Spinetta, 1980): Children under the age of about two years do not understand death as a concept or event. Between the ages of approximately three and five children begin to understand death in terms of something that happens to others and has a relationship to sleep and lack of motion, but they do not understand its permanence. At this age interest and questions concerning dead animals and plants are common and illustrate the manner in which children actively seek to understand the world through observation, direct involvement, and questioning of adults. From about age six there is a growing awareness that death is permanent and will affect those whom the child knows and the child herself. However, only with the acquisition of more complex knowledge and analytic abilities in adolescence does a full understanding develop that death is permanent and affects all living organisms. The process of learning about death is acquired through many incremental steps in knowledge and understanding, yet it also involves qualitative shifts in perception and comprehension. There is also much individual variation in the process, which is affected in part by intellectual ability and experience. Thus, discussions about or explanations of death, as with other topics, must take into account both the child's knowledge and experience and his or her cognitive ability to understand the relevant concepts. There are comparable developmental paths in myriad areas including the understanding of the body and of illness (Garrison & McQuiston, 1989; O'Dougherty, 1983).

When faced with emotional distress from either external events or internal states such as anger or depression, children do not in general tend to verbalize their feelings directly or analyze either the cause or the nature of their distress (Kalter, 1990). Individual responses vary tremendously from child to child and, to a lesser extent, from situation to situation. However, children's verbal responses tend to involve denial that anything is wrong. This denial is often coupled with social and emotional withdrawal, an externalization of blame for the problem, and/or overt behaviors that discharge the emotion and serve as a defense against the psychological pain. Thus, for example, a child who feels angry toward an affected sibling because of a perceived imbalance in parental attention may become socially withdrawn; tease, taunt, or pick fights with the affected child; or have behavioral or academic problems at school. If questioned directly about social withdrawal, if it occurs, the child will very possibly be unable to either explain the underlying cause or describe in any detail his or her emotional state. If questioned directly about the teasing, taunting, or school problems, the child is likely to respond by blaming the sibling or peers, with limited understanding or acceptance of responsibility for the interactions. If adult or peer responses are angry, blaming, or retributive, and if there is no help in adjusting the direction in which the child's mood or behavior is evolving, a cycle may be established in which the child feels increasingly upset, misunderstood, and isolated and in which the problematic behaviors increase.

Given children's limited ability to analyze or verbalize emotional distress and its consequences, thoughtful, empathic, and age-appropriate adult responses to a child's moods and behaviors or in response to known stressors may be very helpful. Validating and addressing the child's emotions and helping the child sort out their origins may reduce the child's sense of isolation, confusion, and being misunderstood and help the child develop a better understanding of and vocabulary for the complex nature of moods and emotional states (Chethik, 1989; Kalter, 1990). As an example, for the young child who is in a funk, the simple question "Are you mad or sad?" may help develop a more articulate understanding of what had been experienced up until that time as only a global sense of being out of sorts. Adult responses that help the child feel understood and accepted, less isolated, and better able to understand his or her own situation may also result in a reduction of unproductive or socially problematic behaviors by helping the child learn to react constructively to the normal vicissitudes of life. Empathic responses are an important component of day-to-day parenting and of the responses of other adults such as caretakers and teachers. Such responses also provide the basic guidelines for adult interventions around acute stressors such as those relevant to genetic counseling.

Children's perceptions of and responses to the world tend to be action and process oriented rather than verbal and analytic. In general, children are very attuned to nonverbal communication and cues and to the mood and implicit meanings of human interactions. Thus, on the one hand, an adult's comments or reassurances that are at odds with his or her actual emotions or nonverbal communications are often discounted or seen through. Conversely, honest concern, empathy, acceptance, and physical responsiveness, such as a hug, can go a long way with a child, even when the adult is unsure how to address an issue verbally.

When a child is present in a genetic counseling session, even if apparently preoccupied by play or other activities, he or she is in all probability very attuned to the proceedings. Even if the child understands relatively little of what is said, much is absorbed about the parents' emotions and about the quality of the parents' interactions with the genetic counselor. If approached by the genetic counselor, the child's responses will depend in substantial part on what he or she has perceived about the genetic counselor and the parents' responses to her. Similarly, through their attention and sensitivity to the emotions and nonverbal communication of adults, children who are seriously or fatally ill are usually aware of the gravity of their situation even when their parents and other adults attempt to "protect" them from the difficult truth (Spinetta, 1980).

Play is a natural activity of childhood that has a central role in psychosocial development. Play combines fantasy and reality, both of which are partly under the child's control and partly outside it (a crashed toy truck may actually break; an angry comment to a doll may induce feelings of guilt or fear of retribution). Through play children learn to imitate and understand elements of the adult world, try out new roles and ways of acting, express their fears and fantasies in a manner that allows some control, and deal with fears and fantasies by assuming roles of power, omnipotence, and bravado that they cannot have in the "real" world. Children's play reveals much about their concerns, fears, emotional state, defenses, and coping mechanisms (Chethik, 1989).

Techniques for Genetic Counseling with Children

For both ethical and therapeutic reasons, genetic counseling with children must be carried out with the permission and participation of the parent or parents. In some instances, issues concerning the adaptation and well-being of children will have been brought up by the parents during an intake phone call or in the session. If the parents do not do so, the genetic counselor may, at an appropriate time, bring up the possibility and potential value of interacting directly with the child. Two ways of requesting parental permission follow:

> *Genetic Counselor (on the telephone):* You've said that your son Bill will be coming with you. In my experience, children are very attentive to what the adults talk about when I meet with their parents, and they often have questions and concerns too. With other families it has been helpful for me to talk to the child, and I could do that with Bill. If you are agreeable, we can keep that as an option.

> *Genetic Counselor (to the parents in the session):* I can see that Jill has been paying attention to what we've been talking about, and I know you've had concerns about how this is affecting her. Based on my experience working with other families, it might be helpful for us to take a few minutes for me to talk to her directly. Would you be comfortable with my giving that a try?

Some parents will accept the offer with little or no further discussion. Others, including some who are aware of the potential value of communicating with the child, will have doubts or concerns. These may arise because the parents are not comfortable discussing the issues with the child, are concerned that discussing them will make the child more anxious or fearful, or have had emotionally difficult experiences attempting to discuss the issues with the child. Unless the parents' response is strongly opposed, the genetic counselor can provide a brief further explanation of the potential value of working with the child. However, it is critical to abide by the parents' wishes and beliefs. Failure to do so will undermine their confidence in the genetic counselor and, if the counselor speaks to the child anyway, may set up a difficult dynamic between parents and child. Even when parents do not accept the offer, the counselor's explanation may lead to a change in the parents' attitude in subsequent sessions, with other professionals or in their approach to the child.

> *Genetic Counselor:* I understand your concern about my discussing this with your son. However, children are very perceptive about their parents' moods and interactions. If he has questions or concerns that don't get discussed, his fears and fantasies could be worse than they would be if he had some adult help in understanding what is going on.

As discussed in the preceding section, children are often highly attuned to what is occurring in the session and this responsiveness provides a potential opening for the genetic counselor. However, even when they have pressing questions and concerns or strong emotions, children may be reluctant to talk to the genetic counselor because they are uncomfortable or frightened about talking to an unfamiliar person. There are the difficulties and inhibitions involved in verbalizing concerns and addressing fears and behaviors that were discussed in the previous section. In addition, anxiety, boredom, or cognitive and behavioral limitations resulting from the genetic disorder may make it difficult for the child to turn his or her attention to a discussion with the genetic counselor.

Several techniques may be used to overcome these barriers. To begin with, it is important that the child perceive that the parents support an interaction with the genetic counselor. Involving the parents, even if briefly, will help convey this message. Furthermore, the parents may assist in bringing the child's attention to the counselor.

> *Genetic Counselor (to parent):* Why don't you ask him to come over and sit by us now.

The counselor should approach the child in an open, empathic manner while gently initiating a discussion of the issues.

> *Genetic Counselor (to a six-year-old child):* I can see that you've been listening to what the grown-ups were talking about. We've been using some pretty big words, and I bet you wonder what some of them mean.

It is often helpful to have one or a few simple, age-appropriate toys. Examples include but are by no means limited to: a small soft ball; small cars, trucks, ambulance, or fire engine; a doll, with or without a baby bottle; a set of family dolls of appropriate ethnicity including a father, mother, boy, girl, and infant; or a simple set of Legos including wheels. These can be used initially to engage the child's interest and attention. As the interaction proceeds, play can be interspersed with talk to limit the emotional impact of what is being discussed. At times, the toys and play may be used to express or work out emotions. For example, while talking about anxiety concerning a forthcoming medical procedure, a child might crash one vehicle into another. This could provide an opportunity for the genetic counselor to comment that the child is angry as well as afraid, thereby facilitating acknowledgment and expression of an emotion that the child had not felt it was safe to express.

It is important to meet the child at his or her level, both literally and figuratively. Thus, in addition to using age-appropriate language and concepts, it is helpful to be physically at the child's level. If the child is playing on the floor, one can squat or kneel to make the initial contact. Leaning forward in a chair, without getting unduly close, also brings the genetic counselor to the child's level. Working on the floor can be very effective. It allows freer play with toys, and it overtly moves the arena of interaction to the child's level and away from the adult sphere. If it is inappropriate or unappealing to work directly on the floor of the counseling or examination room, a small rug may be unrolled for the purpose.

One method for engaging a child in a discussion of difficult material is to make reference to a hypothetical other child.

> *Genetic Counselor:* I knew another boy who had a sister with Down syndrome and he told me . . .

Children are often intrigued by reference to another child in similar circumstances and will listen intently to the genetic counselor's description of that child's feelings or behavior. Not infrequently, the child asks questions that seek further identification with the hypothetical child or a better understanding of his or her circumstances and relationship to the counselor: "What was her name?" "Was he my age?" "How many times did you see her?" "Did his sister have to go to the hospital too?"

Another technique is to engage the child in a guessing game concerning the counselor's knowledge and understanding.

Genetic Counselor: I've worked with other children who had to go to the hospital for tests, and I've learned a lot about how they feel. Let me guess how you feel about different parts of it, and you tell me if I'm right or wrong. First, I bet that sometimes you feel really mad at your parents because all this is happening. Am I right or wrong?

Children enjoy the game-like give and take of this approach and the fact that the genetic counselor seeks their input in order to better understand them and their situation. At the same time, the child's awareness of the genetic counselor's empathic understanding or attempt to understand develops in a step-wise manner. If the initial questions are on the mark and the child acknowledges them as correct, it is useful to add some questions in which the counselor is incorrect. This avoids the appearance of omniscience, "magical" reading of the child's mind, or a fake game in which the counselor doesn't really need the child's answers.

These methods are examples of "displacement techniques," which use indirect and/or nonverbal communication to help a child address emotionally charged issues that it would be difficult or impossible to discuss directly (Kalter, 1990). There are a variety of other such techniques, and many approaches use a combination of two or more. Among those that may be adapted to the genetic counseling situation are drawing, telling a story made up by the genetic counselor or by the counselor and child together, and the use of hand puppets for spontaneous interactions or putting on "plays." In addition, toys may be chosen for their relevance to the issues that need to be addressed. For example, toy doctor's equipment or toy doll figures and hospital furniture may be used with a child who faces medical interventions or hospitalization.

The following example illustrates the possible use of drawing with a five-year-old girl who, the genetic counselor suspects, is afraid that she will "catch" phenylketonuria, by contagion, from an affected brother.

The genetic counselor asks the child to draw a picture of herself and her brother. The counselor then asks her to draw her brother with a cold. If the child is uncertain how to do this, the genetic counselor suggests making the brother's nose red. The counselor then asks her to draw "germs" showing how she could catch a cold from her brother. These might be represented by brown dots drawn between the two figures. The genetic counselor then says, "Another girl I talked to was worried that she would catch PKU from her brother, just like a cold. Have you ever worried about that?" If the girl says yes, the counselor asks her to draw how this could happen, suggesting a different color than brown for the PKU "germs." If the child says no, the counselor draws in a few "germs" in a different color saying, "This is what the other girl thought could happen." After a pause the counselor adds firmly, "But it can't," simultaneously blacking out each of the PKU "germs." With either outcome, the genetic counselor then provides a more extended explanation, as discussed later.

Children frequently respond positively when asked if they like to draw or to the suggestion to make a drawing. However, some older children are self-conscious about their drawing ability and need encouragement or a statement that the genetic counselor is pleased with their effort. Drawing engages the child's attention and may help sustain or deepen the interaction. The process of drawing and the resulting pictures may evoke and illustrate both emotions and information. For example, the child might draw her brother much larger than herself, depicting her feeling that he gets most of the parental attention and she is less significant. The counselor can then comment on and explore this. By referring to the drawing, emotions can be discussed without the need to confront them directly. The drawings may also reveal important aspects of the child's understanding or beliefs. For example, the child might draw the PKU "germs" larger than the cold germs and with heads and legs, thus revealing a fear of their potency and virulence. Finally, the genetic counselor may add to the child's drawing or make one of her own to add emphasis (e.g., blacking out the PKU "germs") or to supplement a verbal explanation.

Factual information should be provided with age-appropriate explanations that draw on the child's experience and use concepts and terminology with which he or she is familiar. Children may deny a concern or fear even though deeply troubled by it. Thus the genetic counselor must use her experience, judgment, and information from the parents in deciding whether to address an issue. When a child has denied concern but seems likely to be troubled by it, a brief discussion may be introduced by saying, "Well, just in case you ever wondered about that, . . ."

The following examples illustrate explanations that might be used with children of ages five, eight, and twelve years, respectively, to address a concern about "catching" phenylketonuria from an affected sibling:

Five-year old: When your brother gets a cold, you can catch it from him. Your mom and dad have told you about that and how to help keep it from happening. Maybe you think it can happen with PKU too. Well, it can't. PKU isn't caused by germs. You can't catch PKU from your brother, and your mom and dad can't either. Nobody ever caught PKU from somebody else.

Eight-year old: Some diseases like colds are caused by germs and you can catch them from other people. Maybe you've wondered if you can catch PKU from your brother. That's a smart question. Doctors wondered about that too, and a long time ago they found out that you can't. Your brother's PKU is caused by something in his body that doesn't work the same as in other people. It isn't caused by germs. You can't catch it from him and neither can anyone else. Nobody ever caught PKU from somebody else.

Twelve-year old: Maybe you've wondered if you can catch PKU from your brother, the way you can catch a cold from him. Well, you can't. Colds are caused by germs, and you can get his cold germs from him. But PKU is very different. You know how your body turns the chemicals in food into muscle and bones and blood to make your body grow. Well, your brother's body can't use one of the chemicals in the food he eats. Instead it turns it into something bad that makes him sick. That's what PHEs [a measure of phenylalanine content] are, they measure how much of that chemical he is eating. His body has been that way since he was born. PKU isn't caused by germs. You can't catch PKU from him and neither can anyone else. Nobody ever caught PKU from somebody else.

The genetic counselor's explanation may repeat, expand on, or complement explanations that the parents have given the child. It is helpful to determine what explanations parents have provided the child, if the child has had other sources of information, and if there are areas in which the parents would like assistance clarifying the child's understanding. It may be useful to include the parents in the discussion. This adds the genetic counselor's authority and clarity to the parents' explanation and demonstrates that the adults are in agreement with regard to factual information and the importance of helping the child understand the situation.

As is the case with adults, children also benefit from the opportunity to express their emotions, to clarify their feelings, and to receive support and reassurance concerning the validity and normality of what they are experiencing. These experiences help reduce the child's sense of isolation and of being different, and they may help reduce feelings of guilt and responsibility (Kalter, 1990). Direct conversation and the displacement techniques discussed earlier may be used to elicit and clarify the child's emotions. Whenever appropriate, the genetic counselor should reassure the child that what he or she is feeling is normal:

It's normal to feel that you want to help and protect your sister, but you also want to have your own life with your friends. Lots of kids I've worked with feel that way.

It's normal to be scared before you go into the hospital, especially when you don't know exactly what's going to happen.

I know another boy with muscular dystrophy, and he told me he gets really mad and sad when he can't play the games his friends play.

The child's initial expression or acknowledgment of emotions opens further opportunities for the genetic counselor to provide support, clarification, and practical suggestions; to elicit further emotions; and to engage the parents in the interaction. Thus, each of the situations just described might be pursued further in the following ways:

Genetic Counselor (taking out a drawing pad and marking pens): Can you draw me a picture of how it feels to be pulled in two directions, wanting to help your sister and wanting to play with your friends?

Siblings of children with Down syndrome draw poignant illustrations of how this feels. These drawings help clarify and validate the child's feelings. They may enlighten even the most perceptive and concerned parents and lead to a discussion of how to better handle the conflicting responsibilities and emotions that the child feels.

Genetic Counselor: When the doctor comes in, we'll ask him to explain as much as he can about what will happen in the hospital. Then you and your parents can talk about ways to help you get ready for each part and how they can help you feel less scared. I've got some ideas that might help too.

Genetic Counselor: I'm sorry you can't do all the things your friends can do. And I know your mom and dad are very sorry too. If you told them how mad you get, then I bet it would be easier to also talk about how sad you get.

Children's feelings of guilt and their beliefs concerning responsibility for events may be carefully hidden from adults and difficult to elicit under the short-term interactions of genetic counseling (Buckman, 1992; Seligman & Darling, 1989). However, the child's mood, such as sadness or withdrawal, parental observations, and the genetic counselor's knowledge and experience provide sources of information about the mistaken beliefs that a child may have. A direct question from the genetic counselor may elicit a denial and create a defensive mind set. It is often more effective to draw reasonable inferences and present the material indirectly.

Genetic Counselor: Some children think that because they were angry at their brother it caused him to get more sick with CF. But it doesn't work that way at all. He got sicker because of changes that are happening in his body. Maybe you feel bad now that you got angry at him. That's normal. But that isn't what made him get sick.

Interventions such as this will not eliminate deep or long-standing feelings of guilt and responsibility. However, they contribute to an ongoing process of support and education by parents and other adults that may help to alleviate such feelings and beliefs.

When more than one child is present, the techniques that have been presented may also be used, although the situation is likely to be more complex. More time will be required, interactions among the children may make it hard to keep a given child's attention focused, and the parents' need to attend to one child may reduce their ability to participate in the discussion or help maintain the attention of another child. When it seems appropriate, these problems may be overcome by asking one parent and child to stay with the genetic counselor while the other parent and children leave. Alternatively, the counselor may schedule an additional session structured to meet the needs of working with one or more child.

The counseling of children with severe disabilities and serious, progressive or fatal illness lies beyond the scope of this discussion. However, the same psychological principles are relevant and may be applied when the genetic counselor has interactions with severely affected children and their families (Spinetta, 1980). Because of their sensitivity to the moods, interactions, and nonverbal communication of adults, children become aware of the gravity of their situation, even when adults attempt to withhold relevant information. Effective communication helps alleviate the child's sense of isolation and fear and allows adults to provide more effective support and appropriate reassurance. In addition, open communication helps reduce self-blame and a sense of being punished for the illness or disability and for medical treatments or other interventions. Because of the central role of the family in the child's life and care, it is essential to attempt to understand the coping mechanisms and the philosophical or religious framework within which the family attempts to make sense of and adapt to the child's situation. Families differ greatly in their ability to communicate openly and effectively, under such circumstances. Thus, the family's ability to do so and the time required for this to take place must be respected.

When there is evidence that a child is experiencing sustained emotional distress, behavioral problems, or social isolation, a referral for counseling is appropriate. Child counseling or therapy must involve the parent or parents and may include other relevant family members. When the child's problems are grounded in family dysfunction or the impact of disease or disability on the family, family therapy may be the most appropriate primary approach or serve a vital adjunct function. Knowledge of the available counseling personnel and resources and of professionals who can provide consultation is important in providing appropriate mental health referrals.

Countertransference in Genetic Counseling with Children

In working with children, the genetic counselor confronts their hopes and fears, anxieties and fantasies, misunderstandings and self-blame, and the impact of disease or disability on their lives. This experience may raise new counter-transference issues or intensify some of those elicited when working with adults (Chethik, 1989; Spinetta, 1980). Certain stages of development may have heightened emotional significance for the genetic counselor, based on her own life experience or that of her siblings or children. This reaction may result in increased sensitivity to the psychosocial tasks of these developmental stages and to the pain, anger, and frustration that arise when development is inhibited. Certain types of abilities or accomplishments may also be of particular personal significance, increasing the emotional impact of some physical or cognitive disabilities as well as specific psychosocial constraints encountered by both affected and unaffected children. Confronting the child's emotions and perceptions in addition to those of the parents may heighten the poignancy of the parents' grief, sadness, or anger.

Inherent aspects of working with children also produce countertransference reactions. Children's communication may be unclear, confusing, or contradictory, raising anxiety on the genetic counselor's part about her ability to work effectively. Children's fears and fantasies may be frightening in their intensity, in their effects on the child, or in the child's view of the world, which they reveal. Behavior that is antisocial, destructive, hyperactive, or withdrawn is difficult to deal with, even when there is compassionate understanding of its origins, and such behavior may evoke strong emotions. Seriously incompetent or abusive parental behavior may be encountered, which raises strong emotions that are enhanced by direct involvement with the child. Such behavior may require social or legal interventions that include reporting child abuse, and these actions can induce intense countertransference. In addition to their inherent aspects, any of the dynamics just discussed may resonate strongly with the genetic counselor's experiences as a child or a parent.

Feelings of sadness, hopelessness, confusion, and anger, and fantasies of protecting or rescuing the child are common countertransference reactions when working with children. These emotions may interfere with the genetic counselor's objectivity or effectiveness or with her own emotional well-being. They may also provide useful sensitivity and insight. For example, the counselor's feelings of confusion and anger in working with a child may help her better understand the parents' emotions and responses to the child and his or her situation. This, in turn, may clarify a deficit in communication between parent and child that can then be addressed.

As in work with adults, consultation and personal counseling or psychotherapy are important resources in dealing with countertransference issues.

Genetic Counseling with Adolescents

Adolescents are directly involved in genetic counseling concerning reproductive issues and when they are affected by a genetic disorder or birth defect. They may be included when another family member is affected by virtue of their ability to participate at the adult cognitive and verbal level in which genetic counseling is ordinarily conducted. However, their cognitive, verbal, and emotional level of development differs from that of adults, as do their psychosocial concerns. Thus, an understanding of adolescent processes and issues facilitates effective genetic counseling with adolescents (Peters-Brown & Fry-Mehltretter, 1996).

Adolescence encompasses the period between the onset of puberty, with the physical, hormonal, and neurological changes it involves, and the establishment of young adult status and autonomy. The age of onset, which is primarily determined biologically, varies substantially in both sexes, although on average it is earlier in girls than in boys. The end of adolescence is defined to a large extent by economic, social, and cultural factors. In some cultures, and for some individuals in many cultures, there is a relatively brief transition from childhood to the responsibilities of adulthood. By contrast, in the United States and other highly economically developed societies, many individuals experience a prolonged period of adolescence due to social and economic factors that include an extended period of education, limited opportunities in the adult work world, and adolescent-oriented recreation and consumption (Johnson, 1989; Sahler & Kreipe, 1991).

Stages of Adolescent Development

Between childhood, with its nearly complete dependence on family and other adults, and adulthood, with its relative independence and multitude of social interactions, adolescence involves changes that profoundly affect the individual and his or her family. The physical, hormonal, emotional, cognitive, and social development that occurs during adolescence alters the individual's perceptions of self, autonomy with respect to parents and family, relationships with peers, and interactions with and expectations of the broader social order. The personal and social changes of adolescence are often conceptualized as "developmental tasks." This term implies that these changes involve challenges that, when adequately negotiated, lead to a relatively well functioning early adulthood and establish the basis for further effective development over the life cycle. Conversely, inadequate resolution of one or more tasks may contribute to problems or deficits at the individual and/or social levels during adolescence and beyond. None of these developments is unique to adolescence. Instead, it is their rapid rate of change and degree of interrelatedness that characterize adolescence (Peters-Brown & Fry-Mehltretter, 1996; Preto, 1989).

The developmental tasks may be grouped into several broad categories:

Developing a sense of self-identity. Physical and cognitive changes are accompanied by a new sense of self, as well as by changes in how one is perceived by others. Sexual development has a major role, leading to an expanded sense of sexual identity. An important aspect of self-identity is body image, which includes the individual's self-perceptions regarding his or her physical and sexual attractiveness and blemishes, physical abilities and limitations, and body integrity and right to privacy. Other developing physical, cognitive, emotional, and social attributes must also be incorporated into the sense of self. The process includes a more mature sense of mastery and creativity and of ideals and values that form a basis for judging oneself, other individuals, and society. The establishment of positive self-identity is grounded in increased physical and cognitive abilities, facilitated by the guidance, support, and respect of others. This process can be a source of newfound excitement, energy, and a sense of self-esteem. However, it may also create conflict for the adolescent and his or her family. If inadequately negotiated or supported, it may lead to anxiety, disappointment, and a sense of failure.

Establishing autonomy from family and other adults. Physical, emotional, and economic separation from the family of origin is a major aspect of the adolescent transition. Separation is facilitated by a flexible family structure that adapts to the adolescent's growing independence and autonomy. A high degree of enmeshment or disengagement, triangles involving the adolescent, and rigidity during times of structural change may all impede the development of autonomy. The child's transition into adolescence affects all relationships within the family, including the parents' relationship as they adapt to this new stage in family life, which may include stresses or disagreements involved in establishing expectations and limits for adolescent behavior. Sibling relationships with parents and the adolescent are also affected, as the siblings respond to their brother's or sister's increasing autonomy (Preto, 1989; Trad, 1993).

These changes often coincide with the parents' transition into midadulthood, which may involve reevaluation of work, life goals, and the marital relationship. In the same period, grandparents may enter later life, with the associated issues of retirement, declining health, and possible increased dependence on the parents. Thus, the adolescent's increasing autonomy parallels other major family changes. It may evoke strong emotions in family members related to change, loss, feelings of abandonment, and the need to reevaluate life goals at a time when these emotions are also heightened by the other family transitions (Preto, 1989). For example, a parent may resist the adolescent's desire for autonomy in an attempt to maintain a close relationship that has helped defend against issues of intimacy with the other parent. In a more general example, if a parent has unresolved issues concerning independence and autonomy, these may be revived by the adolescent's demands and behavior just as the parent is reevaluating life goals and relationships. Thus, a developmental task that was not fully completed during the parent's adolescence affects the comparable family transition one generation later.

Developing appropriate relationships with peers of both sexes. As dependence on the family declines, relationships with peers assume increasing importance. Peers provide companionship, emotional support, and the opportunity to develop and pursue mutual interests. With peers, adolescents can try out new ways of behaving and relating to others and develop new attitudes and values toward the larger society. Peers can provide a critical sense of belonging during a time of great individual change and uncertainty. However, pressure to conform to the values, behavior, and appearance of the group can be intense. Thus, failure to conform, if perceived by either the adolescent or members of the peer group, can lead to intense feelings of rejection, loneliness, isolation, failure, and low self-esteem (Sahler & Kreipe, 1991). In addition, opportunities and social expectations experienced with peers can lead to illegal activities and substance abuse (Emler, 1993).

Peer interactions have a significant role in establishing a sense of sexual identity, and they create impetus and opportunities for developing sexual relationships. Here, too, peer values, expectations, and behaviors may have a facilitating and/or a troubling impact. They may lead to intimate relationships that are sources of support, growth, and self-esteem. However, they may also contribute to sexual exploitation and abuse and to the risk or reality of unintended pregnancy and sexually transmitted diseases including AIDS. Indicative of the interrelationship between the various developmental tasks, these risks are a common source of conflict with parents over issues of autonomy (Kirchler et al., 1993; Preto, 1989).

Establishing a basis for economic independence. This involves identifying career or job goals and developing the necessary knowledge base, skills, and work habits. Entry into the work world supports economic independence and thus autonomy. It may also have a critically important role in developing a sense of productivity, self-esteem, and competence in the social and societal domains (Sahler & Kreipe, 1991).

Establishing a sense of involvement, investment and values concerning the larger society. This involves an understanding and acceptance of social expectations and norms and the development of adequate behavioral constraints against impulsive, emotion-driven, or peer-driven behaviors that are socially unacceptable or harmful. A more solid foundation for these capabilities lies with the acquisition of a set of values and beliefs that supports productive involvement in the larger society (Emler, 1993).

The adolescent's capabilities and the developmental tasks that he or she faces change throughout the transition from childhood to early adulthood. Early adolescence is partly defined by the visible physical changes initiated at the onset of puberty. These are accompanied by increased self-awareness and by a concern for how the individual's physical appearance and abilities compare to those of peers and societal norms. Discrepancies, both real and imagined, can lead to intense feelings of shame and low self-esteem. Increased involvement in formal and informal peer groups promotes autonomy from the family. Peer interactions often place much emphasis on conformity in appearance and behavior. When the adolescent finds acceptance among peers, feelings of physical and social competence are enhanced, identity development is promoted, and concerns with appearance and "fitting in" may be reduced. However, complete or partial exclusion from peer groups, and the comparisons and teasing that occur within them, may contribute to feelings of incompetence, shame, and low self-esteem. Cognitively, the early adolescent retains the relatively concrete, present-oriented, egocentric thinking of childhood. The sense of self as a central figure in the universe contributes to the acute concern that presumed differences or blemishes are apparent and of interest to everyone. At the same time, the early adolescent has difficulty with abstract approaches to understanding the world (Johnson, 1989; Sahler & Kreipe, 1991).

Middle adolescence is marked by an increase in sexuality, both physiologically and emotionally. Concerns with peer acceptance and peer definitions of social norms remain strong, but they are now more focused on the multiple stages of exploring and establishing emotional and physical relationships with sexual-romantic partners. Issues of physical and social attractiveness continue to be important to the development of self-identity, which now more overtly includes sexual identity. Relationships between the adolescent and his or her parents assume a new level of complexity. Potential or explicit sexual attraction involving the opposite sex parent must be accommodated in some manner, which often involves defensive anger, hostility, and emotional distancing. The same-sex parent's standing as a role model often declines as the adolescent increasingly identifies with the peer culture, leading to a more competitive, overtly conflicted relationship. Parental concerns about the adolescent's sexual activities and unresolved sexual issues on the part of the parent may increase the level of discord during this period. With maturing cognitive abilities, the midadolescent begins to perceive larger patterns of interactions and beliefs. However, still limited by concreteness, this perception may result in relatively rigid adherence to newly found beliefs and rejection of parental values. Despite the tensions of this period, the underlying dynamics support the adolescent's transition from primary affiliations within the family to affiliations with peers and adults in the larger world (Preto, 1989; Sahler & Kreipe, 1991).

In late adolescence, issues of integration into the broader social order predominate. Abstract thinking is more fully developed, as is the ability to contemplate and plan for the future. Vocational choice and preparation for or entry into the workplace promote economic and social independence. With job training and experience, an increased ability for abstract thought, and a decline in behaviors that are driven by the need to assert autonomy, the late adolescent can develop a more balanced view of his or her strengths and weaknesses as they relate to the realities of the workplace. Establishing a vocational or professional identity, with attendant responsibilities and rewards, is an important part of overall identity formation. In this same period, other commitments to community and values also develop. With autonomy more firmly established, there is often a softening of attitudes toward parents and reintegration into the family on a basis more consistent with early adult status. All of these steps also contribute to the basis for establishing a long-term emotional commitment to a sexual partner (Johnson, 1989; Trad, 1993).

The Impact of Genetic Diseases and Birth Defects on Adolescents

Genetic disorders and birth defects may affect any of the interrelated developmental processes just discussed. In many instances, the disorder was present at birth or began in childhood. When this is the case, accommodations and coping mechanisms developed during childhood will provide some guidance in meeting the new developmental tasks of adolescence. In other instances, such as type I diabetes, onset may occur in adolescence. In these situations the individual and his or her family experience the early stages of grief, coping, and adaptation at the same time as they meet the new issues that arise in adolescence. However, even when a disorder has been present since childhood, its effects on the individual's life may change with entry into adolescence. For example, physical or cognitive impairments that were reasonably well accepted by childhood peers may present a much greater barrier to adolescent peer interactions, with their emphasis on conformity and on romantic and sexual relationships (Ablon, 1984; Driscoll, 1986).

Visible physical abnormalities and neurological deficits that affect gait, balance, coordination, and other aspects of physical ability may interfere with development of a positive body image or lead to a negative sense of body attractiveness and capabilities. Even when the effects of a disorder are not apparent to others, invasive medical procedures and their sequelae can significantly affect the development of body image. Based on a broad in-depth study,

Seiffge-Krenke (1998, p. 167) states, "Despite [their] good health status, diabetic adolescents showed a more negative body image [than controls]. For example, in the semi-structured interviews, nearly all afflicted adolescents displayed evidence of marked problems in accepting their bodies. Many diabetics also said that they perceived a strong threat to physical identity, caused by the daily self-injury of injections and the related lesions, hardenings, and bruises."

Peer interactions, romantic relationships, and sexual experience are all potentially affected by genetic disorders and birth defects. As discussed previously, visible physical abnormalities or limitations as well as neurological, cognitive, and behavioral deficits may reduce peer acceptance. Special education classes may limit the range of peers who are available as potential friends. School absences due to illness, medical procedures, or hospitalization can constrict the adolescent's sense of membership in the peer community and of keeping up with the activities and opportunities for intellectual and social development in which peers are involved (Hobbs et al., 1985; Miezio, 1983).

Peer interactions and the development of self-image are closely interrelated. Poor self-image may inhibit the adolescent from seeking or accepting involvement with peers. Thus, Seiffge-Krenke (1998, p. 168) continues the preceding quotation by stating, "The experience of one's own body as being deformed and damaged often caused the adolescents to feel so ashamed that they avoided participating in certain activities with their peers, such as visits to the swimming pool." Conversely, the resulting loss of opportunities to learn social skills, the self-fulfilling sense of being socially undesirable, and the lack of support from friends in coping with the effects of the disorder contribute to poor self-image. Furthermore, the delayed physical and sexual maturation associated with disorders such as cystic fibrosis and sickle cell anemia, and the psychosocial delays in achieving autonomy common in individuals with a disability or chronic disease may also have a negative impact on both self-image and peer interactions (Driscoll, 1986; Karlin, 1986).

When physical or cognitive limitations or the need to administer medical treatment create dependence on the family, the process of developing autonomy may be delayed. When full autonomy is not possible, the adolescent may retain some dependence, or care may be transferred outside the family. Even when this is not an issue, family patterns involving dependence, guilt, triangulation, or anxiety about competence and acceptance outside the family may cause parents and/or the adolescent to resist steps toward autonomy. When peer relationships are also limited, their countervailing promotion of autonomy is diminished and the anxieties related to leaving the family may be increased (Seiffge-Krenke, 1998; Seligman & Darling, 1989).

Parental and family support as well as that of that of school and social services have a central role in helping adolescents meet these developmental challenges. The most effective support involves an understanding of the adolescent's specific needs in the context of overall adolescent development. For example, when the adolescent requires assistance with mobility or transportation in order to engage in peer activities, the assistance most effectively promotes self-esteem and peer relations when it respects insofar as possible the needs for privacy and autonomy. With parents in particular, the adolescent may experience ambivalence or anger over the inevitably contradictory roles involved in such assistance. This type of ambivalence and anger arises with all adolescents. It is the parents' ability to understand and accept the emotions while setting appropriate limits to their expression that provides the fundamental parental support for these developmental tasks (Marshak et al., 1999; Rolland, 1994).

Concern with body image, a desire to fit in with peers, and the drive for increased independence may lead to intense resistance or noncompliance with dietary restrictions or medical procedures such as insulin injections or kidney dialysis. Illustrative of the qualitatively different dynamics that emerge in adolescence, noncompliance may occur with adolescents who had previously been compliant and taken age-appropriate personal responsibility. These issues are critical because of the severe implications of noncompliance for physical and mental development or the maintenance of life. As with the preceding issues, understanding and respect for the adolescent's position coupled with firm guidance regarding the necessary behaviors help promote a satisfactory resolution (Hobbs et al., 1985; Seiffge-Krenke, 1998).

Finally, the adolescent's steps toward establishing economic independence and finding a place in the work and social order may be affected, because of both inherent limitations in abilities and accumulative effects of the other developmental processes that have been discussed (Driscoll, 1986; Seligman & Darling, 1989).

This discussion has focused on factors that may impede adolescent development. However, this emphasis must not obscure the fact that many adolescents who have a genetic disease or birth defect adequately master many or all of the tasks of adolescence and establish the basis for an effective entry into early adulthood (Seligman & Darling, 1989). This mastery depends in substantial part on the individual and family strengths and resources discussed in Chapters 1 and 2 (Hobbs et al., 1985; Seiffge-Krenke, 1998). By combining a knowledge of adolescent development, the potential effects of genetic diseases and birth defects during adolescence, and the broader aspects of individual and family dynamics, genetic counselors will be able to most effectively assist adolescents and their families.

Issues in Adolescent Pregnancy

As with adults, myriad factors influence both planned and unplanned adolescent pregnancies. Nevertheless, certain dynamics are more common or influential in adolescence and are thus relevant to genetic counseling with adolescents.

To the extent that the adolescent remains at the stage of concrete and egocentric thinking, many aspects of pregnancy may be affected. The adolescent may believe that she or he is personally exempt from pregnancy following unprotected sex, despite knowing that this does occur to others. These ways of thinking also limit the adolescent's ability to foresee the implications of having a child. This includes difficulty appreciating the level of responsibility, the need for continuous care, and the importance of empathic attention and response to the child's physical and developmental needs (Peters-Brown & Fry-Mehltretter, 1996). Thus, a pregnancy may be initiated or maintained for which the adolescent is inadequately prepared. Under these circumstances, the adolescent's parents may be concerned not only with the well-being of their child and their future grandchild but also with the responsibilities they may incur for the well-being or direct care of their grandchild (Fuller-Thomson et al., 1997). Immature thinking patterns may also limit the adolescent's ability to understand and make decisions about prenatal care, the use of prenatal diagnosis, and the implications of medically positive genetic test or screening results. With all these issues, genetic counseling must take into account the adolescent's level of cognitive and emotional development.

Planned or "accidental" pregnancies may serve a number of adolescent needs. Pregnancy and parenthood may be perceived as one of the few available means for achieving adult status, separating from the family of origin, or making a more general assertion of individuation and autonomy. The future child may be perceived as a way of resolving feelings of loneliness or abandonment, as a focus for giving and/or receiving unequivocal love, or as the one thing the adolescent will have for herself. Furthermore, the developmental needs of the adolescent may interfere with attending to the needs of the pregnancy or the child. Pregnancy involves physical, hormonal, emotional, interpersonal, and social changes. Adaptation to these may be greatly complicated if the pregnant mother is simultaneously struggling with the analogous developmental challenges of adolescence. Once the child is born, comparable issues arise. For example, an adolescent's anger or frustration over her own unresolved need for autonomy may cause her to overlook her role in meeting her infant's analogous stage-specific needs. They may, in fact, lead to conscious or unconscious anger at, rejection of, or competition with the developing child, with attendant risks of neglect and abuse (Peters-Brown & Fry-Mehltretter, 1996; Trad, 1993).

These potential issues do not preclude happy and successful adolescent pregnancy and child rearing. They are of greater significance in earlier adolescence or with adolescents whose emotional or cognitive development is delayed. They do require assessment and attention in genetic counseling with adolescents.

Genetic Counseling Techniques with Adolescents

The issues discussed in the preceding sections also influence the genetic counseling session. From the adolescent's perspective the encounter is inherently unequal. It involves one or more adult professionals and often includes the parents as well. It frequently addresses topics such as medical compliance or pregnancy that are a source of contention with parents or other adults. If the adolescent is shy or self-conscious, has difficulty expressing anxiety and concerns, cannot readily formulate answers to questions, or does not understand or accept the need for the session, it may feel as if the adults are intrusive and demanding. If these factors are not attended to they may lead to withdrawal, anger, silliness, defiance, agreement that masks opposition, and failure to keep appointments or respond to phone calls (Peters-Brown & Fry-Mehltretter, 1996).

As with adults and children, a period of introductions and social warming up is essential. Brief but genuine inquiries about such topics as music, sports, hobbies, or activities with peers are a useful way to get started. They demonstrate the genetic counselor's acceptance of the adolescent's interests and a willingness to devote time to them in a primarily adult-oriented agenda (Hofmann & Greydanus, 1989; Mills, 1985). It may also be helpful to acknowledge the difficulties inherent in the genetic counseling situation.

Genetic Counselor (to a fourteen-year-old boy with diabetes, after an inquiry and brief discussion of the sports team named on his baseball cap): I'm glad we'll have a chance to talk. Maybe you have some questions I can help answer. But I know it's not easy talking to a stranger about these things, and maybe you are wondering what your mom and I discussed when we talked on the phone.

With these remarks the genetic counselor demonstrates her openness to the adolescent's concerns and questions, acknowledges some of the anxiety or defiance he may be feeling, and indicates a sensitivity to parent-adolescent tensions that may exist concerning the session and the topics to be discussed. As the conversation deepens, topics such as the desire for more independence or difficulties with peers are often easier for the adolescent to discuss than issues such as medical compliance or fears about the progression of the disorder. Thus, it is useful to begin with the former and, as a more trusting relationship develops, move on to the latter (Mills, 1985).

It is critically important to avoid appearing judgmental or as though one is siding with the parents or other adult authority figures. Probably no other action so powerfully replicates the problematic aspects of other relationships with adults and evokes defensive responses of withdrawal, anger, defiance, or dismissal. This does not preclude the genetic counselor's expressing a concerned professional position with respect to critical issues. However, this must take the adolescent's perspective into account and avoid being judgmental or preachy (Hofmann & Greydanus, 1989).

> *Genetic Counselor:* I know it's really hard to keep taking the injections now that you want to be with your friends and not feel dependent on your parents. Maybe we can figure out some ways around that. But I'm really concerned about the harm it does to your body when you miss an injection.

Anxiety, fear, and ambivalence often lie beneath a defiant or uninterested attitude. The genetic counselor's nonjudgmental statement of concern and willingness to help may be received with relief by the adolescent, even if he or she is unwilling or unable to so acknowledge (Hofmann & Greydanus, 1989; Peters-Brown & Fry-Mehltretter, 1996).

It is equally important that the genetic counselor respect and support the parents' concerns, adult perspective, and sense of parental responsibilities. Clearly, this attitude addresses the parents' needs. However, if the counselor has been even partially accepted as a fair and nonjudgmental arbiter by the adolescent, thoughtful attention to the parents' concerns may also give them greater value in the adolescent's eyes.

> *Genetic Counselor (to a parent who has just expressed great concern over her daughter's failure to maintain a dietary regimen):* I agree with you. That really is important for Mary's health both now and in the future.
> *Genetic Counselor (to Mary, in an even-tempered tone):* I understand how much you hate the diet. But this is one place where I agree with your parents.

In addition to addressing specific issues, the counselor can model for both parent and adolescent an attitude of respect and fair-minded consideration of the other's point of view. For example, when struggles over independence are described or occur in the session, it can be helpful to acknowledge the legitimacy of both sides and the normality of this process.

> *Genetic Counselor (addressing Mary and her parents):* Mary is at the age when it's appropriate for her to have more autonomy. In fact, getting it in reasonable doses will help her learn how to cope with the situations she'll be running into

as a teenager. But I know that you, as her parents, still have important concerns and responsibilities. (*to Mary*): I'll bet there are times when you feel that you should be able to make these decisions and your parents should butt out. (*to the parents*): And I'm sure there are times when you feel that you really have to exert your parental authority out of your love and concern for your daughter. This can be hard for families, but it's a normal part of growing up.

Meeting alone with the adolescent can bypass his or her need to assert independence in front of the parents or other adults and may facilitate discussion of embarrassing or confidential topics. Sometimes this occurs without the genetic counselor's direct involvement, as when the adolescent comes to prenatal diagnosis counseling accompanied by a friend, sibling, or the father of her child (Peters-Brown & Fry-Mehltretter, 1996). When the adolescent is accompanied by one or both parents, the genetic counselor may suggest the value of meeting separately with the adolescent and with the parents. The suggestion to meet separately demonstrates the counselor's awareness of and respect for the adolescent's developing autonomy. Insofar as is legal and appropriate, he or she should be assured of confidentiality, with the agreement of the parents. This requires that the genetic counselor be knowledgeable about laws related to the emancipation of minors and reporting physical or sexual abuse. When seen alone, adolescents are often much more open and responsive and able to suspend expressions of suspicion or anger (Preto, 1989).

As with children, displacement techniques can help circumvent denial or anxiety about discussing issues directly. One approach is to make an educated guess concerning the adolescent's feelings or concerns and present them as one's own (Hofmann & Greydanus, 1989).

> *Genetic Counselor:* If I were going to have a baby and didn't know how I could support it, I bet I would lie awake at night sometimes wondering how things will work out.

As with all such empathic hunches, if the statement is on target and the counselee is receptive the discussion will move forward with deepened emotional content. However, the only likely outcome of a failure in content or timing is that the statement will be ignored or rejected. Another displacement technique involves asking the adolescent how he or she thinks a peer would perceive the problem or act in such a situation (Peters-Brown & Fry-Mehltretter, 1996).

Genetic Counselor: How do you think your friend Ellen would handle it if she got pregnant?

If the adolescent is withdrawn, angry, or appears to have difficulty formulating responses, closed-ended questions such as "Do you ever feel angry about the way this disease limits you?" can be helpful in getting started. Questions of this sort can be answered with a single word such as "yes" or "no," with a verbally limited response such as a grunt of assent, or with a nonverbal response like a nod. This may facilitate a response because it does not require an extended statement. It may also allow the adolescent to save face because he or she can respond without having to give up an angry or withdrawn demeanor.

A nonjudgmental statement regarding a potentially conflicted situation may also help the adolescent respond. For example, "Many teenagers these days have sex. Are you sexually active?" By "announcing" the existence of the behavior without judgment or expectation concerning the answer, the genetic counselor demonstrates her willingness to take the initiative in raising the issue and to discussing it without judging the adolescent's response or behavior (Johnson & Tanner, 1989).

Several aspects of adolescence affect the processes of presenting technical information, facilitating decision making, and developing plans of action. These include concrete and egocentric thinking, difficulty orienting toward the future, lack of experience with which to understand options and make decisions, limited self-disclosure to adults, and the need to assert independence either overtly or covertly. Technical information, decision options, and long-term plans should all be presented in small steps with careful assessment of understanding. In decision making, the use of scenarios can be made more concrete through the technique of "anticipated regret," in which the counselor presents a potential outcome and then asks closed-ended questions about how the adolescent might feel were the outcome to occur (Peters-Brown & Fry-Mehltretter, 1996).

Genetic Counselor (to a pregnant seventeen-year-old with a family history of spina bifida): If you have the special ultrasound test and your baby does have spina bifida, then you could decide what you want to do. If you don't have the test, you may not find out. Do you think you would feel bad if you didn't have the test and then your baby was born and had spina bifida?

This technique can facilitate a discussion of issues that the adolescent would rather avoid or has difficulty contemplating. However, care must be taken that an emphasis on "regret" does not lead to unintended directiveness toward using tests or an emphasis on the negative aspects of potential outcomes.

Given the adolescent's stage-appropriate concern with body image and autonomy, it is essential that care be taken to respect modesty and privacy as much as possible during physical examinations and presentations of the adolescent for teaching or consultation purposes. This is not only a matter of fundamental respect and decency. It also contributes to the development of a positive body- and self-image, and it may help compensate for previous experiences that the adolescent found embarrassing or demeaning.

As with individuals of other ages, mental health referrals may be valuable. Indications of depression, suicidal ideation, social withdrawal, a rapid decline in mood or school performance, or severe or protracted adolescent–parent conflict are potential indicators (Driscoll, 1986). Initially, adolescents may angrily reject a suggestion concerning referral. However, with the empathic approach discussed in Chapter 3 under Mental Health Referrals, the adolescent and/or the parents may be open to assistance.

Genetic counseling with adolescents can evoke strong countertransference that may involve unresolved issues that remain from the genetic counselor's own adolescence (Peters-Brown & Fry-Mehltretter, 1996; Preto, 1989). For example, the genetic counselor may have strong feelings concerning an adolescent who is demonstrating a level of independence that the counselor did not obtain at the same age. This emotion will be particularly significant if the counselor consciously or unconsciously feels that her subsequent life has been affected in some way as a result. Conversely, genetic counselors who are or have been parents of an adolescent may have strong countertransference concerning parental anxieties, fears, and responsibilities. When such identification with the adolescent or the parent occurs, the countertransference responses may lie in either "direction." For example, if the genetic counselor identifies with the parent, her feelings may be based either on unresolved feelings that she should have established more effective limits with her son or daughter or that her own fears and concerns unduly limited the adolescent's development at that age. When unexamined, such feelings can lead to an overt alliance with the parent or the adolescent or to more subtle but significant differences in how the counselor responds to the concerns and arguments of one compared to the other.

Adolescent pregnancy may also evoke strong countertransference based on the genetic counselor's own life, experiences with her children, situations encountered in professional work, or broader societal issues. In addition, behaviors such as anger, boredom, dismissal, and defiance, which are sometimes expressed by adolescents may elicit strong emotions. These behaviors can be particularly troubling when they come from an individual whom the genetic counselor is attempting to help. As with other forms of countertransference, self-awareness and exploration as well as peer or professional assistance may be of great benefit.

7

THE ETHNOCULTURAL
IMPERATIVE

A S with all aspects of life, health care beliefs and practices, reproductive decisions, and the meanings attributed to children and family are profoundly influenced by the culture of the individuals involved and by counselees' experiences as members of ethnocultural communities. Thus, consideration of the psychosocial aspects of genetic counseling must take culture and ethnic identity into account. The perspectives of the preceding chapters are based primarily on the dominant culture of the United States. Thus, they include, although not without discussion, such fundamental assumptions as the primacy of scientific understanding and the control of natural processes and the potentially healing value of expressing and sharing emotional experiences with professional health care providers. However, these and myriad other values and beliefs relevant to genetic counseling are not, in fact, common to all cultures and communities. It is a principle of fundamental fairness in human interactions and equity in the provision of genetic counseling services that genetic counselors be sensitive to and knowledgeable about ethnocultural issues and be competent in working with individuals from diverse backgrounds.

Cultural beliefs and practices create major barriers to obtaining effective genetic counseling (Lin-Fu, 1990), as do the historical and contemporary experiences of both established and recently immigrant ethnocultural groups. These topics are discussed in more detail later. However, in broad terms,

TABLE 7–1. Resident United States Population, 1997

RACE/ETHNICITY	NUMBERS (MILLIONS)	PERCENT
American Indian, Eskimo, and Aleut	2.0	0.7
Asian and Pacific Islander	9.4	3.5
Black non-Hispanic	32.3	12.1
Hispanic origin	29.3	11.0
White non-Hispanic	194.6	72.7

Data from Statistical Abstract of the United States, 1998, Table 19.

they include differences in language; health care beliefs and practices; attitudes toward time, fate, and human instrumentality; and obligations toward and expectations of children, family, and society. They also involve the multiple effects of racism, exploitation, violence, and prejudice. Unless these factors are understood and appropriately addressed, the ideals and goals of providing accessible, useful services to all who might benefit from them cannot be met.

The figures given in Table 7.1, based on 1995 census data, are one indication of the ethnocultural diversity of the United States. Sixty-nine million people, more than one-quarter of the population, describe themselves as having an ethnocultural identity differing from that of the "majority." Present and predicted patterns indicate that the population will continue to diversify. Both immigration rates and growth rates within the United States are higher for all other groups than for white non-Hispanics (Statistical Abstract of the United States, 1998). In Los Angeles and San Francisco, no ethnocultural group currently has majority status (Viviano, 1988), and some projections indicate this will be true for the United States by the year 2050 (U.S. Bureau of the Census, 1992). Historical patterns and contemporary migration also create situations of great ethnocultural diversity in many other areas of the world. Furthermore, issues of culture and cultural self-identification may be of major importance with respect to sexual orientation, disability, and other criteria by which individuals define themselves. There is no question that genetic counselors must have the knowledge and sensitivity needed to provide effective services to individuals from a wide range of ethnocultural backgrounds.

Culture and Ethnocultural Identity

The term *culture* refers to the socially transmitted values, beliefs, behaviors, customs, social and political institutions, arts, crafts, and science shared by a group of people (Randall-David, 1989). Within this concept of culture there are multiple levels of complexity, which include the following:

The groups to which the term is applied vary greatly. At one end of the spectrum, just below those aspects of culture applicable to all of humanity, lie the largest, most inclusive categories, such as "Asian culture" or "European culture." Within these are multiple cultural groups that reflect geographic, historical, linguistic, and ethnic groupings. The term culture may also be applied to groups of individuals defined by various other criteria, such as the "culture of deafness" (Israel et al., 1992; 1996), the "culture of science" (Rapp, 1993a), and elements of culture and cultural identity associated with characteristics such as sex, sexual orientation, and physical or mental disability (Saxton, 1998; Finucane, 1998a; Ablon, 1984).

Within any such group there is immense diversity in the cultural components themselves, such as beliefs and institutions, and among the individuals who make up the group. Thus, for example, Asian culture includes many countries and ethnic groups that have different histories, language, customs, beliefs, and other elements of culture. Similarly, deaf culture involves individuals from many ethnocultural groups who are also diverse with respect to education, socioeconomic status, language, and communication modes (Israel et al., 1992).

Both the culture of a group and those who identify with it evolve over time and vary depending on context. Historic and contemporary migration and increasingly available means of travel and communication contribute to this process (Laird, 1998). As a large-scale example, the immigration of individuals from countries with Hispanic culture to the United States has introduced millions of people to the dominant culture of the United States, with attendant issues of evolving and fluctuating cultural identification (see Ethnocultural History and Social Experience: Immigration and Acculturation). This has also changed and enriched the dominant U.S. culture with elements of Hispanic culture.

As a smaller-scale example of change and the importance of context, the individual who receives training in genetic counseling enters the conceptual and professional cultures of science and genetic counseling, which are added to the other cultural categories relevant to her. Her cultural identification and her culturally determined behaviors and perceptions may fluctuate depending upon the circumstances. Thus, her identification as a genetic counselor may be strong on the job but limited during a social or family gathering. Similarly, her language, perceptions, and behaviors involving an individual with a disability may differ greatly under these two sets of circumstances. Furthermore, she may feel like an integrated member of the community at work but encounter bewilderment, misunderstanding, or hostility in social settings where genetic counseling is unfamiliar or thought to primarily lead to abortion.

Culture greatly influences perceptions, cognition, and, in broader terms, the manner in which individuals create a relatively cohesive, meaningful world view from the immense complexity of reality (Sue & Sue, 1990). This world view contributes to the sense of belonging and understanding that is often experienced in culturally familiar situations. It is also responsible for the confusion, disorientation, anxiety and sense of loss that one may experience in culturally unfamiliar settings. Because of their pervasive influence, many aspects of an individual's own culture are often largely unconscious and unperceived. The self-evident "rightness" of the way one perceives and responds to the world is not experienced as "culture," but as reality (Lynch, 1998a).

Conversely, components of an unfamiliar culture are often perceived and evaluated in isolation, owing to a failure to understand the broad, integrated features of the culture. The frequently cited characteristic of emotional reticence among people of Asian and Asian American culture provides a useful example. Viewed from the perspective of a different culture, this reticence may be perceived as an inhibition or as an impediment to the receipt of genetic counseling services. However, within the culture, it is part of a far larger, integrated set of personal and social expectations and behaviors. These include a strong sense of responsibility for the well-being of the family or social group, a concern with maintaining social harmony, and sophisticated forms of indirect and nonverbal communication. In addition, in cultures in which there is a high level of expected interpersonal interaction and limited opportunities for physical privacy, withholding the expression of one's emotions may provide a means of maintaining a sense of a protected, private inner self (Nilchaikovit et al., 1993; Sue & Sue., 1990).

The term *ethnicity* refers to membership in a group that is defined by a combination of race, language, culture, religion, and national or geographic origin (Greb, 1998). A sense of ethnic identity is transmitted through the family, through the language, religion, and other aspects of culture, and by identification with others who share common physical traits. It may be reinforced in both negative and positive ways by the larger community. McGoldrick (1989, p. 69) states that ethnicity "involves conscious and unconscious processes that fulfill a deep psychological need for identity and historical continuity. It unites those who conceive of themselves as alike by virtue of their common ancestry, real or factitious, and who are so regarded by others." However, individuals may be largely unaware of elements of their ethnicity, may return to a sense of ethnic identity after one or more generations of assimilation into the larger society, or may denigrate or attempt to deny ethnic identity in order to assimilate into the majority ethnocultural group or in response to prejudice and negative stereotypes promoted by the larger society.

Based on these definitions, the term *ethnocultural* is used in the present discussion to refer, in broad and inclusive terms, to membership, sense of identity, personal and social beliefs and practices, social history, world view, and transmitting mechanisms related to ethnicity and to culture defined at all levels.

The term *race* originated in observed and presumed biological differences among individuals based on geographic origin and physical appearance (Pinderhughes, 1989). The biological basis for the term and for racial classifications is now largely discredited, based in part on ambiguities and difficulties of classification and on extensive evidence that, for the large majority of phenotypic or genotypic characteristics, genetic variability within ethnocultural groups, greatly exceeds the average differences among such groups (Lewontin, 1982). Nevertheless, the term race has social meanings and implications that retain great importance. Historical and contemporary patterns of exploitation, discrimination, stereotyping, and violence against members of specific ethnocultural groups are defining elements of the history and culture and the social, political, and economic institutions of the United States and many other countries. Typified by the term *racism,* these factors must be considered in any discussion of ethnocultural issues.

There has been substantial discussion concerning the most appropriate means by which health care professionals can be educated for and then provide services to counselees whose ethnicity and culture differ from their own. Among the central issues are the relative importance of knowledge about the counselee's culture and ethnicity as opposed to self-awareness and knowledge concerning one's own culture and ethnicity and the dynamics of cross-cultural encounters. In addition, there is a question of the relative importance of human characteristics and behavior at different levels: those that are common to all humanity and thus provide a potential basis for working with any individual; those that are characteristic of or relevant to a given ethnocultural group, which must be acknowledged and taken into account in working with individuals from that group; and those that are specific to the individual, which must also be addressed and not obscured by stereotypes concerning the ethnocultural group to which the individual belongs (Carter & Qureshi, 1995; Ota Wang, 1998b).

The following discussion draws on all the above perspectives. However, there is an explicit premise that ethnocultural issues and cross-cultural counseling must be approached in terms of an interaction or intersection between the ethnicity and culture(s) of the genetic counselor, including the institutions and practices she represents, and those of the counselee (Fadiman, 1997; Ota Wang, 1998a). Stated differently, the impact of the genetic counselor's culture on the counselee and the genetic counseling process is as important as the impact of the counselee's culture on the counselor and the genetic counseling process. This point of view stands in contrast to a unidirectional consideration of the counselee's ethnicity and culture. By their nature, all cultures create a strong tendency for individuals to perceive their own world view as representing reality and civility, and thus to perceive other cultures as encumbered with "beliefs and practices" (Lynch, 1998a; Sue & Sue, 1990). For the genetic counselor, this tendency may be reinforced by the scientific assumptions and successes of Western medicine and by the growing body of information and technology that support genetic counseling (Greb, 1998; Rapp, 1993a). Therefore, explicit attention must be given to the bidirectional, interactional aspects of cross-cultural encounters.

Information concerning any culture, including the dominant culture, must be used with care. On the one hand, it can be critically valuable in understanding the beliefs and practices of the counselee, and thus help guide appropriate responses and interventions. On the other hand, it may contribute to stereotypes that restrict the genetic counselor's thinking, perceptions, and responses. Any such information represents a generalization—an attempt to reduce complex reality to a limited, comprehensible description. The diversity that exists within cultures, among the ethnocultural groups that compose them, among individuals within any such group, and in the particular situation must always be kept in mind. Cross-cultural influences and assimilation into the dominant culture further complicate the situation.

It is useful to consider the analogous situation involved in using psychosocial information in genetic counseling. For example, in counseling a couple whose infant has recently been diagnosed with Down syndrome, the genetic counselor should be aware that anger may be one aspect of the couple's response. An understanding of its psychodynamic origins, its role in the grief and coping process, and the many ways it may be expressed all contribute to effective observation, interpretation, and interventions. However, it would be grossly inappropriate and counterproductive to conduct the session based on a rigid, stereotyped assumption that the counselees *are* angry because of their circumstances and *are* expressing anger directly or indirectly. Similar care must be taken with all ethnocultural information.

This example also illustrates an additional point: There is no clear-cut distinction between "psychosocial" and "ethnocultural" issues or perspectives. From one point of view, a consideration of ethnocultural issues involves, in substantial part, a consideration of psychosocial issues as they pertain to various cultures and ethnocultural groups (Weil & Mittman, 1993). Thus, in the example just cited, the counselees' perceptions of the significance of Down syndrome, their emotional responses to it, and the extent and manner in which anger is experienced and expressed will all be greatly influenced by the counselees' ethnocultural background.

Increasing ethnocultural diversity among the practitioners of genetic counseling would make a critical contribution to addressing the issues involved in cross-cultural genetic counseling. Such diversity would allow counselor and counselee to more frequently share elements of culture and ethnicity and would be of particular value in clinics that serve a high proportion of individuals from ethnocultural groups other than European American (Mittman et al., 1998). Beyond this, the presence of genetic counselors and genetic counseling students of diverse backgrounds enriches the knowledge, sensitivities, and experiences of individual genetic counselors and the profession. Despite continuing efforts and concern, such diversity has not been achieved among master's degree genetic counselors in the United States (Smith et al., 1993). In 1998 the membership of the National Society of Genetic Counselors (NSGC) was approximately 93% white American and 96% female (Schneider & Kalkbrenner, 1998). Ethnocultural diversity is almost certainly limited among other groups of providers as well. Although it lies outside the scope of the present discussion, there is a pressing need to continue to address this situation. However, the issues discussed here are relevant to genetic counselors of all ethnocultural heritages, because all will work with counselees whose backgrounds differ from their own, both within and outside the major ethnocultural group to which the genetic counselor belongs.

Cultures and Cultural Differences

Information, knowledge, sensitivity, and empathy concerning the counselee's culture are critical in any genetic counseling interaction. These are relatively readily achieved to the extent that the counselee's culture is similar to that of the genetic counselor. To the extent that their cultures differ, a more active role is required of the counselor both before and during the encounter.

The information to be presented here addresses the broad issues that are relevant to cross-cultural genetic counseling. However, the genetic counselor should also draw on other sources of information about specific ethnocultural groups to whom services are provided. An illustrative but by no means comprehensive list of references in the professional literature is presented in Table 7.2. However, there are many other ways to obtain information, understanding, and experience that complement and extend what can be obtained from written professional materials. Meeting members of the relevant population, both individually and in community settings such as churches, marketplaces, festivals, and areas of geographic concentration, provides direct experience. It also allows the genetic counselor to learn about characteristics of the local culture, which inevitably vary from location to location and from more general descriptions. Other sources of information and understanding include novels, poetry, movies, videos, folk arts and crafts, anthropological and ethnographic accounts, language study, and travel to foreign countries. (See Lynch, 1998, p. 513 for a suggested list of novels, plays, movies, and other resources.)

Elements of World View

Sue & Sue (1990), drawing on the work of Kluckhohn and Strodtbeck (1961), discuss several elements of overall world view that differ among cultures. Of

TABLE 7–2. References Providing Information About Specific Cultures and Ethnocultural Groups

REFERENCE	CULTURES/ETHNOCULTURAL GROUPS INCLUDED	PROFESSIONAL ORIENTATION
Fisher, 1996a	National, regional	Genetic counseling
Wang & Marsh, 1992	Asian American	Genetic counseling
Lew, 1990	Southeast Asian	Genetic counseling
Israel et al., 1996	Deaf culture	Genetic counseling
Finucane, 1998b	Mild mental retardation	Genetic counseling
Wang, 1993	Major groups	Bibliography (genetic counseling)
Spector, 1996	Major groups	Health care beliefs and practices
Sue & Sue, 1990	Major groups	Counseling
Lynch, 1998	Major groups/regional	Education/health care/social services
Seligman & Darling, 1989	Major groups	Childhood disability
McGoldrick et al., 1996	National, regional	Family therapy
Boyd-Franklin, 1989	African American	Counseling
McAdoo, 1997	African American	Cultural, social, and economic
Lee, 1997	Asian American	Counseling
Daneshpour, 1998	Muslim	Family therapy

these, three are particularly pertinent to genetic counseling. However, before discussing them, one caveat related to the problem of stereotypes must be noted: These and other elements of world view are frequently described in terms of discrete alternatives such as "mastery over nature" versus "harmony with nature." However, each actually involves a complex spectrum or continuum, and cultures as well as individuals are more appropriately considered in terms of their position along such continua (Lynch, 1998b).

Relationship toward nature concerns the extent to which humanity controls, is subject to, or may be in harmony with natural forces and events. The dominant culture of the United States perceives nature as largely subject to human understanding and control. Dominance of nature was an important element in the westward expansion of the United States and the conversion of the land to agriculture and domestic purposes. It is also an underlying premise of contemporary scientific research and its technological and medical applications. It is manifest in many aspects of genetics and genetic counseling, including the techniques and goals of the Human Genome Project and the use of prenatal diagnosis for purposes of elective termination or fetal or neonatal intervention. By contrast, a greater sense of harmony with or acceptance of natural phe-

nomena characterize, in broad terms, the cultures of the other major ethnocultural groups: Native Americans, African Americans, Hispanic Americans,
and Asian Americans. These attitudes toward humankind's relationship to nature do not preclude knowledge or acceptance of science. However, insofar as
individuals hold these views, they may be more accepting of or resigned to human variation and departures from "normal" outcomes, including genetic diseases and birth defects. Complementing this point of view may be reduced acceptance or active disagreement with instrumental goals associated with genetic
counseling such as carrier screening, prenatal diagnosis or screening, and invasive medical interventions (Mittman et al., 1998).

Time orientation. The dominant United States culture places much emphasis on the future, be it planning the next work day or the next vacation, developing a business plan or a research project, or making financial preparations
for children, education, or retirement. There is also a great emphasis on time
as a commodity, to be measured and used, even in "recreation," rather than
allowed to "slip by" and be "wasted." Relatively speaking, Native American and
African American cultures place greater emphasis on the present, with less concern for the passage of time. This attitude may result in more spontaneity and
involvement in the present but less organization or preparation for the future.
In yet another orientation, Hispanic and Asian cultures place value on the past,
history, and tradition, as well as on the present (Sue & Sue, 1990). The veneration of ancestors and the elderly characterizes a number of Asian cultures,
and in China this veneration is coupled with a profound sense of millennia-
long cultural history.

Differences in time orientation may affect various aspects of genetic counseling, from punctuality for appointments to receptiveness to future-oriented
prenatal or presymptomatic testing. As an example, consider the possible effects on a parent's responses to the diagnosis of an infant with a severe genetic
disorder. Future orientation leads to concern for the long-term implications,
including the social and financial impact on the family and the effects the disorder will have on the child's life and accomplishments. Present orientation
will lead to concern for the child's current well-being and may limit acceptance
of the diagnosis if the visible symptoms are mild or obscure. Past orientation
may influence beliefs concerning why the disorder occurred, such as events in
the past, or to anxiety about the impact on the family's social standing and rep-
utation. The danger of stereotyping is evident in this example: Any parent may
have concerns in any or all of these domains. Nevertheless, the extent and intensity of these different concerns will be affected by the time orientation of
the parent's culturally based world view.

Relationships among individuals. Many aspects of the culture of the United
States can be characterized by the term "individualism." Given the heading of

this paragraph, the relative underrepresentation of "relationships" is evident. Individualism envisions much of psychosocial development, consciousness, and responsibility at the level of the individual. Family is defined by genetic relationships, and the functional family is often limited to the two-generation nuclear family augmented somewhat by the parents' first-degree relatives—the grandparents, aunts, and uncles. Most other cultures define human relationships and the family more interactively and broadly, and they perceive human consciousness and experience in more social terms. Many traditional Asian cultures define relatively strict responsibilities and obligations among individuals in different generations. In Native American, Asian, Hispanic, African, African American, and Middle Eastern cultures there is often a strong sense of responsibility for the well-being of members of the extended family. African American culture commonly defines family to include nonbiological relationships (Telfair & Nash, 1996). Thus, for example, a close friend of a parent who provides support and participates in family events may be known to the children as "auntie" and treated as a family member. There are other cultural variables as well. The nature of marital and couple relationships varies from relative equality in emotional, social, and power domains to strongly hierarchical or authoritarian with male dominance. Consanguineous marriages, which are common in a number of Middle Eastern and other cultures, create interlocking family relationships, obligations, and sense of identity (Darr, 1997).

These aspects of family and relationships affect genetic counseling in multiple ways (Greb, 1998). They have a major role in determining the social support available to counselees. They may also intensify feelings of guilt or shame concerning the occurrence and believed causes of genetic disorders and birth defects, insofar as these stigmatize or cast shame on the extended family. Family relationships and obligations can influence decision making and complicate the process of obtaining informed consent as defined in contemporary Western medicine. The counselee may consider the emotions, wishes, advice, and expectations of others, or the well-being and social standing of the family, to be of major importance in reaching a decision. Consanguineous marriages can broaden sources of social support and promote a sense of familial and cultural identity that helps sustain the counselees through difficult times. But such a marriage may also produce distrust, embarrassment, or shame when the counselee confronts the dominant culture and the culture of genetic counseling, which perceive consanguinity in primarily negative, biological terms (Darr, 1997).

The parents of a child with developmental delay of unknown etiology, both of whom were second-generation Middle Eastern Americans, were referred for genetic counseling. A telephone intake interview with the mother included obtaining a pedigree and family medical history. It was only after the genetic counselor commented that she herself had been born in the Middle East that the mother revealed that she and her husband were first cousins.

Language and Communication

Language has a significant role in defining and delimiting cultures and ethnocultural groups. The ability to communicate in a common language promotes a sense of cultural identity and greatly facilitates the exchange of information, ideas, and values. Conversely, the absence of a common language creates a major barrier to communication. Languages structure the individual's world view. This is demonstrated by the difficulty in translating from one language to another when topics such as social interactions, perceptions of the natural world, religious and spiritual beliefs, and esthetics are involved. Within a given language, differences in dialect, accent, and colloquialisms contribute to national, regional, ethnic, and socioeconomic identities and differences (Rauch & Curtiss, 1992). These linguistic differences can have a strong emotional impact. A familiar dialect, accent, or colloquialism may evoke a powerful sense of identity and/or nostalgia. Conversely, unfamiliar usage or that associated with groups other than one's own may evoke fears and uncertainty associated with regional, national, or ethnocultural experiences and conflicts.

Language usage also helps define self-identification with and the world view of other cultural groups. Terms such as "disabled" (Asch, 1989), "little people" (dwarf) (Ablon, 1984), "learning disabled" (mild mental retardation) (Finucane, 1998b), "Deaf" (Israel et al., 1996), and "gay" (male homosexual) illustrate, at the most immediate level, words that have been adopted by individuals in different cultures in the service of self-definition, self-esteem, and advocacy. Language plays a similar role with respect to self-identification and world view in the cultures of science and genetic counseling. Technical terms and their associated acronyms and abbreviations, such as "PCR" (polymerase chain reaction), "cDNA" (complementary DNA), and "u/s" (ultrasound), allow efficient communication based on shared knowledge that is largely impenetrable to those who are unfamiliar with the concepts and terminology. Another component of this scientific culture involves the concept of genetic information. This is exemplified by terms such as "genetic code" and "missense" and "nonsense" mutations, and by the frequently used explanation that "the chromosomes carry the instructions that determine how a person develops." This way of understanding human development and characteristics may seem very foreign to counselees who are unfamiliar with the concepts of contemporary biology, especially if their culture has not yet appropriated the terminology of "information" to describe other aspects of postindustrial, computer-based society.

As discussed in Chapter 4 under Presenting Information: Terminology commonly used clinical terminology such as "a positive family history," "an uneventful pregnancy," and to "appreciate" a sign or symptom have meanings within the culture of clinical genetics and genetic counseling that differ from common, lay culture usage. When the counselee does not understand the terms in the medical-cultural context used by the genetic counselor and instead interprets them in their lay cultural meanings, misunderstanding, anger, or distrust may result. This situation, which is familiar to genetic counselors, is instructive of how similar misunderstandings, with similar consequences, can occur across any linguistic/ethnocultural boundary with respect to both verbal and nonverbal aspects of communication.

Cultures also differ greatly in the extent to which nonverbal communication and contextual cues are used to convey meaning (Lynch, 1998b). European American speech relies heavily on the explicit content of the words used. By contrast, African American speech transmits a greater proportion of its meaning through the context in which it occurs, the direct expression of emotions, and nonverbal behaviors. As discussed earlier, Asian cultures use subtle verbal indirection and nonverbal communication to convey meanings that may be in direct contradiction to the specific word content. Concerning contextual cues, Sue & Sue (1990, p. 58) state:

> [A] normal-stressed "no" by a U.S. American may be interpreted by an Arab as "yes." A real negation in Arab culture would be stressed much more emphatically. In Filipino culture, a mild, hesitant "yes" is interpreted as a polite refusal. In traditional Asian society, to extend an invitation only once for dinner would be considered an affront, because it implies you are not sincere.

Such differences in the meanings of "no" and "yes" can lead to serious misunderstanding when the genetic counselor inquires if an explanation has been understood or seeks a verbal response concerning acceptance or rejection of a procedure such as amniocentesis.

Cultures differ with respect to many other aspects of verbal and nonverbal communication (Lynch, 1998b; Sue & Sue, 1990). These include voice tone and loudness, rate of speaking, inflections and pauses, hand and body movements, extent and circumstances of eye contact, degree of emotional expressiveness, and the physical distance between individuals that feels comfortable. All these factors are powerful determinants of meaning and emotions. For example, the reader is probably familiar with the sense of claustrophobia and being impinged upon that occurs when another person stands too close for comfort during a conversation. Likewise, if the other person stands further away than is socially comfortable, there is a tendency to feel that he or she is not interested or is attempting to avoid or leave the situation. The feelings that arise in these circumstances can be intense, as can those that occur if either member of the dyad moves to correct the distance from his or her perspective.

Socioeconomic Status

Socioeconomic status is an important determinant and component of culture (Seligman & Darling, 1989). Individual, family, and group experiences are profoundly affected by many variables associated with socioeconomic status. These include differences in education; financial resources and security; occupational status including job security, health insurance, disability benefits, and the ability to take time from work for health care matters without loss of income or employment; the nature, quality, and availability of health care services; and multiple aspects of treatment by and access to sources of institutional, financial and political power (Kliman, 1998). These factors lead to differences in world view and other aspects of culture discussed previously. Socioeconomic status is an important cultural variable in its own right. However, given the impact of racism, discrimination, immigration, and other aspects of ethnocultural experience, socioeconomic status is also correlated with, although by no means determined by, ethnocultural identity (see next section, Health Care Beliefs and Practices).

Socioeconomic status influences the accessibility, acceptance, and utilization of health care services including genetic counseling (Hill, 1994; Lemke et al., 1998). In the most general terms, lower socioeconomic status is associated with reduced use and adequacy of health care services. However, the relationships between socioeconomic status, on the one hand, and health care beliefs and practices, on the other, are complex. Rapp (1993a) and Bernhardt and coworkers (1997) have investigated these factors as they relate to genetic counseling. As they point out, caution must be used in generalizing from their specific findings. Nevertheless, their research demonstrates the interacting influences of socioeconomic status, ethnocultural identity, and individual experience on the resulting complex patterns of acceptance, utilization, and expectations of genetic counseling. For example, in focus groups exploring issues related to cancer risk counseling, the findings of Bernhardt and associates (1997) included the following: Compared to women with higher socioeconomic status, women with lower socioeconomic status were more likely to value test information for its presumed predictive value independent of potential health care interventions, to favor testing their children as an aspect of comprehensive medical care, and to prefer risk counseling from a health care provider whom they knew and trusted over an unknown individual with formal expertise.

Health Care Beliefs and Practices

Given the great impact of diseases and birth defects on individuals, families, and society, all cultures have evolved means for understanding, treating, and preventing them. Specific beliefs and practices may directly affect genetic counseling. For example, Mittman and coworkers (1998) reported a belief in the evil eye and the eating of specific foods as causes of birth defects among recent immigrants of both Asian-Pacific and Hispanic origins. The belief among Asian-Pacific counselees that blood and other body fluids carry the essence of life and must be conserved can result in resistance to amniocentesis and diagnostic tests that require blood samples. In addition, lack of familiarity with the fundamentals of biology and Western medicine may lead to disbelief that prenatal tests can predict the future child's health or development (Mittman, 1988; 1990). In traditional Navajo culture, thought and language control the future, and thus discussion of potentially negative outcomes is to be avoided (Carrese & Rhodes, 1995). A wide variety of relevant beliefs and practices have been reported among individuals receiving genetic counseling (Cohen et al., 1998; Greb, 1998; Mittman, 1988; Mittman et al., 1998; Rapp, 1990; Weil, 1991) and in more general cultural descriptions (Fadiman, 1997; Lee et al., 1988; Lew, 1990; Spector, 1996). Knowledge of relevant beliefs and practices and respectful inquiry during genetic counseling are important when working with counselees from cultures that differ from one's own.

For the present discussion, however, it is equally important to recognize that specific beliefs relevant to genetic counseling are integral components of far more general cultural patterns. For example, many Asian beliefs concerning the effect of specific foods in causing birth defects are part of the broad metaphysical concept of opposites, which are called *yin* and *yang* in Chinese. Balance and harmony between these opposing but complementary forms of energy are essential to social as well as personal well-being. Thus, partaking of specific "cold" or "hot" foods that unduly shift the energy balance toward *yin* or *yang*, respectively, can affect the well-being of the fetus, just as comparable imbalances can affect many aspects of human life and fate (Lew, 1990). Many cultures believe in metaphysical and supernatural causes of disease that are part of far broader beliefs concerning the forces and processes that affect human experiences and fate (Mittman et al., 1998; Spector, 1996).

This embeddedness in the broader culture helps explain why health beliefs and practices, including the use of community healers, may remain important despite acculturation and exposure to Western medicine. For recent immigrants, and all who have lived their lives primarily within the traditional culture, these beliefs and practices represent the known world and how to protect oneself and one's family within it. With acculturation, these beliefs and practices may continue to be held for various interrelated reasons. They may be retained because of unsatisfactory experiences with Western medicine or because of barriers in obtaining such medical services. They may be part of a more general adherence to and identification with the culture of origin. They may be espoused or practiced to maintain the support of less acculturated members of the family or community. Even when Western medicine is accepted and utilized, the deep personal and communal roots of these beliefs and practices may cause the individual to turn to them either as insurance, believing they may have some efficacy, or in critical situations that lead to a search for all possible means of prevention or cure. Counselees may be reluctant to reveal such beliefs because of embarrassment, shame, or fear of rejection or disparagement (Rapp, 1993; Mittman et al., 1998). For all these reasons, it is essential that the genetic counselor be respectful of such beliefs and practices and attempt to find ways to include them, as appropriate, in both explanations and interventions.

Within the dominant culture of the United States, various aspects of health care also involve beliefs and practices that lie outside or in equivocal relation to established Western medicine. In terms of general health, many individuals use home remedies that are of varying efficacy and concurrence with established medicine. More relevant to genetic counseling is the growing utilization of health foods and additives and of alternative medical practices, including those such as acupuncture that are established aspects of medical practice in other cultures (Eisenberg et al., 1998). The Internet is a new cultural development that is a growing source of data, information, advice, and social interaction. Increasingly, counselees enter genetic counseling with information obtained on the Internet that is of diverse origins and varying quality. Various dynamics comparable to those discussed earlier with reference to other cultures contribute to these beliefs and practices: cross-cultural exposure, dissatisfaction with the ethos and practice of standard medicine, a desire for health care practices that are more integrated with other aspects of life, and a desire to use all possible options in severe or terminal conditions including genetic diseases, birth defects, and cancer. As with counselees from other cultures, the genetic counselor must strive to understand and acknowledge both the specific beliefs and practices and the dynamics that underlie them.

The perceived consequences of a disease or birth defect are also influenced by cultural factors. Cultures differ in their acceptance of and sense of responsibility for individuals with genetic diseases and birth defects. Cultural differences also influence how specific disorders or disabilities are perceived (Kleinman, 1980). The counselee whose culture and socioeconomic status place a high value on intellectual achievement and cognitive abilities may be most concerned with the impact of mental retardation. For the counselee to whom physical work and participation in social and family life are of greater importance, physical limitations may be of more concern than mild or moderate mental retardation (Hauck & Knoki-Wilson, 1996). When stigmatization or the impact on marriageability is of concern, the visibility of the disorder may be of great importance (Applebaum & Firestein, 1983). Equally significant are differences in the personal and social implications of disabilities. These may involve a primary concern for the physical, social, and medical well-being of the affected individual; a sense of shame and stigmatization of the family; or the impact on the marriageability of the affected individual or his or her siblings (Mittman et al., 1998). Rapp (1999; 1993a) has been particularly effective and eloquent in elucidating the complex interplay of personal, cultural, and socioeconomic factors that contribute to the highly individual responses of women to amniocentesis and the possibility of having an affected child.

Culture also influences the perception of risk and risk figures. Lack of familiarity with predictive Western medicine or with the statistical concepts of probability may cause counselees to misunderstand or discount the occurrence/recurrence risks presented in genetic counseling (Mittman et al., 1998). Even if accepted, the numerical values may have limited impact in comparison to other risks in current life or prior to immigration. As Rapp (1993b, p. 92) so evocatively states, "[F]or those leading very stressful lives under conditions of urban poverty, the risk of losing housing by the end of the year may be as high as 50%, of losing a brother, son or partner to jail or premature death may be as high as 25%, and the risk of running out of food stamps by the end of the month is 100%. So the numbers offered by counselors may seem almost insignificant and distant."

There are also cultural differences in expectations of medical treatment and the role of the health care provider. Counselees may consider the provision of medication or direct therapeutic interventions to be an essential component of any health care encounter. They may anticipate that the health care provider will establish a personal relationship, with overt demonstrations of concern for their well-being and that of their family, before beginning formal diagnosis and treatment. A recitation of family history may be foreign to their experience with health care providers. In some cultures, personal and family problems are carefully withheld from outsiders, and great shame may be associated with revealing relevant information to health care providers (Daneshpour, 1998).

> A recently immigrated Central American woman and her twenty-year-old daughter with Down syndrome were referred for genetic counseling at the request of another daughter who had lived in the United States for eight years and was concerned about recurrence risk. The mother was confused about the reason for the visit "to a doctor" and reticent regarding the family's medical history. However, she was outspoken in her insistence on a full medical examination for herself, stating that she had several health concerns she wanted addressed. This may have reflected her previous experiences and expectations concerning the nature of medical treatment in a clinic or hospital and/or an attempt to obtain primary medical services that she was unable to obtain by other means.

Culturally based expectations for advice, guidance, and directive counseling create a challenge to the ethos of nondirective genetic counseling. As discussed

in Chapter 5, Nondirective Counseling, individual, social, and professional factors have converged in the United States to promote a concept of patient rights
that is accepted by a substantial proportion of the population, in which the individual client has access to all relevant information including risks of procedures and has a central role in decision making that complements that of the
medical professional. These are recent historical developments. As late as the
1960s and 1970s, a more authoritarian, paternalistic form of medicine was practiced by most physicians and accepted by most patients. In many other cultures, the medical professional continues to be seen as the authority who pre-
scribes procedures as well as medications. The idea that decision making
regarding these issues is partially or fully vested in the patient may be very foreign. Thus, attempts to counsel nondirectively may lead to confusion, anger,
or a sense of being inadequately or unprofessionally served (Greb, 1998; Rapp,
1993a).

This issue is discussed in more detail later under Ethnocultural Expectations, Decision Making, and Nondirective Genetic Counseling. However, it is
important to point out here that the use and acceptance of both directive and
nondirective counseling are culturally determined. As Kessler (1992b, p.11)
states from a somewhat different vantage, "[T]here are more similarities [to directiveness and nondirectiveness] than meets the eye. Both are counseling
strategies in which an attempt is made to influence the counselee. . . . In the
case of directiveness, the counselor wishes to influence the counselee's behavior, whereas in the case of nondirectiveness, the counselor attempts to influence the way the counselee thinks about a specific problem."

Ethnocultural History and Social Experience

The history and social experiences of any ethnocultural group have a major impact upon many aspects of its culture. These elements include self-perception
and self-definition, the extent of group identification experienced by different
members, the degree and nature of acculturation, the range and distribution
of socioeconomic status, and a multitude of perceptions, beliefs, and practices
forged from individual and group experiences.

Racism, Discrimination, and Violence

Racism, discrimination, and violence have been significant or central to the experience of all the major "minority" ethnocultural groups in the United States,
as well as for some European American subgroups. Native Americans have
been subjected to systematic murder, dislocation, appropriation of land, and
slavery, as well as to violent suppression of culture that included forcible sep-

aration of young children from their parents and the imposition of "civilized white" culture and religion (Tafoya & Del Vecchio, 1996). African Americans were transported to the United States under unspeakably brutal circumstances into the state of slavery. Emancipation was followed by systematic discrimination, racism, and violence that continue to this day (Black, 1996). For many individuals in other groups as well, racism, discrimination, and violence, both institutional and personal, *de facto* and *de jure*, are daily and lifelong, personal and/or historical facts of life. As one of a multitude of examples, during World War II, 120,000 Japanese American men, women, and children, both citizens and noncitizens, were interned in geographically remote concentration camps. The consequences included not only total dislocation and incarceration under harsh circumstances but also immense losses of property and means of livelihood that remain largely uncompensated (Daniels, 1971; Matsui, 1996).

The attitudes, institutions, and consequences associated with these historical events have also had a profound effect on European Americans. Considering only the more individual issues, unconscious and overt prejudice and stereotyping, fear, guilt, and limitations in understanding the experiences and world view of other groups are, to greater or lesser extent, the inevitable consequences of growing up and living in a society in which racist attitudes and institutions have such a significant role (Batts, 1990; McIntosh, 1998; Pinderhughes, 1989).

Racism, discrimination, and violence result in reduced educational and economic opportunities, poverty, self-doubt and self-denigration, and the destruction of lives, families, and communities. In response to these circumstances, a variety of adaptive family and community resources and structures have developed, as well as ways of viewing the dominant culture and its members. For example, for African Americans, strong community, religious, and extended family support systems help mitigate against forces that have suppressed or forcibly disrupted the nuclear family (McAdoo, 1997). The emotionally expressive, contextually rich communication style may have its origins in African speech and song. But it has evolved under circumstances in which the overt expression of emotions in the presence of European Americans could result in violence or death and in which sensitivity to covert expressions of racism by European Americans was a critical survival skill (Pinderhughes, 1989). The resulting differences in communication patterns can be a source of major misunderstanding. In one direction, the expressive nature of African American speech may be interpreted by European Americans as threatening or as involving an inappropriate introduction of emotions into a factual discussion. In the other direction, the relatively flat delivery of European American speech, with its greater reliance on specific word content, may be perceived as avoiding the issue at hand, substituting empty words for feelings and action, or disguising racist attitudes. With a 350-year history of racism and conflicted "race relations," these differences can evoke strong emotions (Sue & Sue, 1990).

Many African Americans have an appropriate and adaptive distrust of the motives and intentions of individual European Americans and the institutions of the dominant culture (Boyd-Franklin, 1989; Rapp, 1993a). At the individual level, this distrust may involve a period of "testing" at the beginning of a genetic counseling session, in which the counselee or counselees make careful, sometimes probing or provocative assessments of the willingness of the genetic counselor to accept their presentation of the issues and their modes of communication and expression (Pinderhughes, 1989). At the institutional level, the predominant experiences may be of discriminatory, authoritarian institutions and processes, including the welfare, police, and judicial systems as well as those involving health care (Telfair & Nash, 1996).

More specifically relevant to genetic counseling, many African Americans are acutely aware of discriminatory, harmful medical research and public health policies. The preeminent example, well known within the African American community (Duster, 1990; Jones, 1993; Rapp, 1993a), is the infamous United States Public Health Service–sponsored "Tuskegee experiment," so called for the county seat of Macon County, Georgia, where it was conducted. From 1932 to 1972, 399 poor, rural, uneducated African American men with syphilis were "studied" to determine the "natural course" of untreated syphilis infection. The study involved numerous deceptions including the nature of the investigation, the subjects' medical diagnosis, the intent to perform autopsies upon death, and the withholding of medical treatment including penicillin when it became the treatment of choice. The policy of deliberately withholding treatment was implemented by the physicians directly involved in the study and imposed by the United States Public Health Service upon local African American and European American doctors, public health programs administered by the Alabama Health Department in Macon County and in the city of Birmingham 100 miles distant, and the U. S. Army draft board. While scientific reports were regularly published in the medical literature and the first was read at the annual meeting of the American Medical Association in 1936, as many as a third of the subjects died through the direct, agonizing, end-state cardiovascular or central nervous system effects of the disease (Jones, 1993).

There are other examples affecting members of many ethnocultural groups, for example, involuntary sterilization of women from various minority groups (Nsiah-Jefferson, 1993) and research projects in which prisoners, military personnel, or poor individuals, overrepresented by members of minority ethnocultural groups, were the subjects of inappropriately informed or executed research. In the 1970s, many states enacted legislation concerning sickle cell carrier testing that was ill-conceived and discriminatory. In many instances these policies led to individual and institutional confusion between carrier and affected status, and to medically and socially unwarranted employment and insurance discrimination (Bowman, 1977; Hill, 1994). Thus, the burden of proof may lie with the genetic counselor to demonstrate the appropriateness, effectiveness, and nondiscriminatory nature of the medical genetic services that are offered and to acknowledge and address historically based suspicion and fears.

Discrimination, violence, and other forms of oppression have also been the experience of individuals belonging to other groups including women, gays and lesbians, and the physically and mentally handicapped. The culture and sense of individual and group identity of individuals in these and other relevant groups have thus also been influenced by and developed in response to these social and historical experiences.

Immigration and Acculturation

Immigration is a historical reality for all ethnocultural groups. This includes Native Americans, who were forcibly exiled from their native lands into government-controlled reservations that in some instances were hundreds or even thousands of miles distant. For some ethnocultural groups, recent and continuing immigration is the experience of a significant proportion of the current population. In 1996, approximately 38% of Hispanic Americans in the United States were foreign born (U. S. Bureau of the Census, 1998), and most of the immigration from Vietnam, Cambodia, and Laos has occurred since the end of the Vietnam War in 1976 (Lew, 1990).

Emigration precedes immigration, and the severing of physical and emotional ties to the country of origin is one of the central experiences of the process. The events and circumstances prior to physical departure are often complex and may have an important bearing on adaptation in the new country. Economic deprivation, violence, political repression, and forced evacuation may contribute to the decision to emigrate. Some members of a family or social group may have relatively great influence or authority in making the decision. For others, including children and sometimes wives or older parents, there may be little or no choice concerning emigration, or, conversely, the need to remain behind (Falicov, 1998; Berry, 1997).

The loss of cognitive and emotional sources of meaning and identification in the country of origin may be unsettling or traumatic. Familiar and loved people, sights and sounds, foods and holidays, ways of interacting, language and shared world view, which all support a sense of competence, orientation, and emotional connectedness, are to greater or lesser extent lost. The impact is likely to be greatest on older members of the emigrating generation. For them, maintaining language, customs and beliefs, cultural contacts and participation, and the hope or dream of return to the country of origin may be particularly essential to maintaining mental health (Jalali, 1988; Lynch, 1998a).

For many individuals, including contemporary immigrants from Southeast Asia and Central America, immigration was preceded or accompanied by violence and loss. Severe economic deprivation, civil war, systematic murder and torture, rape, and wholesale killing of families may have occurred in the country of origin or at intermediate locations during migration (Lew, 1990). Violence, robbery, and rape may occur during entry or upon arrival (Falicov, 1998). Great sensitivity must be used when there is the possibility that counselees have had such experiences. Inquiries concerning family history and pedigrees may evoke exceedingly painful memories and emotions. Even when all family members survived, the loss of contact with and information about those who did not immigrate may be very painful.

Many factors determine the nature and magnitude of the changes involved. Individuals and families vary immensely in the economic and social resources with which they enter the new country, including whether the family is intact or fragmented and the degree of empowerment or loss of control that is experienced concerning the act of immigration (Falicov, 1998). Other factors include the nature and extent of differences between the new and old cultures and languages, experience with the new language and culture prior to immigration, the availability of an ethnocultural community in the new country, and the attitude of members of the new country toward the immigrant's ethnocultural group and toward immigration and immigrants in general (Jalali, 1988). For many new immigrants and ethnocultural groups, economic hardship or poverty is their lot.

Initially, a general sense of disorientation and lack of competence is a common experience, in which even the most simple or fundamental activities require new learning and understanding. Again, older members of the immigrating generation are likely to be most affected. Those who immigrate as children or adolescents, or who are born in the new country, face different circumstances. Whatever their identification with the old culture, they do not have the same lived experience of the country of origin. They are also likely, by exposure and developmental flexibility, to be more fully integrated into the new culture. For them, the concurrent pulls of the two cultures may be intense and lead to difficult issues of loyalty and identity (Lynch, 1998a).

The process of acculturation is multidimensional. A given individual may integrate some elements of the new culture relatively readily, while others, owing to lack of exposure, difficulty of assimilation, and/or desire to retain old ways, are subject to limited change (Anderson et al., 1993). Family members may differ significantly, as when the husband works in the larger community, the wife stays at home in the local community, and the children attend school. Intergenerational stresses and conflicts are common, involving issues such as demonstrations of respect toward adults, gender role expectations, dress, sexual and romantic relationships, and choice of marital partner. In cultures based on a hierarchical relationship between the generations, the more rapid acculturation of the children may cause a disruptive inversion of generational interactions. For example, a parent may experience shame and a sense of being disrespected when the child acts as interpreter in the new language or demonstrates greater facility with money or the public transportation system (McGoldrick, 1989).

Marital and couple relationships may also be stressed by the gender role and marital expectations of the new culture. Men from cultures that value male authority and responsibility may feel particularly threatened or disempowered if they experience a loss of authority and respect in many areas of their lives in addition to the couple relationship (Falicov, 1998). The retention of elements of the old culture over long periods of time and multiple generations leads to complicated cultural patterns that can create both adaptive flexibility and stress (Berry, 1997). Couples and marriages involving individuals from different cultures require that cross-cultural issues be addressed and negotiated within intimate relationships (Crohn, 1998). The children of such relationships may have complex issues of self-definition and ethnocultural identity.

It is essential that genetic counselors appreciate the temporal, interpersonal, and cultural complexity of acculturation and cross-cultural interactions. The concept of "acculturation" should not be treated as a unidimensional metric used to assess or predict the counselee's understanding and acceptance of Western medicine or any other specific issue relevant to genetic counseling (Wang & Marsh, 1992; Anderson et al., 1993). A multitude of relevant issues may arise in genetic counseling, including perceptions of disabilities and risks; the individual, family, and social resources that are available to cope with difficult situations; attitudes toward and use of both traditional and Western medicine; and issues concerning who should participate in decision making and the interpersonal dynamics involved (Greb, 1998). As the preceding discussion demonstrates, when these issues arise in genetic counseling they may have a depth and intensity grounded in the profoundly significant issues of identity, adaptation, and survival that are a consequence of the historical and social experiences of individuals and families in any ethnocultural group.

A Southeast Asian couple was referred to prenatal diagnosis counseling for advanced maternal age. The husband had been in the United States 12 years, spoke excellent English, was financially secure, and wished to obtain amniocentesis for his wife. The wife had immigrated two years previously and spoke limited English. Although confused and concerned about the nature of the clinic visit, she indicated a desire to have a "medical test" that would help determine if her baby was normal. On the previous evening, her mother, who lived in the home, had first instructed and then implored her not to attend the clinic, stating that it would bring bad luck to the pregnancy. The husband felt the decision should be up to his wife and himself. The wife was far more ambivalent. On the one hand, she wished to comply with her husband's beliefs about who should make the decision, which she saw as part of his generally successful, secure, moderately acculturated life. On the other hand, she retained a strong sense of filial obedience, based both on the culture she had only recently left and on a sense of obligation to her mother, whose efforts had made their immigration possible. Multiple issues related to acculturation, immigration, family relationships, and health care beliefs influence this couple's decision-making process.

Institutional and Social Barriers to Services

Barriers to services also occur at institutional and societal levels, many related to low socioeconomic status, poverty, or immigrant status (Greb, 1998). Language barriers may extend beyond direct conversation to include a lack of written materials in the counselee's language concerning genetic counseling services, specific procedures and disorders, or informed consent (Mittman, 1990). For this and many other reasons, individuals and communities may lack information or have misinformation about clinical genetics and genetic counseling (Mittman, 1998; Rapp, 1998). Physical access to services may be limited by distance and isolation in rural areas, exacerbated by poverty, unreliable or nonexistent means of personal transportation, and poor or absent public transportation (Gettig et al., 1987; Telfair & Nash, 1996). In urban areas, comparable barriers arise when a lack of personal transportation is coupled with public transportation that is inadequate or absent, unfamiliar to counselees, or not useful because of clinic location. Equally constraining, clinic hours may not accommodate counselees who have low status jobs from which they cannot take time off without an unacceptable loss of income or a threat or certainty of job loss (Mittman et al., 1998).

Many poor, low income, and immigrant individuals have neither private nor government-sponsored health insurance. Even with insurance, there may be limited coverage of services or limitations with respect to participating health care professionals and clinics (Nsiah-Jefferson, 1993). Use of medical services may be largely confined to emergency rooms or to public clinics in which services are limited or fragmented (Telfair & Nash, 1996). Prenatal care may not begin until late in pregnancy (Lemke et al., 1998). For all these reasons, counselees may fail to receive timely information or referrals for genetic screening, medical genetics, and genetic counseling. When referrals are made to counselees, the impediments to obtaining services may lead to failure to follow through. When referrals are acted upon, counselees may have little or no information or understanding of either the reason for the referral or the nature of the services that are available (Mittman, 1998).

In her investigation of prenatal diagnosis counseling provided to the heterogeneous populations served by public and private clinics in New York City, Rapp (1993a) found that the quality of service was a major determinant of counselee responses. Acceptance rates for amniocentesis among African American and Hispanic American women varied widely among institutions. Discussing the disparate acceptance rates at two clinics she states,

> We could go fishing for a cultural explanation about pregnancy beliefs, or medical attitudes. A simpler observation, however, is this: The first prenatal clinic is a stable and welcoming environment; women tend to be very comfortable there, and to trust the nurses. By the time they arrive for an appointment with a genetic counselor, they have usually talked with a favorite nurse, often in Spanish, and feel competent to accept or reject the test. In contrast, the second hospital has been a site of struggle over services for many years, and the prenatal clinic is a difficult environment in which to receive health care. Women (and often their young children) feel imprisoned in uncomfortable waiting rooms where they routinely spend 2–3 hours before being seen. By that time, the level of anger and frustration, as well as the lack of communication, makes it much more likely that a woman will break a counseling appointment, or sit through it in a state of distrust. (p. 186)

Genetic counselors can help alleviate institutional and social barriers: by understanding the limitations under which many counselees attempt to obtain services, by providing direct assistance and support where appropriate, by working to change institutional policies and procedures, by collaborating in the development of clinical programs and sources of financial support, by providing community outreach, and by addressing the broader issues through social and political activities.

> A monolingual Hispanic family whose seven-year-old son had a provisional diagnosis of Duchenne muscular dystrophy was referred by a local clinic in the family's rural community 80 miles from the genetics clinic. The family did not arrive for two sequential clinic appointments. Each time a family member telephoned several days later, with the help of a bilingual acquaintance, to explain that their car had broken down. Although the genetic counselor cognitively understood the plausibility of this explanation, she also recognized growing feelings of annoyance and distrust concerning the "failed" appointments and the repetitive explanation. On the third appointment, which the genetic counselor felt was a "last chance or last try," the family arrived on time. They expressed their appreciation for the genetic counseling services that were available for their son, about whom they were very concerned. They were accompanied by the child's teacher, who had taken an unpaid day off from work to drive them and who told the genetic counselor that she too was very concerned for the boy's well-being.

Ethnocultural Self-awareness

Awareness of one's own ethnocultural identity, values, and circumstances is essential to providing informed, sensitive, culturally appropriate genetic counseling. Such ethnocultural awareness is central to a number of interrelated issues. First, as with psychosocial issues, sensitivity and empathy are more genuinely available when the genetic counselor has acknowledged and addressed the emotional impact of comparable events and circumstances in her own life. For example, a consideration of the immigration experiences of one's own family will provide a deeper understanding of the counselee's relevant experiences, even when the circumstances and passage of time differ greatly. Second, examination of one's own ethnocultural identity, culture, and history is essential to recognizing the values, assumptions, limitations, stereotypes, and biases that are the inevitable underpinnings of one's own world view (Ota Wang, 1994; Rauch & Curtiss, 1992). As Lynch (1998, p. 497) states: "Until one understands the impact of his or her own culture, language, race, and ethnicity on attitudes, beliefs, values, and ways of thinking and behaving, it is not possible to fully appreciate the cultures of others. . . . Thus, examining one's own roots is the place to begin any journey toward increased cross-cultural competence."

At a more fundamental level, ethnocultural self-awareness is essential to the premise stated in the introductory section of this chapter: Ethnocultural issues and cross-cultural counseling must be approached in terms of the intersection between the ethnicity and culture(s) of the genetic counselor and those of the counselee, in contrast to a unidirectional consideration of the counselee's ethnicity and culture. Genetic counseling takes place within the sociopolitical structures and institutions of the dominant culture. It is physically located in clinics or hospitals that embody the premises and practices of Western medicine. It is based on the concepts, information, and procedures of clinical genetics and genetic counseling. And the cultures of the genetic counselor and other medical staff members predominate within the counseling session. It is only through ethnocultural self-awareness that the genetic counselor can understand, at least in part, the impact of these multiple forms of "legitimated power" (Wang, 1993, p. 13) upon the counselee, and thus appropriately address the counselee's needs within the context of his or her ethnocultural values, beliefs, and experiences (Fadiman, 1997; Greb, 1998).

Areas of Ethnocultural Self-awareness

Self-exploration and the development of ethnocultural self-awareness are lifelong processes that involve many sources of information, guidance, and insight. All aspects of culture and ethnocultural experience discussed in the previous sections are potentially relevant, and the many components are highly interrelated. The following questions provide one way of approaching such exploration (Greb, 1998; Lynch, 1998b; Wang, 1993).

Ethnocultural identity
- How do you define your ethnocultural identity in terms of country or countries of origin, language, ethnicity, race, religion, and socioeconomic status?
- How uniform versus mixed are you and your family with respect to each of these characteristics?
- How strongly do you identify at present with each of these characteristics? That is, do you speak the language or languages of your forebears; do you identify yourself as having the ethnicity of your forebears, etc.?
- What ceremonies, customs, holidays, foods, and social practices do you or your family practice or retain that reflect your ethnocultural origins and identity?
- What other characteristics such as sex, sexual orientation, disability, or professional training are important to your sense of self-definition and place in the social order?

Immigration and acculturation
- When did you or your family immigrate to your present country of residence?
- How many generations have passed since immigration? What "generation" of immigrant do you consider yourself (i.e., first, second, "$2^1/_2$," etc.)?
- What were the circumstances that led to emigration and immigration?
- Were emigration and immigration voluntary or involuntary? How do you define "voluntary" and "involuntary" for these purposes?
- What information do you and your family have concerning the process of establishing yourselves in your present country of residence?
- What stories or family myths do you and your family have concerning the process of establishing yourselves in your present country of residence?
- How much contact or affiliation do you retain with your country of origin, including family who remained there? Have you visited your country of origin?
- What aspects of your ethnicity and culture are/were helpful or supportive in establishing yourself or your family in your present country of residence?
- What aspects were impediments or made the process more difficult?
- How do/did the attitudes and behaviors of people in your country of residence toward individuals with your ethnocultural identity affect you or your family?
- How do/did the institutions and laws in your country of residence relevant to individuals with your ethnocultural identity affect you or your family?

World view: values and beliefs

- What do you define as the central or most important beliefs, attitudes, behaviors, and values of your world view?
- How do you describe your world view with respect to issues such as the nature and importance of interpersonal relationships, attitudes toward nature and natural phenomena, and the meaning and passage of time?
- How and to what extent is your world view influenced by that of your family?
- How and to what extent is your world view influenced by the ethnocultural group(s) with which you identify?
- What do you consider to be the strengths or positive aspects of your world view and that of your ethnocultural heritage?
- What do you consider to be the weaknesses or negative aspects of your world view and that of your ethnocultural heritage?
- How does your world view influence your perceptions of and interactions with individuals from other ethnocultural groups?
- How does your world view influence your work as a genetic counselor?

Racism, Oppression, and Power

Racism is pervasive in the culture and history of the United States, and it is a major factor in many other countries as well. Racism involves the exploitation, oppression, and domination of one ethnocultural group by another through unequal access to power, resources, and political representation. This is implemented and maintained through a multitude of interlocking individual, institutional, and legal mechanisms, which often include various levels of official and unofficial violence. In its overt forms, racism is based on explicit assumptions about the cultural, biological, cognitive, and/or moral superiority of one ethnocultural group compared to another. However, there are also many less overt forms of racism that involve the attitudes and behaviors of individuals who consider themselves to be unprejudiced or actively supportive of racial equality and civil rights (Rauch & Curtiss, 1992; Telfair & Nash, 1996).

Batts (1990) discusses five manifestations of these more covert forms of "modern racism":

1. Helping people of color under the assumption that they cannot help themselves or in a manner that limits their ability to help themselves.
2. Ignoring the impact of racism in a manner that blames people of color for their social and economic situation.
3. Avoiding interactions with people of color and opportunities to learn about conditions in their communities.

4. Denying physical, behavioral, and cultural differences and discounting the importance of culture and ethnocultural experiences.
5. Denying or minimizing the impact of differences in social, political, and economic power and resources on individuals and communities of different ethnocultural identities.

In addition, it is often difficult for people who benefit from the differential distribution of power and resources to recognize and acknowledge the many, far-reaching forms of privilege that they experience as a result (McIntosh, 1998).

These characteristics of racism are also relevant to other situations in which prejudice, oppression, and the unequal distribution of power and resources affect individuals and communities with identifiable characteristics such as sex, socioeconomic status, sexual orientation, and disabilities (Asch, 1989; Kliman, 1998). As with racism, these analogous situations may also involve both overt and covert attitudes, behaviors, stereotypes, and institutional barriers, often coupled with defensive denial by those who benefit from them of their existence and impact.

McIntosh (1995; 1998) writes movingly of how, in the process of attempting to address unacknowledged male privilege within the academic setting, she came to recognize comparable elements of white privilege from which she benefited.

> I have come to see white privilege as an invisible package of unearned assets that I can count on cashing in each day, but about which I was "meant" to remain oblivious. White privilege is like an invisible weightless knapsack of special provisions, assurances, tools, maps, guides, codebooks, passports, visas, clothes, compass, emergency gear, and blank checks. Since I have had trouble facing white privilege, and describing its results in my life, I saw parallels here with men's reluctance to acknowledge male privilege. (McIntosh, 1995, pp. 76–77)

As an exercise in self-awareness she listed 46 "special circumstances and conditions I experience that I did not earn but that I have been made to feel are mine by birth, by citizenship, and by virtue of being a conscientious law-abiding 'normal' person of goodwill." (McIntosh, 1995, p. 78). Among these were the following (pp. 79–80):

> I can turn on the television or open to the front page of the paper and see people of my race widely and positively represented.

> I can swear, or dress in secondhand clothes, or not answer letters, without having people attribute these choices to the bad morals, the poverty, or the illiteracy of my race.

> I can do well in a challenging situation without being called a credit to my race.

If a traffic cop pulls me over or if the IRS audits my tax return, I can be sure I haven't been singled out because of my race.

McIntosh's papers illustrate several critical points. First, there is frequently a strong, defensive denial of the existence of privilege by those who benefit from it through racism or other forms of oppression, and this denial is actively supported by the world view of the dominant group to which the individual belongs. Second, attaining increased self-awareness of this and other aspects of covert racism or other forms of oppression may involve an intense, painful process. Third, a given person may benefit from one oppressive situation (e.g., racism) while suffering the personal and group limitations and disadvantages of another oppressive situation (e.g., sexism).

These issues must be addressed if the genetic counselor is to provide ethnoculturally appropriate and sensitive genetic counseling. On the one hand, the genetic counselor's biases, stereotypes, and fears concerning individuals from other groups, as well as the privileges attendant on her group memberships, must be acknowledged and addressed. Without this, inevitable elements of covert, "modern racism" and its analogs will enter the genetic counselor's interactions with the counselee (Browner & Preloran, 1999; Greb, 1998). Equally important, an awareness of discrepancies in power and resources and of the many aspects of institutional racism and other forms of institutionalized oppression are essential to achieving an adequate understanding of the experience of counselees in the social world at large and in the genetic counseling process (Rauch & Curtiss, 1992).

Methods for Increasing Self-awareness

Self-exploration in the areas of racism and of ethnocultural identity, experience, and world view is a complex, ongoing process. Difficult emotions and discoveries concerning self and family may be involved (Akamatsu, 1998; Yamoto, 1988). On the subject of self-exploration of racism, Pinderhughes (1989, p. 73) states the following:

> [T]here is none of the levity and pleasure that characterize the search for ethnic understanding. Instead, the mood is one of discomfort, struggle, and pain. For Whites, the work requires breaking through the denial, projection, rationalization, and other defenses that have maintained the stereotypes and then enduring the anxiety and psychological pain they have served to ward off. For people-of-color it also means enduring the pain and anger which an exploration of racial dynamics inevitably mobilizes.

The topics and questions presented here provide limited direction for such efforts. More extensive discussions, suggestions, and questions for self-exploration can found be in Greb (1998), Akamatsu (1998), McIntosh (1995), Wang

(1993), Batts (1990), Pinderhughes (1989), and Randall-David (1989). Interactive classes or workshops as well as discussion and consultation with colleagues belonging to different ethnocultural or other groups can be very helpful. They can assist the individual in addressing the inevitable limitations to individual self-exploration due to culture-specific world view, psychological defenses, conflicted and frightening emotions, and the continuing presence of racism and other forms of oppression in the environments in which people grow up, live, and work. Whatever the approaches used, it is essential that the development of cultural competence be approached as a lifelong, career-long effort that requires humility as well as honesty and commitment (Tervalon & Murray-García, 1998).

Cross-Cultural Genetic Counseling Techniques

Despite the complexity of cross-cultural genetic counseling, certain general principles and approaches can be identified. In the most broad terms, these approaches use the psychosocial principles and practices discussed in the preceding chapters informed by the culture-specific information and understanding available to the genetic counselor. Underlying this procedure is the essential element of respect for the counselee and his or her culture and ethnocultural history and experiences.

Establishing and Maintaining Trust

Establishing trust, which is central to all genetic counseling (Kessler, 1979b), assumes additional importance when there are issues of different health care beliefs, practices, and expectations; shame at seeking professional help for family issues; unfamiliarity with Western medicine; or mistrust of Western medicine, genetics, or the institutions of the dominant culture (Daneshpour, 1998; Nilchaikovit et al., 1993). The genetic counselor should take time to greet each family member respectfully, beginning with those in the older generation. The use of surnames and the titles "Mr.," "Mrs.," and "Miss" or "Ms." will preclude erring in the direction of culturally inappropriate informality (Telfair & Nash, 1996). Even a brief period spent inquiring as to the family's general health, country or locale of origin, or experiences in reaching the genetics clinic will indicate the personal concern for the family and its well-being that is an expectation in many cultures. When members of the extended family or the community are present, their inclusion should be specifically noted, as an indication of respect for the counselee's definitions of family, interpersonal support, and potential breadth of decision making.

It is helpful, early in the session, to inquire as to the counselee(s)' understanding of the nature of the problem or situation, its possible causes if relevant, the reason for referral, and steps taken so far to address it. Allowing the counselee to tell his or her own "story" serves several purposes (Djurdjinovic, 1998). It demonstrates the genetic counselor's respect for the counselee's culture and world view as they influence understanding, expectations, and means for addressing the problem. The counselee's responses provide useful information about each of these issues, including how comfortable he or she is discussing these matters and revealing relevant information. This information then establishes the basis for potential further exploration. Counselees may be reluctant to discuss their beliefs or those of their culture concerning the causes of birth defects and genetic diseases, because they fear their beliefs will be dismissed or ridiculed. A respectful inquiry may help overcome such fears and, more generally, increase the sense of trust and openness.

Genetic Counselor: How does your culture understand what causes cleft lip?
Counselee (with considerable hesitation and embarrassment): Well, . . . some people in my country think it happens because the mother used a pair of scissors when she was pregnant.
[This is an indirect acknowledgment of belief.]
Genetic Counselor: So women in your country must try to be very careful about that while they are pregnant.
[This statement validates the significance of the belief. By using the word "try," the genetic counselor also implies that there may be inevitable, understandable lapses in behavior.]
Counselee (slightly more relaxed): Yes they do. But sometimes you forget.
Genetic Counselor (thoughtfully): Yes, that can happen to anyone. *(pause)* How do you feel about that explanation for your son's cleft lip?
Counselee: Well, my mother thinks that is what caused it. I look at things differently now that I have been in this country for three years, but it still worries me sometimes.
Genetic Counselor: It's perfectly understandable that you would still think about that. And you must also be concerned about what your mother thinks, especially if it means she blames you. This is very important, and we will talk about it more after I have explained how we understand what causes cleft lip.

By referring to the medical genetic etiology as "how we understand what causes cleft lip," the genetic counselor continues to validate the counselee's cultural beliefs, treats the issue as an intersection between two cultures, but also indicates that the services to be provided are based on different premises and understandings. (See further discussion later under Alternate Health Care Beliefs and Practices.)

Confusion or mistrust concerning the genetic counseling process should be addressed as early in the session as possible. Some counselees will require an explanation of the nature of genetic counseling and/or the procedures that will be followed (Wang, 1993).

Genetic Counselor: Your doctor was concerned that your child's problem might be caused by something that runs in your family. Sometimes that happens even though no one else in the family is affected. We don't know yet. But that is the sort of disease (or condition) that we specialize in here, so we may be able to give you some helpful information.

[By speaking in provisional language, the genetic counselor attempts to avoid undue initial shock or stigmatization while at the same time indicating the reason for the referral and the orientation of the clinic.]

Counselee distrust should be validated nondefensively, with an indication of willingness to present the case for the services that are offered.

Genetic Counselor (to an African American counselee who has expressed strong, explicit mistrust, citing "the shit they pulled at Tuskegee"): What happened at Tuskegee was terrible. And there are other reasons to be mistrustful too. Let me explain to you and your wife how we handle things here. Then the two of you can decide how it sounds, and whether we might be of help to you.

Pedigree and Family Medical History

Several issues may arise during the process of obtaining a pedigree and family medical history. Information may be unavailable or withheld because of shame, mistrust, lack of information, lack of medical diagnosis, absence of a relevant diagnosis under the health care beliefs and practices in the country of origin, concerns about confidentiality, or unfamiliarity with the relevance of a family medical history to medical treatment (Greb, 1998). Elements of family medical history or relationships may have been withheld or altered during the process of gaining entry to the country of immigration, as when an unrelated individual is reported to be genetically related to obtain entry. Counselees may be fearful of providing alternate, correct information, especially in an "official" setting (Lum & Whipperman, 1987). As discussed earlier under Ethnocultural History and Social Experience: Immigration and Acculturation, questions concerning family history may be very painful for counselees whose families have experienced severe violence or multiple deaths.

The process of obtaining an accurate pedigree and family medical history may be facilitated by scheduling it relatively late in the session, when there has been an opportunity to develop trust and answer counselees' questions. More specific steps can also be taken to help overcome potential impediments. For example, the genetic counselor should explain the relevance and importance of a family's medical history to the genetic counseling process, provide appropriate assurance concerning confidentiality, and give such detailed guidance as is needed concerning the types of information that are desired (Nilchaikovit et al., 1993).

Alternate Health Care Beliefs and Practices

It is very important that the counselee's culturally based health care beliefs and practices be acknowledged and respected. This acknowledgment is an important element in building trust and allowing the counselee to feel heard, understood, and respected and helps open the way for acceptance of the medical-genetic explanation and the services offered through genetic counseling (Cohen et al., 1998). As demonstrated in the example of cleft lip given earlier, such beliefs may be validated in terms of the counselee's own beliefs, in terms of "covering all bases" in a critical situation, and/or in terms of family and community cohesion and interactions. When the beliefs in question are of a religious or spiritual nature, such as "It is God's will," they can be accepted as representing a different level of explanation from that provided by clinical genetics: The religious/spiritual beliefs address the existential question, "Why did this happen to me and my family?", while the medical-genetic etiology provides a mechanistic explanation (Panter-Brick, 1992). This technique of distinguishing between the explanatory levels of religion and genetics is not without its limitations and potential problems, especially if a recurrence risk involving probabilities is to be presented. Nevertheless, I believe that the counselee's receptiveness to genetic counseling explanations and services is enhanced by the genetic counselor's open-minded acknowledgment and acceptance of the counselee's beliefs.

Some counselees, especially relatively new immigrants, may adhere to alternative beliefs, coupled with disbelief or distrust concerning the explanations and procedures of clinical genetics and genetic counseling (Mittman, 1990). In such circumstances, the best approach is to offer the services in the spirit of "how we understand" the disorder or circumstances and "the way(s) in which we can be of help to you." This was illustrated and discussed in the previous scenario involving cleft lip. This approach offers the services of the genetics clinic in terms of the assumptions and procedures involved without insisting they represent the only legitimate set of beliefs or health care practices. It respects the counselee's culture and beliefs but is equally forthright with respect to the nature of the services offered.

When the counselee is unfamiliar with human anatomy and physiology as they are understood by Western medicine, or with the concepts of genes, chromosomes, embryogenesis, etc. (Mittman et al., 1998), the genetic counselor must attempt to explain the relevant structures and processes without overwhelming the counselee with facts or concepts. Although care must be taken not to underestimate the counselee's ability to understand these concepts, simple explanations may be the most appropriate under such circumstances. In cases such as this, it must be kept in mind that the defining element of genetic counseling is the provision of useful services concerning genetic disorders and birth defects, not the provision of a scientific explanation at some given level of complexity.

> *Genetic Counselor (to a recently immigrated rural Cambodian couple whose infant has been diagnosed with hemoglobin E/α-thalassemia disease):* As we understand it, both parents pass a material along to the child that causes this disorder. It isn't one parent or the other alone, but the fact that both parents happened to pass it on to the same child.

It is important to be aware of beliefs and practices that may directly interfere with or be negatively affected by genetic counseling. For example, the belief in many Asian cultures that blood and other bodily fluids are vital and irreplaceable can lead to resistance to amniocentesis, blood draws for diagnostic tests, and blood transfusions (Mittman et al., 1998). As with other beliefs and practices, the genetic counselor should acknowledge the counselee's concerns and then explain Western medicine's understanding that these fluids are replaced naturally in a brief period of time and that the procedure has been used many times without ill effects of the sort that are feared. In a number of cultures, bad thoughts concerning a pregnancy are believed to cause birth defects. When this belief is held, great care must taken to avoid a disrespectful, counterproductive outcome. For example, when providing prenatal diagnosis counseling to Chinese Americans who retain traditional beliefs, the genetic counselor should avoid showing pictures of children with Down syndrome or at least inquire beforehand about the appropriateness of doing so. In discussing how a medically positive outcome might be received, the genetic counselor can pose the question in terms of a hypothetical family rather than explicitly with respect to the counselee(s) (N. Chow, 1998, personal communication). The broad prohibition in Navajo culture against thinking negative thoughts can lead to refusal of genetic counseling, ultrasound, prenatal diagnosis, and even prenatal care in which pregnancy risks are discussed. When such services are accepted, the discussion of risks that is required to obtain informed consent may be experienced as detrimental. Thus, careful evaluation of the counselee's beliefs is essential. It may be possible, with the collaboration of a Navajo healer, to combine genetic counseling and Navajo rituals related to positive thinking in a manner that is acceptable (Olney & Olney, 1993).

It is also important to be aware of and avoid social behaviors that are proscribed or considered harmful in a given culture. Examples include the belief among Southeast Asian cultures that a child's head is the seat of the primary soul and should not be touched (N. Chow, 1998, personal communication), and the prohibition in Hispanic culture against admiring, praising, or looking directly at a child without touching him or her, which can place a spell of *mal de ojo*, or evil eye, on the child (Lopez-Rangel, 1996).

Ethnocultural Expectations, Decision Making, and Nondirective Genetic Counseling

A quandary arises when the counselee's cultural expectations and experiences lead to a desire for advice, direction, or prescription that is at odds with the ethos of nondirective genetic counseling. For counselees from a number of cultures, the genetic counselor, serving as the medical professional, may be considered the appropriate authority in whom medical decision making is vested. These expectations may be part of a broad hierarchical approach to issues of authority and responsibility, the result of social and political forces that suppress individual autonomy, or relate more narrowly to expectations about decision making in medical matters. When the expected authoritative advice is not provided, the counselee may be left feeling confused; at a loss as to how to proceed; at risk of making a shameful, stigmatizing error; or denied the services he or she expects from a medical professional. Given expectations of directive counseling, the counselee may infer directiveness from a counseling approach that is intended to be nondirective. There may be a loss of trust and respect for the genetic counselor, who is perceived as incompetent, rude, or shirking responsibility. In some instances, the counselee may respond by seeking more culturally acceptable directive advice from family members, religious or community figures, other health care professionals or community healers, all of whom are presumably less knowledgeable concerning the genetics of the situation (Mittman et al., 1998; Rapp, 1993a; Wang & Marsh, 1992).

Situations of this sort raise major issues concerning cross-cultural communication, respect for cultural as well as individual values and autonomy, and the ability to obtain informed consent. Despite the complexities involved, I believe that the approaches discussed in Chapter 5 under Nondirective Genetic Counseling: Critiques of Nondirective Genetic Counseling provide a framework for addressing these issues. General guidance comes from the broad definition of nondirective counseling as a means for promoting counselee autonomy. From this perspective, it is counterproductive to adhere to a narrow definition of nondirectiveness that leaves the counselee feeling unsupported, unrespected, deprived of professional services, or with an otherwise diminished sense of efficacy and ability to act in accordance with cultural as well as individual values (Greb, 1998).

In terms of specific counseling approaches, the genetic counselor should begin by addressing the situation in terms of a counseling impasse, attempting to determine its nature and origins, and responding appropriately. Given the many potentially relevant psychosocial dynamics and great variability in the nature and extent of counselee acculturation, it is important to avoid prematurely classifying the impasse as resulting from cultural expectations for directive counseling. The genetic counselor should assess the relevance of other reasons for the impasse and address them appropriately. Two dynamics are particularly relevant in cross-cultural situations. First, the counselee may believe that a procedure for which she has been referred to genetic counseling, such as expanded alphafetoprotein screening or prenatal diagnosis, is mandatory. Thus, the counselee is confused when asked to make an independent decision (Mittman et al., 1998). This misunderstanding requires careful clarification that referral does not compel acceptance, which may be an unfamiliar concept for the counselee. Second, the counselee may feel under pressure to reach an individual decision when he or she feels that family members or other individuals should also be included in the process (Greb, 1998). If the counselee is unable to consciously articulate this concern, or feels constrained from doing so because of the perceived authority of the genetic counselor in requiring an individual decision, the counselee may request that the counselor make the decision. When this is the case, the time available for making the decision should be clearly articulated and provisions made for the counselee to include the other individuals in consultation or deliberation.

When the impasse appears to be based on the counselee's cultural expectations for directive genetic counseling, the best approach is to elicit, insofar as possible, the counselee's beliefs, values, fears, and concerns related to each of the possible options and then make a recommendation based on these. To the extent consistent with the counselee's cultural expectations, the genetic counselor should be explicit that this is a recommendation and that it is based on what has been expressed by the counselee. In so doing, the genetic counselor distances as much as is appropriate from a completely directive stance and introduces the idea of a decision grounded in the counselee's beliefs and values.

> *Genetic Counselor (to a couple referred for prenatal diagnosis counseling):* From what we have discussed, I can see that you are concerned about the possibility of a miscarriage. However, it seems that for you the most serious outcome would be having a child with Down syndrome or another severe detectable disorder. Based on that, I recommend that you have amniocentesis.

This approach has its limitations. The genetic counselor may misunderstand or misinterpret the counselee's values and concerns, thus making a recommendation that does not represent the counselee's most desirable or risk aversive course of action. In general, the greater the cultural and linguistic differences between the counselor and the counselee, the greater the possibility of this happening. Furthermore, the likelihood that the counselee will accept the recommendation despite a misinterpretation presumably increases to the extent that the counselee expects directive counseling or perceives medical decision-making authority to lie with the genetic counselor. Nevertheless, I believe this represents the most effective compromise between the counselee's culturally based need for an authoritative decision and the counselor's culturally based ethos of promoting a decision that supports counselee efficacy and autonomy and is as consistent as possible with the counselee's beliefs, values, and wishes.

A different culturally based situation arises when the locus of decision making is perceived to lie with a broader group of individuals than the single counselee or couple. In many such situations the inclusion of other individuals is a matter of cultural norms concerning the relationships among family members. Although the genetic counselor may perceive this broader concept of decision making as limiting individual autonomy, it may have important social and cultural roles. It may elicit and strengthen family and/or social supports, including a diffusion of responsibility for decision making. It may involve obtaining the advice or sanction of religious, spiritual, or community leaders or advisers (Foster, et al., 1999; Greb, 1998; Rapp, 1993a). It may also be based on fundamental aspects of world view concerning the relationship between the individual and larger social entities. As Wang and Marsh (1992, pp. 85–86) state,

> The concept of autonomy among the Asians springs from the perspective of a collective group, the family, rather then the individual, as emphasized in Western thought. Therefore, to refer to an individual's health and welfare independent of the health and welfare of the family unit would be out of context. . . . Understanding the phenomenon of shame and stigma is also essential in counseling and treating the Asian patient and accepting the notion of collective autonomy. . . . In Asian culture, dishonorable situations such as infertility and ill health diminish not only the individual but the entire family. Perceived failures may not be directly associated with the individual's conduct, but may be viewed as reflections of the family's collective conscience.

In general, the genetic counselor should support and facilitate the inclusion of other relevant individuals in the decision-making process. This may involve their inclusion in the counseling session, inquiries as to who else should be included or consulted, information and reassurance concerning the time interval available for making a decision, and/or referral or a suggestion to consult with religious, spiritual, or community leaders or advisers. However, tension or disagreement about decision making may occur among the individual counselee and her spouse, partner, or extended family, or among the couple and members of the extended family (Rapp, 1998). These tensions may arise within any culture, but they may also be related to differing degrees of acculturation into the dominant culture. Speaking to the primary counselee or counselees in a separate segment of the session or by telephone may help elicit such concerns and provide support for relatively greater individual or couple autonomy. These situations can generate strong countertransference. It is important to avoid unconscious, directive interventions that may have the effect of increasing tension for the primary counselee(s) or subjecting them to the possibility of social stigmatization or violence.

Working with Interpreters

When the counselor and counselee do not speak a common language, use of an interpreter is mandatory. However, even when there is partial cross-fluency, the use of an interpreter should be carefully considered. It is always useful for a genetic counselor to have some facility in the counselee's language. However, the ability to convey and understand the complex information and subtle psychosocial meanings involved in genetic counseling should not be overestimated. Comparable considerations arise when the counselee has limited fluency in the language of the genetic counselor. Furthermore, in highly emotional, anxiety-provoking, or crisis situations, individuals with limited fluency may experience a reduced ability to express themselves or to understand upsetting information in the non-native language (Haffner, 1992; Lum & Whipperman, 1987). When some family members can speak the language of the genetic counselor but others can not, those who can must assume the potentially conflicting multiple roles of interpreter, family member, and counselee (see later under Working with Interpreters).

Cross-lingual interactions are always cross-cultural. Thus, the interpreter has a critical role in determining how well or poorly technical information and concepts, subtle nuances of language and meaning, and other elements of culture and ethnocultural experience are communicated from the counselee to the genetic counselor and vice versa (Lynch, 1998b). The most effective interpreter is a bilingual, bicultural genetic assistant or counselor, who is a member of the genetics clinic staff or has experience working with genetic counselors. Training individuals to serve in this capacity is extremely important (Mittman et al., 1998; Dixson et al., 1992; Lum & Whipperman, 1987). When the clinic does not have the services of such an individual, a professional interpreter, preferably with medical experience, should be used if at all possible. When a professional interpreter is not available, great care should be taken in choosing, orienting, and working with the individual who will provide this crucial service.

A number of potential issues arise in using nonprofessional interpreters such as hospital or clinic staff, a member of the ethnocultural community, or a friend or acquaintance who accompanies the counselee. The individual may be unacquainted with the medical-genetic terms and concepts that must be conveyed. He or she may feel uncomfortable about or censor questions and information concerning personal matters such as sexuality and reproduction. The interpreter may have a personal agenda or personal beliefs and behaviors concerning cultural values or directive decision making that are inconsistent with nondirective, information-based genetic counseling. Censoring or altering information from counselor to counselee or vice versa, changing the emotional tenor in which statements are made, or making opinionated or directive statements to the counselee may result. The counselee may be embarrassed or inhibited about discussing personal issues under such circumstances or worry about confidentiality being maintained within the ethnocultural community. Communication and trust may also be compromised by differences between the counselee and the interpreter in age, sex, social class, position within the community or the country of origin, or involving regional, national, linguistic, or political divisions and conflicts (Fisher, 1996b).

There are additional complexities when a family member serves as interpreter. At the most general level, this requires the individual to be involved in two very different, potentially competing or conflicting roles: interpreter, with the need to understand and translate complex terms and concepts under conditions that may strain fluency and rapidity of translation; and family member/counselee, with the need to understand and process complex information, deal with difficult emotions, and participate in decision making. Specific family or couple relationships may also be affected. When a child or adolescent serves as translator, the discussion of intimate parental emotions, sexuality, and reproduction is either inhibited or revealed under circumstances that may be embarrassing, shame-inducing, or harmful to family relations. The child's greater proficiency in the language may also invert the generational hierarchy in ways that are shaming or embarrassing. When one spouse or member of a couple interprets for the other, couple dynamics are affected by the inequality introduced by the translator's ability to serve as "gatekeeper" of communication in both directions. This can be particularly problematic for the genetic counselor when the man is both translator and the apparently dominant member of the couple, since the counselor is severely limited in her ability to directly address the woman (Haffner, 1992; Wang, 1993).

The genetic counselor can help minimize these potential problems in two ways: by influencing the choice and use of an interpreter and by addressing relevant issues with the interpreter before or at the beginning of the counseling session (Fisher, 1996b; Greb, 1998). When the services of an interpreter are needed, all appropriate efforts should be made to engage a professional. If this is not possible, careful consideration should be given to the issues just discussed in selecting an individual to serve as interpreter. When, in the genetic counselor's judgment, the counselee's fluency is an issue or when one family member offers to serve as interpreter, the counselor should attempt to obtain agreement or permission to engage a professional interpreter. The most problematic situations occur when the counselee or family member construes the suggested use of an interpreter as questioning, criticizing, or challenging his or her language proficiency or role in the family. This problem is best addressed by stressing the other important roles and responsibilities the individual has for the family in the session, which he or she can more effectively exercise when the responsibilities of interpretation are left to another person.

Genetic counselor (to the English-speaking husband of a couple referred for prenatal diagnosis counseling): I know that you speak English very well. That's clear from our conversation. My concern is that you be able to give full attention to discussing the issues with your wife, so that the two of you can make the most appropriate decision.

A brief discussion with the interpreter at the beginning of the session may reduce or prevent later problems that interfere with the counseling process and may be time consuming as well. The genetic counselor should acknowledge the importance of the interpreter and thank him or her for providing the services. This helps establish rapport and a sense of working together. The genetic counselor should also inform the interpreter about aspects of genetic counseling with which he or she may be unfamiliar. These may include the importance of obtaining family information, the personal health and reproductive issues that may be discussed, the genetic counselor's concern with addressing psychosocial issues, and the intention to be nondirective with respect to decision making. It may be helpful to indicate the goals of the session, including limitations such as the fact that a decision need not be reached during the session (Lynch, 1998b).

Genetic Counselor (to a family friend who will serve as interpreter): Thank you so much for coming today. Your help is very important. I will need to ask some questions about Mr. and Mrs. Chan's family, as well as about whether they have had any miscarriages or stillbirths themselves. These are rather personal questions, but the answers are very important in trying to understand what is going on. They don't need to make a decision today—there is plenty of time for that later. But I do want to talk about the choices and how they feel about them, so they will have as much information as possible to help them make a decision.

Brief introductory comments to the counselee(s), through the interpreter, are also useful. These involve acknowledging the complications of using an interpreter, asking the counselee to please alert the counselor if something is confusing or unclear, and acknowledging the interpreter's services (Lum & Whipperman, 1987).

> *Genetic Counselor:* It's always more difficult when people don't understand the same language. I really appreciate that your friend is able to help us today by interpreting. I will go slowly and try to make sure that you understand what I say and that I understand what you say. But if something isn't clear, please let me know. That's the best way for me to be as helpful as possible.

During the session, primary attention and eye contact should be directed toward the counselee, to whom comments and questions are addressed. This establishes the primacy of the genetic counselor–counselee interaction. It also allows the counselor to observe and respond appropriately to nonverbal behaviors and interactions, thus reducing communication errors and encouraging emotional expressiveness. However, brief interactions with the interpreter are appropriate to clarify issues, indicate respect and appreciation, and avoid the interpreter feeling slighted or treated disrespectfully in the eyes of the counselee. The terminology and length of statements should be adjusted so that the interpreter is able to understand and translate them. If the interpreter appears to be altering or censoring communication or engaging in untranslated discussion with the counselee, the situation should be respectfully addressed with reference to the initial conversation with the interpreter. It is helpful if the genetic counselor knows some elements of the language, including statements that indicate lack of understanding. It is also helpful if the counselor is familiar with relevant medical-genetic terms in the counselee's language and can provide assistance to the interpreter if needed. It should be kept in mind that some languages may not have words for technical terms such as chromosome or prenatal diagnosis, and thus the interpreter must present a more extended explanation (Lynch, 1998b).

Discussion among health care providers can create discomfort or concern when the counselee is unable to understand. This may occur when the medical geneticist is discussing the case with the genetic counselor, during consultation or teaching involving more than one physician or other professional, and if the counselee or family are presented to a staff conference or other group such as a craniofacial or tumor panel. Under these circumstances verbatim interpretation or a summary explanation in the counselee's language should be provided. Professional interpreters should be asked to do this if they do not do so spontaneously. Nonprofessional interpreters who are unfamiliar with the medical procedures and terminology often need the assistance of the genetic counselor, who should give an explanation or summary to be translated.

Genetic counselor (to a family friend acting as interpreter): The doctors are talking about whether the baby's fingernails and toenails are as large as they would expect. That's not a major thing by itself, but it might help them understand why the baby has the more serious problems.

The need for interpreting and translating services does not end with the session. Letters and follow-up phone calls must also bridge the language barrier. In addition, if possible, educational materials, consent forms, and any other relevant written materials should be available at an appropriate reading level in the language of the counselee (Lum & Whipperman, 1987).

Reducing Institutional and Social Barriers

Many institutional and social barriers limit the provision of effective genetic services to underserved ethnocultural groups. Genetic counselors can make significant contributions through efforts to reduce such barriers. There are many published examples in which genetic counselors have had a major role in planning, obtaining funding, and implementing relevant programs and activities. These include, but are by no means limited to, direct services such as rural clinics (Gettig et al., 1987; Olney & Olney, 1993), urban clinics oriented to underserved ethnocultural groups (Lemke et al., 1998; Mittman et al., 1998; Punales-Morejon & Penchaszadeh, 1992), training and utilization of bilingual, bicultural counselors (Dixson et al., 1992; Mittman et al., 1998), community outreach (Lemke et al., 1998; Mittman 1998), training lay health workers and community-based care providers to enhance referrals for genetic counseling (Bridge et al., 1998), and the development of educational materials, clinic forms, and questionnaires in the language of counselees (Mittman et al., 1998; Simpson et al., 1994). Examples also include activities such as efforts to recruit and support members of underrepresented ethnocultural groups into genetic counseling (Smith et al., 1993), the training and education of genetic counselors with respect to ethnocultural issues (Ota Wang, 1998a; Punales-Morejon & Rapp, 1993; Wang, 1993; Weil & Mittman, 1993), research concerning ethnocultural beliefs and practices and means for improving services (Brensinger & Laxova, 1995; Cohen et al., 1998; Finucane, 1998a; Israel et al., 1996; Lemke et al., 1998; Mittman et al., 1998; Olney & Olney, 1993), national conferences (Biesecker et al., 1987; Goldstein & Biesecker, 1993; Mittman & Secundy, 1998b) and journal issues on ethnocultural issues in genetic counseling, (Biesecker, et al., 1987; Goldstein & McQuiston, 1993; Mittman & Secundy, 1998a; Ota Wang, 1998b), and conferences and communication concerning genetic counseling as practiced internationally (Kuliev et al., 1992).

Activities such as these involve professional opportunities to improve the equity and efficacy of genetic counseling and are consistent with the ethical principles and standards of practice of organizations such as the National Society of Genetic Counseling (NSGC) (National Society of Genetic Counselors, 1992) and The International Society of Nurses in Genetics (ISONG) (International Society of Nurses in Genetics, 1998).

8

GENETIC COUNSELING
IN AN EXPANDING
SOCIAL CONTEXT

G ENETIC counseling occurs within and contributes to a rapidly changing
world. Genetic concepts, information, and techniques have increasing importance in medicine, public health, and reproduction. There is a growing emphasis on the demonstrated or presumptive genetic contribution to a wide range
of human characteristics and behaviors, including such common sources of concern as obesity, depression, and attention deficit disorder. The Human Genome
Project exemplifies government and social commitment to pursuing information about the nature and role of human heredity. Yet this growing body of
knowledge, when coupled with developments in genetic screening and testing,
reproductive technologies, the genetic engineering of agricultural organisms,
and the cloning of mammals, has raised profound ethical and existential concerns. Some individuals have deep reservations about and resistance to these
rapid changes and the expansion of scientific and technological control into
new domains of life.

Detailed consideration of the broad range of medical, social, ethical, legal,
and practical issues raised by these developments lies beyond the scope of this
book. However, I do choose to address the relevant issues from two perspectives. The first involves the research and interpretations of sociologists and
other social analysts concerning genetic screening, testing, and prenatal diagnosis as they relate to reproductive issues. The second draws on the views of

individuals who are directly affected by genetic disorders, birth defects, and disabilities, either in their own lives or in those of their children. As with the assimilation of psychosocial and ethnocultural perspectives into genetic counseling, these viewpoints also broaden the range of human experience that is included within the theory and practice of genetic counseling (Kessler, 1980; Ota Wang, 1994).

Resistance to Genetic Screening, Testing, and Counseling for Reproductive Issues

The investigation of resistance to genetic counseling is important because it identifies values and world views that are seldom fully expressed in clinical settings. Beeson and Doksum (in press) conducted in-depth interviews with the family members of individuals diagnosed with or having carrier status for sickle cell disease and cystic fibrosis. These are the most common potentially lethal autosomal recessive disorders affecting African Americans and European Americans, respectively. Of particular interest were the family members' beliefs and practices concerning the use of carrier screening, prenatal diagnosis, and abortion of affected fetuses. Although the interviews identified many instances in which genetic services were accepted and utilized, the research focused on the less thoroughly investigated issue of resistance to the use of these services. This resistance involved "reluctance or refusal to use genetic testing as a basis for making decisions about partner selection or pregnancy". In analyzing the interviews Beeson and Doksum distinguished three categories of resistance based on family members' predominant beliefs and values. For the most part, these different forms of resistance were not correlated with ethnicity.

Religious values often led to resistance to selective abortion for genetic reasons. Some individuals who expressed religious beliefs did use prenatal diagnosis to prepare for the possible birth of an affected child. However, others rejected prenatal diagnosis. They saw no practical value in it other than selective abortion, which was inconsistent with their fundamental religious acceptance of the outcome of the pregnancy, whatever it might be.

Resistance based on *romantic love* was demonstrated by the belief that carrier testing and other practical matters should not interfere with the search for love and thus are inappropriate considerations in selecting a partner. However, individuals expressing these values often had no problem with using carrier testing for reproductive planning, with or without subsequent prenatal diagnosis and abortion.

According to Beeson and Doksum *experiential resistance* "is apparent among those who are, or in the past have been, particularly close to someone with a genetic condition. . . . [It involves] a moral commitment not to allow intimate relationships to be determined by genetic factors even when threats to health may result. Experiential resistance may be more apparent in deeds than words, reflecting embodied habits, perceptions, and values not easily verbalized". Although not closely related to formal religious beliefs, this set of values was often expressed in terms of moral or ethical principles supporting the unconditional acceptance of parenthood, children, and individuals with disabilities. It was also based on an understanding of the rich, multidimensional aspects of the affected individual's life and contribution to the family.

Several aspects of Beeson and Doksum's findings have particular relevance to the social context in which genetic counseling occurs and identify issues about which genetic counselors must be sensitive. First, family members who had had multiple interactions with genetic counselors or other clinical professionals often responded, early in the interviews, with rather abstract statements supporting the importance and utility of carrier screening and prenatal diagnosis. It was only as the interviews progressed and the interviewees described their own behaviors and interactions with family members that moral concerns and sources of resistance emerged. Thus, the clinical interactions they had experienced and their initial responses to the university-based interviewers inhibited the expression of beliefs and values discordant with a medical-genetic perspective. This finding suggests that, unless genetic counselors exercise relevant skills and sensitivities, such critical beliefs and values may go unexpressed or be actively withheld during genetic counseling.

Second, family members whose resistance was based on religious values or romantic love were able to express themselves in terms of social and moral concepts that have general acceptance in the dominant culture. In contrast, the interviews revealed that it was more difficult for family members to articulate and justify experiential resistance. Although there is social support for the intense emotions and experiences on which experiential resistance is based, there is not a readily available vocabulary or set of explicit moral principles with which to describe it. Thus, this type of resistance may require more sensitive exploration and articulation if it is to be adequately addressed in genetic counseling.

Third, the interviews indicated that experiential resistance was not based on ignorance of genetic risks, patterns of inheritance, or available testing and reproductive options. Instead, it grew out of rational consideration of values, moral principles, and lived experience. Beeson and Doksun conclude "Our data suggest that these family members are refusing to apply genetic criteria to future offspring, because to do so would be to deny the value of another significant part of their experience as family members." This suggests that genetic counselors must be careful not to attribute decisions and behaviors based on experiential resistance to counselees' ignorance or lack of concern. To do so seriously misrepresents the basis for these decisions and behaviors and thus limits the effectiveness of genetic counseling.

Fourth, resistance was often limited to specific aspects or applications of clinical genetics and genetic counseling. Examples included using carrier testing for reproductive decisions but not partner selection, and using prenatal diagnosis while ruling out selective abortion. Thus, what is involved is not a blanket acceptance or rejection of genetic counseling but, rather, careful and specific consideration of "just how far into private life this 'scientific rationalism' or instrumental rationality should extend." This suggests that attention to the limits that counselees place on the use of scientific instrumentality in the realms of family life and reproduction will facilitate more appropriate decision making.

Finally, Beeson and Doksum conclude that interviewees often expressed resistance by *not* seeking testing, *not* using test results in mate selection or reproductive planning, or *forgetting* or *not* communicating test results when they had the most relevance from a medical-genetic perspective. This interpretation suggests that genetic counselors must exercise caution in attributing resistant behaviors of this sort to "psychological defenses," "medical noncompliance," or even "beliefs and values." In making such attributions, genetic counselors may fail to recognize the essential elements of rational thought, moral concerns, and lived experience upon which counselees' resistance is based.

Similar research results and interpretations have been reported by others (Rapp, 1999; Hill, 1994; Lippman, 1994; Parsons & Atkinson, 1993; Rothman, 1986). Taken together, this work defines several broad interrelated areas of relevance to genetic counseling. First, there is resistance on the part of some individuals to the changes in values and world view involved in applying the scientific instrumentality of medical genetics and genetic counseling to partner selection, reproduction, and parenting. Second, some individuals feel that the reproductive quandaries created by genetic information and techniques extend beyond the difficult decisions themselves to include responsibility for defining the moral basis upon which such decisions are made. Finally, for some individuals, the reasons for resisting genetic counseling lie in emotions and experiences that are not readily articulated in terms of accepted vocabulary or frames of reference.

Critiques

The research discussed in the previous section is part of a larger body of investigation and analysis that is concerned with the social and ethical consequences of using genetic concepts and techniques to address issues involving reproduction and the occurrence of disease and disabilities. One area of concern involves the social contexts within which reproductive options are considered and the types of information upon which decisions are based. Genetic technologies provide increased opportunities for choice and control of reproduction. However, as the discussion that follows indicates, various factors may limit the choices that are considered to be acceptable, or they may introduce more fundamental limitations to the range of options considered or the manner in which decisions are reached (Stacey, 1997).

The institutional settings from which referrals are made or services offered may create strong messages. The fact that genetic screening programs and prenatal diagnosis are offered through departments of public health and provided in hospitals and medical clinics implies strong institutional support for the genetic definition of disease and disability, with a genetic-technological means for addressing them (Clarke, 1991; Press & Browner, 1997). Medical referrals based on the explicit or implicit assumption that screening or testing is the only appropriate, expected course of action may have a similar impact (Press & Browner, 1993; Rothman, 1986). The definition of "advanced maternal age" at a specific and essentially arbitrary point, such as thirty-five years, on the smoothly increasing age-risk curve implies a qualitative, scientifically identified change in status that merits a medical-genetic intervention (Bosk, 1993a; Lippman, 1994). On the other hand, if maternal age thirty-five is chosen because it is the age at which the probability of having an affected fetus exceeds the probability of a procedure-induced spontaneous abortion, then, as Markens and colleagues (1999) point out, the "risk" of "advanced maternal age" is as much a property of the test as it is of the counselee.

When procedures are described in predominantly technical terms, their rational basis and place within existing medical practice or public health is stressed while the emotional, social, and moral implications of their use are neglected or downplayed. A similar bias may occur in the discussion of reasons for questioning or declining their use. For example, when the possibility of a procedure-induced miscarriage is the major countervailing argument discussed during prenatal diagnosis counseling, the objective medical aspects of the procedure are again stressed in comparison with other reasons to consider whether or not to use it (Browner & Press, 1995; Press & Browner, 1993).

These potential sources of institutional pressure and limited consideration of options occur within a broader social context. There is constant media attention to new developments in medical genetics, a general increase in the extent to which genetic facts and concepts are invoked to explain a wide variety of health, behavioral, and even social issues, and a strong ethos of information utilization in some sectors of society. Consistent with this, there is a common expectation among individuals in some social/professional strata that amniocentesis and selective abortion will be used and are appropriate means for fulfilling both personal and social responsibilities (Kolker & Burke, 1994; Press & Browner, 1997).

A second aspect of this analysis concerns the ethical and moral issues confronting those who use these genetic technologies. The issues take a number of forms. For counselees who receive medically positive screening or test results, there are direct decisions such as whether to marry, have children, or continue a pregnancy. However, there are broader underlying concerns that often are characterized as moral in nature: the meaning of life, the nature of love and commitment, the social construction of disability (see next section), and the acceptability of genetic technologies with the information they produce and the dilemmas and responsibilities they create (Rapp, 1999; Sandelowski & Jones, 1996; Rothman, 1986). That this characterization is consistent with the views expressed by at least some women who have faced these issues is illustrated in the following quotations from interviews:

> While on the one hand I feel opposed to abortion and would tend to be open and accepting to any baby I carry, I am also aware of the incredible "burden" a severely defective child would be, and how reluctant I would be to take that on. . . . But . . . where do you draw the line? If there is *any* chance for creative potential do I have the right to take the life of a fetus? (Rothman, 1986, p. 70) (ellipsis points in original)

> It's not in me to make a decision about who lives. I don't think it is unnatural for people to be challenged emotionally or physically or mentally. What does seem unnatural is to try and engineer some subjective view of perfection. . . . I think disease prevention is fine. I think palliating symptoms is fine, but I'm against discrimination and I'm personally against abortion. I'm very, very much in support of a woman's decision to abort. I'm not at all in support of the medical community advising abortion on the basis of amniocentesis. I don't want to sound like I'm a proselytizing right to lifer. That's not where I come down on this at all. I understand that people would make those decisions. But I would want someone to make a decision knowing that there are alternatives available to them in the community for support, because I believe life has meaning. (Beeson & Doksum, in press) (ellipsis points in original)

To the extent that individuals draw on religious principles to address these issues or accept the medical-technological rationale for these interventions, they have the benefit of an organized and socially accepted system of moral values. However, for many individuals these systems are insufficient or unacceptable as guides, and there is little in the way of organized or articulated moral reasoning or authority on which to rely (Beeson & Doksum, in press; Rothman, 1986). In addition, a number of factors tend to put the burden of responsibility on the individual or the immediate family.

Ethical, legal, and procedural aspects of genetic counseling may have this effect. The emphasis on privacy and confidentiality tends to contain the discussion within the immediate set of counselees. The requirement for individual informed consent places the burden of choice, both practically and by implication, on the individual counselee. In addition, to the extent that technical aspects of the genetic diagnosis, potential interventions, and specific procedures predominate in the discussion, the emphasis is at the individual level, and broader social and ethical perspectives are underemphasized or overlooked completely (Bosk, 1993a; Rapp, 1988).

Nondirective genetic counseling, especially if it follows the nonprescriptive, value-neutral model, may reinforce the sense of isolation, because it does not provide social context or guidance (Beeson & Doksum, in press). Similarly, when counselee anxiety, confusion, avoidance, or resistance are conceptualized in terms of individual psychodynamics, their nature and causes are defined without reference to the social factors contributing to them (Rothman, 1986). As Rapp (1988, p. 108) states, "each woman is seen, and sees herself, as an individual patient rather than as a member of a larger group of women confronting a new technological possibility or coping with grief."

These aspects of genetic counseling occur, in turn, within the larger social context. This includes how issues of reproduction, disease, and disability are conceptualized and discussed, as well as the limitations in emotional, moral, and practical support given to the women who confront these issues and to the individuals whose lives are affected by disabilities. Rothman (1986, p. 189) summarizes her perception of the situation as follows:

> [The women who make these reproductive decisions] are the victims of a social system that fails to take collective responsibility for the needs of its members, and leaves individual women to make impossible choices. We are spared collective responsibility, because we individualize the problem. We make it the woman's own. She "chooses" and so we owe her nothing. Whatever the cost, she has chosen, and now it is her problem, not ours.

A final aspect of this analysis involves concern for what is perceived to be the growing hegemony of a technological-medical-genetic perspective in the conceptualization of issues and the methods used to address them (Duster, 1990; Lippman, 1994). This perspective includes reproduction, birth defects, and genetic counseling as discussed earlier. However, it extends to other medical and social issues, such as attention deficit disorder, academic performance, and violence. To the extent that the genetic component of these issues is overemphasized or attributed in a scientifically unsound manner, an inappropriately reductionist perspective is introduced, which may limit consideration of and support for environmental and socially oriented means for addressing these issues. In addition, as with any ascendant aspect of culture, the world view promoted by this perspective begins to be taken as fact, and unexpressed alternative viewpoints are no longer perceived to be missing. This is one reason that the critiques that have been discussed and the individual voices they represent have great importance (Beeson & Doksum, in press; Rapp, 1998).

A critical evaluation of this research and analysis lies beyond the present discussion (but see e.g., Parsons, 1997; Wertz & Fletcher, 1993). However, this work does identify important issues that affect genetic counseling at a number of levels. At the broadest level it draws attention to genetics and genetic counseling as agents of social change with profound influence on how pregnancy, reproduction, disease, disability, human variability, and social issues are perceived and addressed. Clearly, many who analyze, criticize, or resist these social changes do so from principled, thoughtful alternative perspectives, whether complexly articulated, as in the case of the writings cited previously, or primarily lived out in the perceptions, values, and actions of individuals who are directly affected. Furthermore, despite criticism or resistance toward the changes involved, there is general recognition of the scientific validity and medical effectiveness of genetic information and technology, coupled with broad support for the right of individual women to chose to use them (Lippman, 1993; Rapp, 1990).

These points of view should continue to be incorporated into the body of knowledge and perceptions considered integral to genetic counseling, in a manner analogous to psychosocial and ethnocultural perspectives. To do so is to assume greater responsibility for the socially transforming aspects of genetic counseling and the larger medical-scientific endeavor of which it is a part, commensurate with the concern given to its scientific validity. This responsibility in turn will more fully inform the internal development of the profession, public outreach and education, and the individual and organizational positions taken in response to legal, social, and public health issues.

In direct work with counselees the effectiveness of genetic counseling is reduced when the reasons for resistance or avoidance are misunderstood. If resistance to genetic instrumentality is misconstrued as involving only individual psychodynamic issues, ignorance, or vaguely defined "noncompliance," the possibility of fruitful engagement with individuals, families, and communities is reduced, as are opportunities to develop services that meet their needs.

These critiques also elucidate some of the limitations of a primary emphasis on technical information as well as in the concept of nondirective counseling. To the extent that issues of morals, ethics, and scientific instrumentality are not actively introduced by the genetic counselor when relevant, matters that are of fundamental importance to the counselee may be overlooked or avoided. I suggest that, when judged relevant to the counselee and the issues under discussion, these topics should be introduced into the counseling session. Again, there are analogies with psychosocial and ethnocultural perspectives. On the one hand, the genetic counselor need not be an expert on the specific issues, should not be an advocate for a particular position, and should confer with and refer to others when appropriate. On the other hand, knowledge, sensitivity, empathy, and experience in raising the issues and facilitating their exploration are the relevant counseling skills.

The issue of scientific instrumentality could be addressed by raising the issue when it seems relevant, asking appropriate questions, exploring sources of
information and perceptions, and inquiring about pertinent values and beliefs.
The following are examples of these approaches in the case of a couple considering whether to have amniocentesis following a screen positive low expanded alphafetoprotein result:

Genetic Counselor: Perhaps you are wondering whether you want the information that amniocentesis would provide.

Genetic Counselor: Some people are concerned about the moral issues they will
face if amniocentesis shows their developing child has Down syndrome. So thinking about whether they want that information is an important part of deciding
what to do. I wonder if questions like that are part of what you are thinking about?

Genetic Counselor: Is there anyone else, such as a trusted friend or your clergyperson, who might help you think about whether this is information you want
to bring into your lives, or whether it is more consistent with your values to continue your pregnancy without this information?

Concerns of this sort should also be added to the list of possible issues underlying the direct or indirect question, "What would you do?" (see Chapter 5
under Decision Making: *"What Would You Do?"*). A potential rephrasing of
the question in terms of this issue might be:

Please help me think about whether this entire approach is one I want to bring
into my life and pregnancy.

or more fundamentally

I am confused and troubled by an uneasy feeling about bringing this approach
into my life and pregnancy.

Several genetic counseling techniques may help alleviate feelings of isolation
and individual responsibility in the face of ethical and moral dilemmas. These
techniques include inquiry into who among family, friends, clergy, or others
might be of assistance; referral to another family who has faced a similar situation; and referral to a support group. However, the counselor might also ad-

dress this issue more directly in the counseling session, in a manner similar to other issues, including identifying or asking questions about the feelings that are involved and facilitating their expression and exploration. The genetic counselor may draw on her experience with other counselees in normalizing these feelings:

> *Genetic Counselor:* In my experience, many people, like you, have found that this decision brings up really difficult questions about what they believe in and how they want to live their lives.

However, as discussed earlier, feelings of isolation may also arise because the circumstances and contexts that create the sense of individual responsibility are unrecognized. Bringing these to consciousness might also be helpful. Thus, the genetic counselor might address the potential impact of confidentiality and informed consent as follows:

> *Genetic Counselor:* We are very careful in genetic counseling to protect your privacy and confidentiality. And for legal reasons, we must get your individual informed consent. But I want to make sure this doesn't stand in the way of your speaking to other people who might be helpful, or of our discussing whether there are ways you could get help and support with this difficult decision.

The genetic counselor might also address the broader social issues.

> *Genetic counselor (to a woman whose fetus has been diagnosed with trisomy 21):* One of the reasons it can be so hard to make the decision between terminating your pregnancy and having a child with Down syndrome is that there is not much social support to draw on. On the one hand, the message from society seems to be, "You made the decision to have amniocentesis, now you have to decide what to do with information that science has provided." On the other hand, there is limited support for families who have a child with a disability. There's nothing we can do about all that here and now. But I find it sometimes helps the people I work with to understand that these are some of the reasons that this seems like such a lonely process, with so much individual responsibility.

These approaches, while potentially helpful to individual counselees, do not address the underlying systemic issues. Indeed, critics might argue that, by alleviating pain and confusion at the individual level, the genetic counselor supports and sustains the status quo by reducing the pressures for change. However, I believe a counterargument is also potentially valid: By helping to bring these issues to consciousness for counselees, and through the genetic counselor's greater focus on them in her clinical work and professional development, increased awareness and motivation to advocate for change might also result.

The Voices of Individuals Affected by Genetic Disease, Birth Defects, and Disabilities

Those individuals whose lives are directly affected by disabilities also present important viewpoints. Their lived experience includes those disorders with which medical genetics and genetic counseling are concerned and those aspects of human variability to which genetic screening, prenatal diagnosis, and selective abortion are directed. They are members of a large minority group, comprising by some estimates more than 40 million people, or approximately 15% of the U.S. population. This group encompasses the broad spectrum of other demographic variables including sex, age, ethnocultural identity, socioeconomic class, sexual orientation, religious affiliation, and attitudes toward genetic screening, prenatal diagnosis, and selective abortion. However, because of both the causes and consequences of disabilities, this group is weighted in the direction of older age and lower socioeconomic status compared to the general population (Asch, 1989; Kaplan, 1993; Saxton, 1998).

Many of those who speak and write on these issues do so from the perspective of the disability rights movement. This movement arose in conjunction with other social-political movements of the 1960s and 1970s and builds, in part, on increases in health, mobility, communication, and life span that are the consequences of technological and medical developments. It involves a growing sense of community, a challenge to and rejection of many assumptions and stereotypes concerning individuals with disabilities, and social-political activism. The 1973 Federal Rehabilitation Act Amendments, which prohibit discrimination against disabled individuals in federally funded programs, and the 1990 Americans with Disabilities Act, which provides broad civil rights protection to individuals with disabilities, are examples of social and political change brought about in substantial part through the activities of individuals affiliated with this movement. In achieving these accomplishments and addressing the many social, political, and physical barriers they still face in the United States and elsewhere, Saxton states, "Today, many disabled people view themselves as part of a distinct minority and reject the pervasive stereotypes of disabled people as defective, burdensome, and unattractive" (Saxton, 1998, p. 375).

There are three major facets to the critique and analysis of prenatal diagnosis and selective abortion presented from the perspective of the disabilities rights movement. The first involves the quality of life of individuals with disabilities, as well as perceptions and stereotypes of individuals with disabilities that influence both popular discourse and public policy. Those who address this issue from this perspective speak passionately about the quality of life of many individuals with disabilities and the important contributions that individuals with disabilities make in many walks of life. Kaplan (1993, p. 607) states,

> [P]eople with disabilities are finding that, with advances in the availability of assistive technology, accessible environments, and appropriate social services, these [previously discussed] widespread negative assumptions are not necessarily true. For many persons with a variety of disabilities, their own experience of the quality of their lives is positive. Persons with very significant disabilities now attend regular schools, colleges, and universities where they receive advanced degrees, find challenging jobs, get married, and live fairly normal lives.

And Saxton (1984 pp. 307-308) writes:

> There is no doubt that there are disabled people who 'suffer' from their physical conditions. There are even those who may choose to end their lives rather than continue in pain or with severe limitations, but is this not obviously as true for nondisabled people who suffer from emotional pain and limitation of resource? [*sic*] As a group, people with disabilities do not 'suffer' any more than any other group or category of humans. Our limitations may be more outwardly visible, our need for help more apparent, but, like anybody else, the 'suffering' we may experience is a result of not enough human caring, acceptance, and respect.

This analysis extends to the parents and family members of individuals with disabilities. Both systematic and anecdotal data demonstrate that the complex effects of the birth and raising of a child with a disability span the spectrum from largely negative and disruptive to experiences of joy, richness, and even personal transformation (Retsinas, 1991). Authors representing the disabilities rights perspective argue that the many positive reports and self-evaluations should not be overlooked, underestimated, or dismissed as romanticized or rationalized accounts.

The second facet of this critique involves an analysis of the factors responsible for the *disabling* aspects of disability. At one level this involves distinguishing the effects of the inherent biological impairment or impairments from the limitations imposed by the socially determined lack of compensatory aids and the presence of physical or technological barriers. For example, the primary disabling aspects of paraplegia are seen to reside, not in the requisite use of a wheelchair, but in the technological limitations of wheelchair design, the economic impediments to obtaining good equipment, and the limitations to wheelchair use imposed by physical barriers and the absence of ramps. Each of these limiting factors, and many others, arise from social-political decisions concerning the importance to be accorded to the needs of disabled individuals and the resulting allocation of resources (Asch, 1989; Kaplan, 1993).

At another level, the more profoundly disabling aspects of disability are due to the social responses to individuals with disabilities. These include neglect, avoidance, hurtful or inept interactions, discrimination, prejudice, and stigmatization. Insofar as these are not counteracted with individual and social-political resources and responses, they can result in social isolation, reduced economic resources, and lowered self-esteem and sense of competence. This analysis can be extended to the difficulties involved in raising a child with a disability, in which limitations in financial resources and support, social acceptance and support, medical treatment and appropriate educational resources contribute to the burden imposed on the individual family (Saxton, 1988; Rothman, 1986; Zola, 1985).

In large part, the disability rights movement arose in response to, and has identified and attempted to address, these multiple aspects of the social construction of disability. From that perspective, insofar as prenatal diagnosis and selective abortion are presented and discussed in terms of a medical-biological model of disability, without reference to or exploration of the attendant social components, counselees are not provided the full context within which to make decisions about bearing and raising a child with a disability.

The third facet of this analysis addresses the broader potential implications of genetic testing and selective abortion on attitudes and policies relevant to individuals with disabilities (Asch, 1989; Saxton, 1998). There is concern that programs and policies that support the abortion of fetuses with abnormalities, when coupled with the expectations for "perfect" children that arise in response to genetic technologies, will reduce support for services that assist individuals with disabilities and parents who have affected children. These same factors may also lead to reduced acceptance of and empathy for human variability. At the same time, there is concern that the emphasis on genetic methods for reducing the birth of affected children will decrease support for medical, social, and economic programs that would more broadly improve prenatal care and reduce birth defects and childhood disabilities. And, as has been pointed out, sustaining and increasing support for individuals with disabilities is relevant not only to those currently affected but to the substantial proportion of currently unaffected individuals who will experience disability during their lifetimes as a result of injury, illness, or age.

These critiques and analyses are open to counterarguments, to empirical validation of the hypothesized effects on public opinion and policy, and to evaluation as a function of the nature and severity of different genetic diseases and birth defects. For example, issues related to quality of life, burden, and personal growth differ greatly between disorders such as Tay-Sachs disease or trisomy 13, on the one hand, and spina bifida, cystic fibrosis, or sickle cell anemia, on the other. However, these critiques and analyses introduce a perspective that has a number of important implications for genetic counseling. As with the issues discussed in the preceding section, they bring to genetic counseling perspectives from a highly relevant aspect of human life and experience.

Continuing and increasing contacts among genetic counselors, individuals with disabilities, and disabilities rights activists are of great importance (Asch, 1989). Such interactions provide an opportunity for genetic counselors to explain the purposes and ethos of genetic counseling. They allow genetic counselors to learn more about the lives of individuals with disabilities and their attitudes and concerns regarding genetic counseling. They also reduce the misunderstandings that exist on both sides and help bridge the differences in perspectives and agendas (Biesecker et al., 1996). In my experience, involving people with disabilities in the training and continuing education of genetic counselors, as well as meetings between genetic counselors and disabilities activists, are valuable and enlightening for members of both groups.

Prenatal diagnosis counseling and decisions concerning the information to be imparted under various circumstances should be informed and guided by the following factors:

- information and knowledge about the lives of individuals, and their families, who are affected by the disorders involved
- information about sources of social and educational support as well as laws pertaining to the rights of and services for people with disabilities (Asch, 1989)
- consideration of the extent to which lack of information, misinformation, or outdated information and stereotypes held by a counselee require addressing in order for there to be informed decision making and meaningful informed consent
- careful attention to countertransference issues, including the role of denial or avoidance of vulnerability and disability, stereotypes, and formative experiences (Saxton, 1988)
- careful attention to the manner in which both individual and institutional agendas influence the information provided and issues raised, including differences between preprocedure counseling and counseling following the identification of an affected fetus (Brunger & Lippman, 1995; Lippman & Wilfond, 1992)

Genetic Counseling: Content and Context

The preceding critiques and analyses are primarily concerned with prenatal diagnosis, selective abortion, and genetic screening related to reproductive decisions. In concluding this book, it is useful to redirect thought and attention to the full spectrum of clinical genetics and genetic counseling, which includes an ever broadening array of genetic testing, medical diagnosis and treatment, psychosocial support, assistance in decision making, advocacy, and referral. Each of these areas has its medical, ethical, legal, social, and practical issues, both current and emerging. In addressing these issues, two broad principles from the preceding discussion are relevant. First, the role of medical genetics and genetic counseling as agents of broad social change must be considered in its full complexity. Second, it is essential that the effects of clinical genetics and genetic counseling on the individuals whose lives they affect be carefully and empathically assessed, drawing on resources both within and outside the profession.

REFERENCES

Ablon, J. (1984). *Little People in America: The Social Dimensions of Dwarfism*. New York: Praeger.

Abromovsky, I., Godmilow, L., Hirschorn, K., & Smith, H. (1980). Analysis of a follow-up study of genetic counseling. *Clin Genet*, 17:1–12.

Ad Hoc Committee on Genetic Counseling (1975). Genetic counseling. *Am J Hum Genet*, 27:240–242.

Akamatsu, N. N. (1998). The talking oppression blues: Including the experience of power/powerlessness in the teaching of "cultural sensitivity." In M. McGoldrick (Ed.), *Re-visioning Family Therapy: Race, Culture, and Gender in Clinical Practice*. New York: Guilford, pp. 129–143.

American Society of Human Genetics, Social Issues Subcommittee on Familial Disclosure (1998). ASHG Statement: Professional disclosure of familial genetic information. *Am J Hum Genet*, 62:474–483.

Anderson, J., Moeschberger, M., Chen, M. S., Jr, Kunn, P., Wewers, M. E., & Guthrie, R. (1993). An acculturation scale for Southeast Asians. *Soc Psychiatry Psychiatr Epidemiol*, 28:134–141.

Applebaum, E. G., & Firestein, S. K. (1983). *A Genetic Counseling Casebook*. New York: Free Press.

Asch, A. (1989). Reproductive technology and disability. In S. Cohen & N. Taub (Eds.), *Reproductive Laws for the 1990s*. Clifton NJ: Humana, pp. 69–124.

Ayme, S., Macquart-Moulin, G., Julian-Reynier, C., Chabal, F., & Giraud, F. (1993). Diffusion of information about genetic risk within families. *Neuromuscul Disord*, 3:571–574.

Baker, D. L. (1998). Interviewing techniques. In D. L. Baker, J. L. Schuette, & W. R. Uhlmann (Eds.), *A Guide to Genetic Counseling*. New York: Wiley-Liss, pp. 55–73.

Bartels, D. M., LeRoy, B. S., McCarthy, P., & Caplan, A. L. (1997). Nondirectiveness in genetic counseling: A survey of practitioners. *Am J Med Genet*, 72:172–179.

Batts, V. A. (1990). An experiential workshop: Introduction to multiculturalism. In G. Stricker, E. Davis-Russell, E. Bourg, E. Duran, W. R. Hammond, J. McHolland, K. Polite, & B. E. Vaught (Eds.), *Toward Ethnic Diversification in Psychology Education and Training*. Washington: American Psychological Association, pp. 9–16.

Baty, B. J., Venne, V. L., McDonald, J., Croyle, R. T., Halls, C., Nash, J. E., & Botkin, J. R. (1997). BRCA1 testing: Genetic counseling protocol development and counseling issues. *J Genet Counsel*, 6:223–244.

Baumeister, R. F. (1993). Understanding the inner nature of low self-esteem: Uncertain, fragile, protective, and conflicted. In R. F. Baumeister (Ed.), *Self-esteem: The Puzzle of Low Self-regard*. New York: Plenum, pp. 201–218.

Baumeister, R. F., Stillwell, A. M., & Heatherton, T. F. (1994). Guilt: An interpersonal approach. *Psychol Bull*, 115:243–267.

Baumiller, R. C., Cunningham, G., Fisher, N., Fox, L., Henderson, M., Lebel, R., McGrath, G., Pelias, M. Z., Porter, I., Seydel, F., & Wilson, N. R. (1996). Code of ethical principles for genetics professionals: An explication. *Am J Med Genet*, 65:179–183.

Beeson, D., & Doksum, T. (in press). Family values and resistance to genetic counseling. In B. Hoffmaster (Ed.), *Bioethics in Context*. Philadelphia: Temple.

Beeson, D., & Golbus, M. S. (1985). Decision making: Whether or not to have prenatal diagnosis and abortion for X-linked conditions. *Am J Med Genet*, 20:107–114.

Benkendorf, J. L. (1987). Grieving and believing: Helping parents through imperfect beginnings. *Birth Defects*, 23(6):25–35.

Bennett, R. L. (1999). *The Practical Guide to the Genetic Family History*. New York: Wiley-Liss.

Bernhardt, B. A., Geller, G., Strauss, M., Helzlsouer, K. J., Stefanek, M., Wilcox, P. M., & Holtzman, N. A. (1997). Toward a model informed consent process for BRCA1 testing: A qualitative assessment of women's attitudes. *J Genet Counsel*, 6:207–222.

Berry, J. W. (1997). Immigration, acculturation, and adaptation. *Applied Psychology: An International Review*, 46:5–34.

Bibring, G. L., Dwyer, T. F., Huntington, D. S., & Valenstein, A. F. (1961). A study of the psychological processes in pregnancy and of the earliest mother-child relationship: I. Some propositions and comments. *Psychoanal Study Child*, 16:9–72.

Biesecker, B., Magyari, P. A., & Paul, N. W. (1987). Strategies in genetic counseling: II. Religious, cultural and ethnic influences on the counseling process. *Birth Defects*, 23(6).

Biesecker, B. B., Chen, L., Israel, J., Fine, B., & Mittman, I. (1996). Seeking common ground: Dialogue between disability rights & genetics. *Perspectives in Genetic Counseling*, 18(3):1, 8.

Black, L. (1996). Families of African origin: An overview. In M. McGoldrick, J. Giordano, & J. K. Pearce (Eds.), *Ethnicity and Family Therapy*. (2nd ed.) New York: Guilford, pp. 57–84.

Black, R. B. (1991). Women's voices after pregnancy loss: Couples' patterns of communication and support. *Soc Work Health Care*, 16(2):19–36.

Black, R. B. (1993). Psychosocial issues in reproductive genetic testing and pregnancy loss. *Fetal Diagn Ther*, 8(suppl 1):164–173.

Bloch, E. V., DiSalvo, M., Hall, B. D., & Epstein, C. J. (1979). Alternative ways of presenting empiric risks. *Birth Defects*, 15(5C):233–244.

Bloch, M., Adam, S., Wiggins, S., Huggins, M., & Hayden, M. R. (1992). Predictive testing for Huntington disease in Canada: The experience of those receiving an increased risk. *Am J Med Genet*, 42:499–507.

Blumberg, B. (1984). The emotional implications of prenatal diagnosis. In A. E. H. Emery & I. M. Pullen (Eds.), *Psychological Aspects of Genetic Counseling*. London: Academic Press, pp. 201–217.

Blumenthal, D., Heimler, A., Edelman, C., Engleberg, J., Feldman, B. D., & Sitron, N. (1990). A protocol for genetic counseling following abnormal prenatal diagnosis. *Birth Defects*, 26(3):157–160.

Bohart, A. C. (1995). The person-centered psychotherapies. In A. S. Gurman & S. B. Messer (Eds.), *Essential Psychotherapies: Theory and Practice*. New York: Guilford, pp. 85–127.

Bosk, C. (1993a). *All God's Mistakes*. Chicago: Chicago Press.

Bosk, C. (1993b). The workplace ideology of genetic counselors. In D. M. Bartels, B. S. LeRoy, & A. L. Caplan (Eds.), *Prescribing Our Future: Ethical Challenges in Genetic Counseling*. New York: Aldine de Gruyter, pp. 25–37.

Bowman, J. E. (1977). Genetic screening programs and public policy. *Phylon*, 38:117–142.

Boyd-Franklin, N. (1989). *Black Families in Therapy: A Multisystems Approach*. New York: Guilford.

Brensinger, J. D., & Laxova, R. (1995). The Amish: Perceptions of genetic disorders and services. *J Genet Counsel*, 4:27–48.

Bridge, M., Iden, S., Cunniff, C., & Meaney, F. J. (1998). Improving access to and utilization of genetic services in Arizona's Hispanic population. *Community Genet*, 1:166–168.

Browner, C. H., & Preloran, H. M. (1999). Male partners' role in Latinas' amniocentesis decisions. *J Genet Counsel*, 8:85–108.

Browner, C. H., & Press, N. A. (1995). The normalization of prenatal diagnostic screening. In F. D. Ginsburg & R. Rapp (Eds.), *Conceiving the New World Order: The Global Politics of Reproduction*. Berkeley: University of California Press, pp. 307–322.

Brunger, F., & Lippman, A. (1995). Resistance and adherence to the norms of genetic counseling. *J Genet Counsel*, 4:151–168.

Buckman, R. (1992). *How to Break Bad News: A Guide for Health Care Professionals*. Baltimore: Johns Hopkins University Press.

Bukatko, D., & Daehler, M. W. (1992). *Child Development: A Topical Approach*. Boston: Houghton Mifflin.

Burke, B. M., & Kolker, A. (1994a). Directiveness in prenatal genetic counseling. *Women Health*, 22:31–53.

Burke, B. M., & Kolker, A. (1994b). Variation in content in prenatal genetic counseling interviews. *J Genet Counsel*, 3:23–38.

Butani, P. (1974). Reactions of mothers to the birth of an anomalous infant: A review of the literature. *Matern Child Nurs J*, 3:59–76.

Caplan, A. L. (1993). Neutrality is not morality: The ethics of genetic counseling. In D. M. Bartels, B. S. LeRoy, & A. L. Caplan (Eds.), *Prescribing Our Future: Ethical Challenges in Genetic Counseling*. New York: Aldine de Gruyter, pp. 149–165.

Carrese, J. A., & Rhodes, L. A. (1995). Western bioethics on the Navajo Reservation: Benefit or harm? *JAMA*, 274:826–829.

Carter, B., & McGoldrick, M. (1989). The changing family life cycle: A framework for family therapy. In B. Carter & M. McGoldrick (Eds.), *The Changing Family Life Cycle: A Framework for Family Therapy*. (2nd ed.) Boston: Ilyn and Bacon, pp. 3–28.

Carter, R. T., & Qureshi, A. (1995). A typology of philosophical assumptions in multicultural counseling and training. In J. G. Ponterotto, J. M. Casas, L. A. Suzuki, & C. M. Alexander (Eds.), *Handbook of Multicultural Counseling*. Thousand Oaks: SAGE, pp. 239–262.

Chapple, A., Campion, P., & May, C. (1997). Clinical terminology: Anxiety and confusion amongst families undergoing genetic counseling. *Patient Education and Counseling*, 32:81–91.

Chapple, A., May, C., & Campion, P. (1995). Parental guilt: The part played by the clinical geneticist. *J Genet Counsel*, 4:179–192.

Chase, G. A., Faden, R. R., Holtzman, N. A., Chwalow, A. J., Leonard, C. O., Lopes, C., & Quaid, K. (1986). Assessment of risk by pregnant women: Implications for genetic counseling. *Soc Biol*, 33:57–64.

Chethik, M. (1989). *Techniques of Child Therapy: Psychodynamic Strategies*. New York: Guilford.

Chodoff, P., Friedman, S. B., & Hamburg, D. A. (1964). Stress, defenses and coping behavior: Observations in parents of children with malignant disease. *Am J Psychiatry*, 120:743–749.

Clarke, A. (1991). Is non-directive genetic counseling possible? *Lancet*, 338:998–1001.

Cohen, L. H., Fine, B. A., & Pergament, E. (1998). An assessment of ethnocultural beliefs regarding the causes of birth defects and genetic disorders. *J Genet Counsel*, 7:15–29.

Costello, A. (1987). Psychosocial management of patients in a fetal medicine and surgery program. *Birth Defects*, 23(6):62–74.

Crohn, J. (1998). Intercultural couples. In M. McGoldrick (Ed.), *Re-visioning Family Therapy: Race, Culture, and Gender in Clinical Practice*. New York: Guilford, pp. 295–308.

Dallaire, L., Lortie, G., des Rochers, M., Clermont, R., & Vachon, C. (1995). Parental reaction and adaptability to the prenatal diagnosis of fetal defect or genetic disease leading to pregnancy interruption. *Prenat Diagn*, 15:249–259.

Daly, M., Farmer, J., Harrop-Stein, C., Montgomery, S., Itzen, M., Costalas, J. W., Rogatko, A., Miller, S., Balshem, A., & Gillespie, D. (1999). Exploring family relationships in cancer risk counseling using the genogram. *Cancer Epidemiology, Biomarkers and Prevention*, 8:393–398.

Daneshpour, M. (1998). Muslim families and family therapy. *J Marital Fam Ther*, 24:355–390.

Daniels, R. (1971). *Concentration Camps USA: Japanese Americans and World War II*. Hinsdale IL: Dryden Press.

Darling, R. B. (1991). Initial and continuing adaptation to the birth of a disabled child. In M. Seligman (Ed.), *The Family with a Handicapped Child*. (2nd ed.) Boston: Allyn and Bacon, pp. 55–90.

Darr, A. (1997). Consanguineous marriage and genetics: A positive relationship. In A. Clarke & E. Parsons (Eds.), *Culture, Kinship and Genes: Towards Cross-Cultural Genetics*. New York: St. Martin's, pp. 83–96.

Denayer, L., Welkenhuysen, M., Evers-Kiebooms, G., Cassiman, J.-J., & Van den Berghe, H. (1997). Risk perception after CF carrier testing and impact of the test result on reproductive decision making. *Am J Med Genet*, 69:422–428.

Dixson, B., Dang, V., Cleveland, J. O., & Peterson, R. M. (1992). An educational program to overcome language and cultural barriers to genetic services. *J Genet Counsel*, 1:267–274.

Djurdjinovic, L. (1997). Generations lost: A psychological discussion of a cancer genetics case report. *J Genet Counsel*, 6:177–180.

Djurdjinovic, L. (1998). Psychosocial counseling. In D. L. Baker, J. L. Schuette, & W. R. Uhlmann (Eds.), *A Guide to Genetic Counseling*. New York: Wiley-Liss, pp. 127–166.

Driscoll, P. T. (1986). Early adolescence: Identity formation. In E. V. Lapham & K. M. Shevlin (Eds.), *The Impact of Chronic Illness on Psychosocial Stages of Human Development*. Washington, DC: Dept. of Social Work, Georgetown University Hospital and Medical Center, pp. 67–75.

DudokdeWit, A. C., Tibben, A., Frets, P. G., Meijers-Heijboer, E. J., Devilee, P., Klijn, J. G. M., Oosterwijk, J. C., & Niermeijer, M. F. (1997). BRCA1 in the family: A case description of the psychological implications. *Am J Med Genet*, 71:63–71.

Duster, T. (1990). *Backdoor to Eugenics*. New York: Routledge.

Duvall, E. M. (1977). *Marriage and Family Development*. (5th ed.). Philadelphia: Lippincott.

Eisenberg, D. M., Davis, R. B., Ettner, S. L., Appel, S., Wilkey, S., Van Rompay, M., & Kessler, R. C. (1998). Trends in alternative medicine use in the United States, 1990–1997: Results of a follow-up national survey. *JAMA*, 280:1569–1575.

Elson, M. (1987). *The Kohut Seminars on Self Psychology and Psychotherapy with Adolescents and Young Adults*. New York: W.W. Norton.

Emler, N. (1993). The young person's relationship to the institutional order. In S. Jackson & H. Rodriguez-Tomé (Eds.), *Adolescence and Its Social Worlds*. Hove UK: Lawrence Erlbaum, pp. 229–250.

Eunpu, D. L. (1997a). Generations lost: A cancer genetics case report commentary. *J Genet Counsel*, 6:173–176.

Eunpu, D. L. (1997b). Systemically-based psychotherapeutic techniques in genetic counseling. *J Genet Counsel*, 6:1–20.

Evers-Kiebooms, G. (1987). Decision making in Huntington's disease and cystic fibrosis. *Birth Defects*, 23(2):115–149.

Evers-Kiebooms, G., Denayer, L., & Van den Berghe, H. (1990). A child with cystic fibrosis: II. Subsequent family planning decisions, reproduction and use of prenatal diagnosis. *Clin Genet*, 37:207–215.

Fadiman, A. (1997). *The Spirit Catches You and You Fall Down: A Hmong Child, Her American Doctors, and the Collision of Two Cultures*. New York: Farrar, Straus & Giroux.

Falek, A. (1984). Sequential aspects of coping and other issues in decision making in genetic counseling. In A. E. H. Emery & I. M. Pullen (Eds.), *Psychological Aspects of Genetic Counseling*. London: Academic Press, pp. 23–36.

Falicov, C. J. (1998). *Latino Families in Therapy: A Guide to Multicultural Practice*. New York: Guilford.

Fanos, J. H. (1996). *Sibling Loss*. Mahwah NJ: Lawrence Erlbaum.

Fanos, J. H., & Johnson, J. P. (1995). Barriers to carrier testing for adult cystic fibrosis sibs: The importance of not knowing. *Am J Med Genet*, 59:85–91.

Fine, B. A. (1993). The evolution of nondirectiveness in genetic counseling and implications of the human genome project. In D. M. Bartels, B. S. LeRoy, & A. L. Caplan (Eds.), *Prescribing Our Future: Ethical Challenges in Genetic Counseling*. New York: Aldine de Gruyter, pp. 101–117.

Finucane, B. (1998a). Acculturation in women with mental retardation and its impact on genetic counseling. *J Genet Counsel*, 7:31–47.

Finucane, B. (1998b). *Working with Women Who Have Mental Retardation: A Genetic Counselor's Guide*. Elwyn PA: Elwyn.

Fisher, N. L. (Ed.). (1996a). *Cultural and Ethnic Diversity: A Guide for Genetics Professionals*. Baltimore: Johns Hopkins University Press.

Fisher, N. L. (1996b). Introduction. In N. L. Fisher (Ed.), *Cultural and Ethnic Diversity: A Guide for Genetics Professionals*. Baltimore: Johns Hopkins University Press, pp. xiii–xxi.

Fonda Allen, J. S., & Mulhauser, L. C. (1995). Genetic counseling after abnormal prenatal diagnosis: Facilitating coping in familes who continue their pregnancies. *J Genet Counsel*, 4:251–266.

Foster, M. W., Sharp, R. R., Freeman, W. L., Chino, M., Bernsten, D., & Carter, T. H. (1999). The role of community review in evaluating the risks of human genetic variation research. *Am J Hum Genet*, 64:1719–1727.

Frets, P. G., Duivenvoorden, H. J., Verhage, F., Niermeijer, M. F., van den Berghe, S. M. M., & Galjaard, H. (1990a). Factors influencing the reproductive decision after genetic counseling. *Am J Med Genet*, 35:496–502.

Frets, P. G., Duivenvoorden, J. H., Verhage, F., Ketzer, E., & Niermeijer, M. F. (1990b). Model identifying the reproductive decision after genetic counseling. *Am J Med Genet*, 35:503–509.

Frets, P. H., & Niermeijer, M. F. (1990c). Reproductive planning after genetic counseling: A perspective from the last decade. *Clin Genet*, 38:295–306.

Fuller-Thomson, E., Minkler, M., & Driver, D. (1997). A profile of grandparents raising grandchildren in the United States. *The Gerontologist*, 37:406–411.

Gabbard, G. O. (1995). Theories of personality and psychopathology: Psychoanalysis. In H. I. Kaplan & B. J. Sadock (Eds.), *Comprehensive Textbook of Psychiatry*. Baltimore: Williams & Wilkins, pp. 431–486.

Gallup, G. H., Jr (1996). *Religion in America 1996*. Princeton: Princeton Religion Research Center.

Garrison, W. T., & McQuiston, S. (1989). *Chronic Illness During Childhood and Adolescence: Psychological Aspects*. Newbury Park CA: SAGE.

Geller, G., Strauss, M., Bernhardt, B. A., & Holtzman, N. A. (1997). "Decoding" informed consent: Insights from women regarding breast cancer susceptibility testing. *Hastings Cent Rep*, 27(2):28–33.

Gervais, K. G. (1993). Objectivity, value neutrality, and nondirectiveness in genetic counseling. In D. M. Bartels, B. S. LeRoy, & A. L. Caplan (Eds.), *Prescribing Our Future: Ethical Challenges in Genetic Counseling*. New York: Aldine de Gruyter, pp. 119–130.

Gettig, E., Hannig, V., & Westphal-Fitzgerald, J. (1987). Rural genetic counseling: Working in the field. *Birth Defects*, 23(6):214–225.

Goldstein, M. A., & Biesecker, B. B. (1993). Introduction to 1992 Asilomar conference papers. *J Genet Counsel*, 2:153–154.

Greb, A. (1998). Multiculturalism and the practice of genetic counseling. In D. L. Baker, J. L. Schuette, & W. R. Uhlmann (Eds.), *A Guide to Genetic Counseling*. New York: Wiley-Liss, pp. 171–198.

Green, J., Murton, F., & Statham, H. (1993). Psychosocial issues raised by a familial ovarian cancer register. *J Med Genet*, 30:575–579.

Green, J., Richards, M., Murton, F., Statham, H., & Hallowell, N. (1997). Family communication and genetic counseling: The case of hereditary breast and ovarian cancer. *J Genet Counsel*, 6:45–60.

Green, R. (1992). Letter to a genetic counselor. *J Genet Counsel*, 1:55–70.

Greenspan, S. I. (1991). *The Clinical Interview of the Child*. (2nd ed.). Washington, DC: American Psychiatric Press.

Grobstein, R. (1979). Amniocentesis counseling. In S. Kessler (Ed.), *Genetic Counseling: Psychological Dimensions*. New York: Academic Press, pp. 107–113.

Guerin, P. J., Jr., Fay, L. F., Burden, S. L., & Kautto, J. G. (1987). *The Evaluation and Treatment of Marital Conflict: A Four-Stage Approach*. New York: Basic Books.

Gurman, A. S., & Messer, S. B. (Eds.). (1995). *Essential Psychotherapies: Theory and Practice*. New York: Guilford.

Haffner, L. (1992). Translation is not enough: Interpreting in a medical setting. *West J Med*, 157:255–259.

Hallowell, N., Statham, H., & Murton, F. (1998). Women's understanding of their risk of developing breast/ovarian cancer before and after genetic counseling. *J Genet Counsel*, 7:345–364.

Hand-Mauser, M. E. (1989). Techniques in systemic family therapy: Applications for genetic counseling. In N. J. Zellers (Ed.), *Strategies for Genetic Counseling*. New York: Human Sciences, Vol. 2, pp. 93–120.

Hauck, L., & Knoki-Wilson, U. M. (1996). Culture of Native Americans of the Southwest. In N. L. Fisher (Ed.), *Cultural and Ethnic Diversity: A Guide for Genetics Professionals*. Baltimore: Johns Hopkins University Press, pp. 60–85.

Hill, S. A. (1994). Motherhood and the obfuscation of medical knowledge: The case of sickle cell disease. *Gender & Society*, 8:29–47.

Hines, P. M. (1998). Climbing up the rough side of the mountain. In M. McGoldrick (Ed.), *Re-visioning Family Therapy: Race, Culture, and Gender in Clinical Practice*. New York: Guilford, pp. 78–89.

Hobbs, N., Perrin, J. M., & Ireys, H. T. (1985). *Chronically Ill Children and Their Families*. San Francisco: Jossey-Bass.

Hodge, S. E. (1998). A simple, unified approach to Bayesian risk calculations. *J Genet Counsel*, 7:235–261.

Hof, L., & Treat, S. R. (1989). Marital assessment: Providing a framework for dyadic therapy. In G. R. Weeks (Ed.), *Treating Couples: The Intersystem Model of the Marriage Council of Philadelphia*. New York: Brunner/Mazel, pp. 3–21.

Hoffman, L. (1981). *Foundations of Family Therapy: A Conceptual Framework for Systems Change*. New York: Basic Books.

Hofmann, A. D., & Greydanus, D. E. (1989). Principles of psychosocial evaluation and counseling. In A. Hofmann & D. Greydanus (Eds.), *Adolescent Medicine*. (2nd ed.) Norwalk CT: Appleton & Lange, pp. 533–551.

Hopwood, P. (1997). Psychological issues in cancer genetics: Current research and future priorities. *Patient Education and Counseling*, 32:19–31.

Humphreys, P., & Berkeley, D. (1987). Representing risks: Supporting genetic counseling. *Birth Defects*, 23(2):227–250.

Imber-Black, E. (1986). Toward a resource model in systemic family therapy. In M. A. Karpel (Ed.), *Family Resources: The Hidden Partner in Family Therapy*. New York: Guilford, pp. 148–174.

Imber-Black, E. (1989). Idiosyncratic life cycle transitions and therapeutic rituals. In B. Carter & M. McGoldrick (Eds.), *The Changing Family Life Cycle: A Framework for Family Therapy*. (2nd ed.) Boston: Allyn and Bacon, pp. 149–163.

International Society of Nurses in Genetics. (1998). *Statement on the Scope and Standards of Genetics Clinical Nursing Practice.* Washington: American Nurses Publishing.

Israel, J., Cunningham, M., Thumann, H., & Arnos, K. S. (1992). Genetic counseling for deaf adults: Communication/language and cultural considerations. *J Genet Counsel*, 1:135–153.

Israel, J., Cunningham, M., Thumann, H., & Arnos, K. S. (1996). Deaf culture. In N. L. Fisher (Ed.), *Cultural and Ethnic Diversity: A Guide for Genetics Professionals.* Baltimore: Johns Hopkins University Press, pp. 220–239.

Jalali, B. (1988). Ethnicity, cultural adjustment, and behavior: Implications for family therapy. In L. Comas-Diaz & E. E. H. Griffith (Eds.), *Clinical Guidelines in Cross-Cultural Mental Health.* New York: John Wiley, pp. 9–32.

Johnson, R. L. (1989). Adolescent growth and development. In A. Hofmann & D. Greydanus (Eds.), *Adolescent Medicine.* (2nd ed.) Norwalk CT: Appleton & Lange, pp. 9–15.

Johnson, R. L., & Tanner, N. M. (1989). Approaching the adolescent patient. In A. Hofmann & D. Greydanus (Eds.), *Adolescent Medicine.* (2nd ed.) Norwalk CT: Appleton & Lange, pp. 21–32.

Jones, J. H. (1993). *Bad Blood: The Tuskegee Syphilis Experiment.* New York: Free Press.

Kalter, N. (1990). *Growing Up with Divorce.* New York: Free Press.

Kaplan, D. (1993). Prenatal screening and its impact on persons with disabilities. *Clin Obstet Gynecol*, 36:605–612.

Karlin, V. L. (1986). Late adolescence: Identity formation. In E. V. Lapham & K. M. Shevlin (Eds.), *The Impact of Chronic Illness on Psychosocial Stages of Human Development.* Washington, DC: Dept. of Social Work, Georgetown University Hospital and Medical Center, pp. 79–87.

Karp, J., Brown, K. L., Sullivan, M. D., & Massie, M. J. (1999). The prophylactic mastectomy dilemma: A support group for women at high genetic risk for breast cancer. *J Genet Counsel*, 8:163–173.

Kaslow, L. (1986). School age: Making, doing, achieving. In E. V. Lapham & K. M. Shevlin (Eds.), *The Impact of Chronic Illness on Psychosocial Stages of Human Development.* Washington, DC: Dept. of Social Work, Georgetown University Hospital and Medical Center, pp. 55–63.

Kaufman, G. (1985). *Shame: The Power of Caring.* (2nd ed.). Cambridge MA: Schenkman Books.

Kaufman, G. (1996). *The Psychology of Shame: Theory and Treatment of Shame-Based Syndromes.* (2nd ed.). New York: Springer.

Kelly, P. T. (1977). *Dealing with Dilemma: A Manual for Genetic Counselors.* New York: Springer-Verlag.

Kelly, P. T. (1991). *Understanding Breast Cancer Risk.* Philadelphia: Temple University Press.

Kenen, R. H. (1984). Genetic counseling: The development of a new interdisciplinary occupational field. *Soc Sci Med*, 18:541–549.

Kessler, S. (1979a). The counselor-counselee relationship. In S. Kessler (Ed.), *Genetic Counseling: Psychological Dimensions.* New York: Academic Press, pp. 53–63.

Kessler, S. (1979b). The genetic counseling session. In S. Kessler (Ed.), *Genetic Counseling: Psychological Dimensions.* New York: Academic Press, pp. 65–105.

Kessler, S. (Ed.). (1979c). *Genetic Counseling: Psychological Dimensions.* New York: Academic Press.

Kessler, S. (1979d). The genetic counselor as psychotherapist. *Birth Defects*, 15(2):187–200.

Kessler, S. (1979e). The processes of communication, decision making and coping in genetic counseling. In S. Kessler (Ed.), *Genetic Counseling: Psychological Dimensions*. New York: Academic Press, pp. 35–51.

Kessler, S. (1979f). The psychological foundations of genetic counseling.. In S. Kessler (Ed.), *Genetic Counseling: Psychological Dimensions*. New York: Academic Press, pp. 17–33.

Kessler, S. (1980). The psychological paradigm shift in genetic counseling. *Soc Biol*, 27:167–185.

Kessler, S. (1989). Psychological aspects of genetic counseling: VI. A critical review of the literature dealing with education and reproduction. *Am J Med Genet*, 34:340–353.

Kessler, S. (1992a). Process issues in genetic counseling. *Birth Defects*, 28(1):1–10.

Kessler, S. (1992b). Psychological aspects of genetic counseling. VII. Thoughts on directiveness. *J Genet Counsel*, 1:9–18.

Kessler, S. (1992c). Psychological aspects of genetic counseling. VIII. Suffering and countertransference. *J Genet Counsel*, 1:303–308.

Kessler, S. (1997a). Psychological aspects of genetic counseling. XI. Nondirectiveness revisited. *Am J Med Genet*, 72:164–171.

Kessler, S. (1997b). Psychological aspects of genetic counseling. X. Advanced counseling techniques. *J Genet Counsel*, 6:379–392.

Kessler, S. (1998). Psychological aspects of genetic counseling. XII. More on counseling skills. *J Genet Counsel*, 7:263–278.

Kessler, S. (1999). Psychological aspects of genetic counseling: XIII. Empathy and decency. *J Genet Counsel*, 8:333–343.

Kessler, S., & Bloch, M. (1989). Social system responses to Huntington disease. *Fam Process*, 28:59–68.

Kessler, S., Kessler, H., & Ward, P. (1984). Psychological aspects of genetic counseling. III. Management of guilt and shame. *Am J Med Genet*, 17:673–697.

Kessler, S., & Levine, E. K. (1987). Psychological aspects of genetic counseling. IV. The subjective assessment of probability. *Am J Med Genet*, 28:361–370.

Kirchler, E., Palmonari, A., & Pombeni, M. L. (1993). Developmental tasks and adolescents' relationships with their peers and their family. In S. Jackson & H. Rodriguez-Tomé (Eds.), *Adolescence and Its Social Worlds*. Hove UK: Lawrence Erlbaum.

Kleinman, A. (1980). *Patients and Healers in the Context of Culture: An Exploration of the Borderland Between Anthropology, Medicine, and Psychiatry*. Berkeley: University of California Press.

Kliman, J. (1998). Social class as a relationship: Implications for family therapy. In M. McGoldrick (Ed.), *Re-visioning Family Therapy: Race, Culture, and Gender in Clinical Practice*. New York: Guilford, pp. 50–61.

Kluckhohn, F. R., & Strodtbeck, F. L. (1961). *Variations in Value Orientations*. Evanston IL: Row, Patterson.

Kohut, H. (1966). Forms and transformations of narcissism. *J Am Psychoanal Assoc*, 14:243–272.

Kolker, A., & Burke, B. M. (1993). Grieving the wanted child: Ramifications of abortion after prenatal diagnosis of abnormality. *Health Care for Women International*, 14:513–526.

Kolker, A., & Burke, B. M. (1994). *Prenatal Testing: A Sociological Perspective*. Westport CT: Bergin & Garvey.

Kroeber, T. C. (1964). The coping functions of the ego mechanisms. In R. W. White & K. F. Bruner (Eds.), *The Study of Lives: Essays on Personality in Honor of Henry A. Murray*. New York: Atherton Press, pp. 179–198.

Kubler-Ross, E. (1969). *On Death and Dying*. New York: Macmillan.

Kuliev, A., Greendale, K., Penchaszadeh, V., & Paul, N. W. (1992). Genetic services provision: An international perspective. *Birth Defects*, 28(3).

Laborde, P. R., & Seligman, M. (1991). Counseling parents with children with disabilities. In M. Seligman (Ed.), *The Family with a Handicapped Child*. (2nd ed.) Boston: Allyn and Bacon, pp. 337–368.

Laird, J. (1998). Theorizing culture: Narrative ideas and practice principles. In M. McGoldrick (Ed.), *Re-visioning Family Therapy: Race, Culture, and Gender in Clinical Practice*. New York: Guilford, pp. 20–36.

Lazarus, R. S. (1999). *Stress and Emotion: A New Synthesis*. New York: Springer.

Lee, E. (Ed.). (1997). *Working with Asian Americans: A Guide for Clinicians*. New York: Guilford.

Lee, R. V., d'Alauro, F., White, L. M., & Cardinal, J. (1988). Southeast Asian folklore about pregnancy and parturition. *Obstet Gynecol*, 71:643–645.

Lemke, A. A., Dayal, S., & Geibel, L. J. (1998). Preconception genetic counseling: Three years of experience at a community-based health center. *J Genet Counsel*, 7:71–85.

Lerman, C., Lustbader, E., Rimer, B., Daly, M., Miller, S., Sands, C., & Balshem, A. (1995). Effects of individualized breast cancer risk counseling: A randomized trial. *J Natl Cancer Inst*, 87:286–292.

Lew, L. S. (1990). Understanding the Southeast Asian health care consumer: Bridges and barriers. *Birth Defects*, 26(2):147–154.

Lewis, F. M. (1996). The impact of breast cancer on the family: Lessons learned from the children and adolescents. In L. Baider, C. L. Cooper, & A. K. De-Nour (Eds.), *Cancer and the Family*. Chichester: Wiley, pp. 271–287.

Lewontin, R. (1982). *Human Diversity*. New York: Scientific American Books.

Lin-Fu, J. S. (1990). Responses to the keynote address. *Birth Defects*, 26(2):21–24.

Lippman, A. (1993). Prenatal genetic testing and geneticization: Mother matters for all. *Fetal Diagn Ther*, 8(suppl 1):175–188.

Lippman, A. (1994). Prenatal genetic testing and screening: Constructing needs and reinforcing inequities. In A. Clarke (Ed.), *Genetic Counseling: Practice and Principles*. London: Routledge, pp. 142–186.

Lippman, A., & Wilfond, B. S. (1992). Twice-told tales: Stories about genetic disorders. *Am J Hum Genet*, 51:936–937.

Lippman-Hand, A., & Fraser, F. C. (1979a). Genetic counseling: Parents' responses to uncertainty. *Birth Defects*, 15(5C):325–339.

Lippman-Hand, A., & Fraser, F. C. (1979b). Genetic counseling: Provision and reception of information. *Am J Med Genet*, 3:113–127.

Lippman-Hand, A., & Fraser, F. C. (1979c). Genetic counseling: The postcounseling period. I. Parent's perceptions of uncertainty. *Am J Med Genet*, 4:51–71.

Lippman-Hand, A., & Fraser, F. C. (1979d). Genetic counseling: The postcounseling period. II. Making reproductive choices. *Am J Med Genet*, 4:73–87.

Lopez-Rangel, E. (1996). Latino culture. In N. L. Fisher (Ed.), *Cultural and Ethnic Diversity: A Guide for Genetics Professionals*. Baltimore: Johns Hopkins University Press, pp. 19–35.

Lubinsky, M. S. (1993). Scientific aspects of early eugenics. *J Genet Counsel*, 2:77–92.

Lubinsky, M. S. (1994). Bearing bad news: Dealing with the mimics of denial. *J Genet Counsel*, 3:5–12.

Lum, R. G., & Whipperman, L. (1987). Practical methods in reaching and counseling the new American. *Birth Defects*, 23(6):188–205.

Lynch, E. W. (1998a). Conceptual framework: From culture shock to cultural learning. In E. W. Lynch & M. J. Hanson (Eds.), *Developing Cross-Cultural Competence: A Guide for Working with Children and Their Families*. (2nd ed.) Baltimore: Paul H Brookes, pp. 23–45.

Lynch, E. W. (1998b). Developing cross-cultural competence. In E. W. Lynch & M. J. Hanson (Eds.), *Developing Cross-Cultural Competence: A Guide for Working with Children and Their Families*. (2nd ed.) Baltimore: Paul H Brookes, pp. 47–86.

Lynch, E. W. & Hanson, M. J. (Eds.). (1998). *Developing Cross-Cultural Competence: A Guide for Working with Children and Their Families*. (2nd ed.). Baltimore: Paul H Brookes.

Lynch, H. T., Lemon, S. J., Durham, C., Tinley, S. T., Connolly, C., Lynch, J. F., Surdam, J., Orinion, E., Slominski-Caster, S., Watson, P., Lerman, C., Tonin, P., Lenoir, G., Serova, O., & Narod, S. (1997). A descriptive study of BRCA1 testing and reactions to disclosure of test results. *Cancer*, 79:2219–2228.

Magyari, P. A., Wedehase, B. A., Ifft, R. D., & Callanan, N. P. (1987). A supportive intervention protocol for couples terminating a pregnancy for genetic reasons. *Birth Defects*, 23(6):75–83.

Markens, S., Browner, C. H., & Press, N. (1999). 'Because of the risks': How US pregnant women account for refusing prenatal screening. *Soc Sci Med*, 49:359–369.

Marks, J. H. (1993). The training of genetic counselors: Origins of a psychosocial model. In D. M. Bartels, B. S. LeRoy, & A. L. Caplan (Eds.), *Prescribing Our Future: Ethical Challenges in Genetic Counseling*. New York: Aldine de Gruyter, pp. 15–24.

Marks, J. H., Heimler, A., Reich, E., Wexler, N. S., & Ince, S. E. (1989). Genetic counseling principles in action: A casebook. *Birth Defects*, 25(5).

Marshak, L. E., Seligman, M., & Prezant, F. (1999). *Disability and the Family Life Cycle*. New York: Basic Books.

Marteau, T. M., & Slack, J. (1992). Psychological implications of prenatal diagnosis for patients and health professionals. In D. J. H. Brock, C. H. Rodeck, & M. A. Ferguson-Smith (Eds.), *Prenatal Diagnosis and Screening*. Edinburgh: Churchill Livingstone, pp. 663–673.

Marymee, K., Dolan, C. R., Pagon, R. A., Bennett, R. L., Coe, S., & Fisher, N. L. (1998). Development of the critical elements of genetic evaluation and genetic counseling for genetic professionals and perinatologists in Washington state. *J Genet Counsel*, 7:133–165.

Matloff, E. T. (1997). Generations lost: A cancer genetics case report. *J Genet Counsel*, 6:169–172.

Matsui, W. T. (1996). Japanese families. In M. McGoldrick, J. Giordano, & J. K. Pearce (Eds.), *Ethnicity and Family Therapy*. (2nd ed.) New York: Guilford, pp. 268–280.

McAdoo, H. P. (Ed.). (1997). *Black Families*. (3rd ed.). Thousand Oaks CA: SAGE.

McGoldrick, M. (1989). Ethnicity and the family life cycle. In B. Carter & M. McGoldrick (Eds.), *The Changing Family Life cycle: A Framework for Family Therapy*. (2nd ed.) Boston: Allyn and Bacon, pp. 69–90.

McGoldrick, M. (1993). Ethnicity, cultural diversity, and normality. In F. Walsh (Ed.), *Normal Family Processes*. (2nd ed.) New York: Guilford, pp. 331–360.

McGoldrick, M., Gerson, R., & Shellenberger, S. (1999). *Genograms: Assessment and Intervention*. (2nd ed.). New York: W. W. Norton.

McGoldrick, M., Giordano, J., & Pearce, J. K. (Eds.). (1996). *Ethnicity and Family Therapy* (2nd ed.). London: Guilford.

McIntosh, P. (1995). White privilege and male privilege: A personal account of coming to see correspondences through work in Women's Studies. In M. L. Andersen & P. H. Collins (Eds.), *Race, Class, and Gender: An Anthology*. (2nd ed.) Belmont CA: Wadsworth, pp. 76–87.

McIntosh, P. (1998). White privilege: Unpacking the invisible knapsack. In M. McGoldrick (Ed.), *Re-visioning Family Therapy: Race, Culture, and Gender in Clinical Practice*. New York: Guilford, pp. 147–152.

McKinney, M. K., Tuber, S. B., & Downey, J. I. (1996). Multifetal pregnancy reduction: Psychodynamic implications. *Psychiatry*, 59:393–407.

Meyers, M., Diamond, R., Kezur, D., Scharf, C., Weinshel, M., & Rait, D. S. (1995a). An infertility primer for family therapists. I. Medical, social, and psychological dimensions. *Fam Process*, 34:219–229.

Meyers, M., Weinshel, M., Scharf, C., Kezur, D., Diamond, R., & Rait, D. S. (1995b). An infertility primer for family therapists. II. Working with couples who struggle with infertility. *Fam Process*, 34:231–240.

Middleton, W., Raphael, B., Martinek, N., & Misso, V. (1993). Pathological grief reactions. In M. S. Stroebe, W. Stroebe, & R. O. Hansson (Eds.), *Handbook of Bereavement: Theory, Research, and Intervention*. Cambridge UK: Cambridge University Press, pp. 44–61.

Miezio, P. M. (1983). *Parenting Children with Disabilities: A Professional Source for Physicians and Guide for Parents*. New York: Marcel Dekker.

Mills, M. C. (1985). Adolescents' reactions to counseling interviews. *Adolescence*, 20:83–95.

Mintzer, D., Als, H., Tronick, E. Z., & Brazelton, T. B. (1984). Parenting an infant with a birth defect. *Psychoanal Study Child*, 39:561–589.

Minuchin, S. (1974). *Families and Family Therapy*. Cambridge MA: Harvard University Press.

Minuchin, S., & Fishman, H. C. (1981). *Family Therapy Techniques*. Cambridge MA: Harvard University Press.

Mittman, I. (1988). Conflict between ancient culture and modern technology. *Perspectives in Genetic Counseling*, 10:3–4.

Mittman, I. (1990). Immigration and the provision of genetic services. *Birth Defects*, 26(2):139–146.

Mittman, I., Crombleholme, W. R., Green, J. R., & Golbus, M. S. (1998). Reproductive genetic counseling to Asian-Pacific and Latin American immigrants. *J Genet Counsel*, 7:49–70.

Mittman, I. S. (1998). Genetic education to diverse communities employing a community empowerment model. *Community Genet*, 1:160–165.

Mittman, I. S., & Secundy, M. G. (1998a). Introduction. *Community Genet*, 1:115–117.

Mittman, I. S., & Secundy, M. G. (1998b). A national dialogue on genetics and minority issues. *Community Genet*, 1:190–200.

Murphy, E. A., & Chase, G. A. (1975). *Principles of Genetic Counseling*. Chicago: Year Book Medical Publishers.

National Society of Genetic Counselors. (1992). Code of ethics. *J Genet Counsel*, 1:41–43.

Nilchaikovit, T., Hill, J. M., & Holland, J. C. (1993). The effects of culture on illness behavior and medical care: Asian and American differences. *Gen Hosp Psychiatry*, 15:41–50.

Nixon, C. D., & Singer, G. H. S. (1993). Group cognitive-behavioral treatment for excessive parental self-blame and guilt. *Am J Ment Retard*, 97:665–672.

Nsiah-Jefferson, L. (1993). Access to reproductive genetic services for low-income women and women of color. *Fetal Diagn Ther*, 8(suppl 1):107–127.

O'Dougherty, M. M. (1983). *Counseling the Chronically Ill Child: Psychological Impact and Intervention*. Lexington MA: Lewis Publishing Co.

Olney, P. N., & Olney, R. S. (1993). Harlequin ichthyosis among the Navajo: Counseling issues. *J Genet Counsel*, 2:3–8.

Ota Wang, V. (1994). Cultural competency in genetic counseling. *J Genet Counsel*, 3:267–279.

Ota Wang, V. (1998a). Curriculum evaluation and assessment of multicultural genetic counselor education. *J Genet Counsel*, 7:87–111.

Ota Wang, V. (1998b). Introduction. *J Genet Counsel*, 7:3–13.

Oyama, O., & Koenig, H. G. (1998). Religious beliefs and practices in family medicine. *Arch Fam Med*, 7:431–435.

Palmer, C. G. S., & Sainfort, F. (1993). Toward a new conceptualization and operationalization of risk perception within the genetic counseling domain. *J Genet Counsel*, 2:275–294.

Panter-Brick, C. (1992). Coping with an affected birth: Genetic counseling in Saudi Arabia. *J Child Neurol*, 7(suppl):S69–S72.

Pargament, K. I. (1997). *The Psychology of Religion and Coping: Theory, Research, Practice*. New York: Guilford.

Parsons, E. (1997). Culture and genetics: Is genetics in society or society in genetics? In A. Clarke & E. Parsons (Eds.), *Culture, Kinship and Genes: Towards Cross-Cultural Genetics*. New York: St. Martin's, pp. 245–260.

Parsons, E., & Atkinson, P. (1993). Genetic risk and reproduction. *Sociological Review*, 41:679–706.

Parsons, E. P., & Clarke, A. J. (1993). Genetic risk: Women's understanding of carrier risks in Duchenne muscular dystrophy. *J Med Genet*, 30:562–566.

Pearn, J. H. (1973). Patients' subjective interpretation of risks offered in genetic counselling. *J Med Genet*, 10:129–134.

Peters, J. A. (1994a). Familial cancer risk part II: Breast cancer risk counseling and genetic susceptibility testing. *Journal of Oncology Management*, Nov/Dec:14–22.

Peters, J. A. (1994b). Suicide prevention in the genetic counseling context. *J Genet Counsel*, 3:199–214.

Peters, J. A., & Stopfer, J. E. (1996). Role of the genetic counselor in familial cancer. *Oncology*, 10:159–166.

Peters-Brown, T., & Fry-Mehltretter, L. (1996). Genetic counseling for pregnant adolescents. *J Genet Counsel*, 5:155–168.

Phipps, S., & Zinn, A. B. (1986). Psychological response to amniocentesis: I. Mood state and adaptation to pregnancy. *Am J Med Genet*, 25:131–142.

Pinderhughes, E. (1989). *Understanding Race, Ethnicity, and Power*. New York: Free Press.

Ponder, M., Murton, F., Hallowell, N., Statham, H., Green, J., & Richards, M. (1998). Genetic counseling, reproductive behavior and future reproductive intentions of people with neurofibromatosis type 1 (NF1). *J Genet Counsel*, 7:331–344.

Press, N., & Browner, C. H. (1997). Why women say yes to prenatal diagnosis. *Soc Sci Med*, 45:979–989.

Press, N. A., & Browner, C. H. (1993). 'Collective fictions': Similarities in reasons for accepting maternal serum alpha-fetoprotein screening among women of diverse ethnic and social class backgrounds. *Fetal Diagn Ther*, 8(suppl 1):97–106.

Preto, N. G. (1989). Transformation of the family system in adolescence. In B. Carter & M. McGoldrick (Eds.), *The Changing Family Life Cycle: A Framework for Family Therapy*. (2nd ed.) Boston: Allyn and Bacon, pp. 255–283.

Pryde, P. G., Drugan, A., Johnson, M. P., Isada, N. B., & Evans, M. I. (1993). Prenatal diagnosis: Choices women make about pursuing testing and acting on abnormal results. *Clin Obstet Gynecol*, 36:496–509.

Punales-Morejon, D., & Penchaszadeh, V. B. (1992). Psychosocial aspects of genetic counseling: Cross-cultural issues. *Birth Defects*, 28(1):11–15.

Punales-Morejon, D., & Rapp, R. (1993). Ethnocultural diversity and genetic counseling training: The challenge for a twenty-first century. *J Genet Counsel*, 2:155–158.

Randall-David, E. (1989). *Strategies for Working with Culturally Diverse Communities and Clients*. Bethesda: Association for the Care of Children's Health.

Rando, T. A. (1983). An investigation of grief and adaptation in parents whose children have died from cancer. *J Pediatr Psychol*, 8:3–20.

Rando, T. A. (1985). Bereaved parents: Particular difficulties, unique factors, and treatment issues. *Soc Work*, 30:19–23.

Raphael, B., Middleton, W., Martinek, N., & Misso, V. (1993). Counseling and therapy of the bereaved. In M. S. Stroebe, W. Stoebe, & R. O. Hansson (Eds.), *Handbook of Bereavement: Theory, Research, and Intervention*. Cambridge UK: Cambridge University Press, pp. 427–453.

Rapp, R. (1988). The power of "positive" diagnosis: Medical and maternal discourses on amniocentesis. In K. L. Michaelson (Ed.), *Childbirth in America: Anthropological Perspectives*. South Hadley MA: Bergin & Garvey, pp. 103–116.

Rapp, R. (1990). Constructing amniocentesis: Maternal and medical discourses. In F. Ginsburg & A. L. Tsing (Eds.), *Uncertain Terms: Negotiating Gender in American Culture*. Boston: Beacon Press, pp. 28–42.

Rapp, R. (1993a). Amniocentesis in sociocultural perspective. *J Genet Counsel*, 2:183–196.

Rapp, R. (1993b). Sociocultural differences in the impact of amniocentesis: An anthropological research report. *Fetal Diagn Ther*, 8(suppl 1):90–96.

Rapp, R. (1998). Refusing prenatal diagnosis: The meanings of bioscience in a multicultural world. *Science, Technology & Human Values*, 23:45–70.

Rapp, R. (1999). *Testing Women, Testing the Fetus: The Social Impact of Amniocentesis in America*. New York: Routledge.

Rauch, J. B., & Curtiss, C. R. (1992). *Taking a Family Health/Genetic History: An Ethnocultural Learning Guide and Handbook*. Baltimore: University of Maryland at Baltimore School of Social Work.

Reed, S. (1974). A short history of genetic counseling. *Soc Biol*, 21:332–339.

Resta, R. G. (1997). Eugenics and non-directiveness in genetic counseling. *J Genet Counsel*, 6:255–258.

Retsinas, J. (1991). The impact of prenatal technology upon attitudes toward disabled infants. *Research in the Sociology of Health Care*, 9:75–102.

Richards, M. (1996). Families, kinship and genetics. In T. Marteau & M. Richards (Eds.), *The Troubled Helix: Social and Psychological Implications of the New Human Genetics*. Cambridge UK: Cambridge University Press, pp. 249–273.

Richards, M. P. M., Hallowell, N., Green, J. M., Murton, F., & Statham, H. (1995).

Counseling families with hereditary breast and ovarian cancer: A psychosocial perspective. *J Genet Counsel*, 4:219–233.

Robinson, J., Tennes, K., & Robinson, A. (1975). Amniocentesis: Its impact on mothers and infants. A 1-year follow-up study. *Clin Genet*, 8:97–106.

Rokeach, M. (1960). *The Open and Closed Mind: Investigations Into the Nature of Belief Systems and Personality Systems*. New York: Basic Books.

Rolland, J. S. (1994). *Families, Illness, and Disability: An Integrative Treatment Model*. New York: Basic Books.

Rosenblatt, P. C. (1988). Grief: The social context of private feelings. *Journal of Social Issues*, 44:67–78.

Rosenblatt, P. G., & Burns, L. H. (1986). Long-term effects of perinatal loss. *Journal of Family Issues*, 7:237–253.

Rothman, B. K. (1986). *The Tentative Pregnancy: Prenatal Diagnosis and the Future of Motherhood*. New York: Penguin.

Rubin, L. B. (1983). *Intimate Strangers: Men and Women Together*. Cambridge MA: Harper & Row.

Rubin, S. S. (1993). The death of a child is forever: The life course impact of child loss. In M. S. Stroebe, W. Stoebe, & R. O. Hansson (Eds.), *Handbook of Bereavement: Theory, Research, and Intervention*. Cambridge UK: Cambridge University Press, pp. 285–299.

Sagi, M., Shiloh, S., & Cohen, T. (1992). Application of the health belief model in a study on parents' intentions to utilize prenatal diagnosis of cleft lip and/or palate. *Am J Med Genet*, 44:326–333.

Sahler, O. J. Z., & Kreipe, R. E. (1991). Psychological development in normal adolescents. In W. R. Hendee (Ed.), *The Health of Adolescents: Understanding and Facilitating Biological, Behavioral, and Social Development*. San Francisco: Jossey-Bass, pp. 58–88.

Sandelowski, M., & Jones, L. C. (1996). 'Healing fictions': Stories of choosing in the aftermath of the detection of fetal anomalies. *Soc Sci Med*, 42:353–361.

Saxton, M. (1984). Born and unborn: The implications of reproductive technologies for people with disabilities. In R. Arditti, R. D. Klein, & S. Minden (Eds.), *Test-tube Women: What Future for Motherhood?* Boston: Pandora, pp. 298–312.

Saxton, M. (1988). Prenatal screening and discriminatory attitudes about disability. In E. H. Baruch, A. F. J. D'Adamo, & J. Seager (Eds.), *Embryos, Ethics, and Women's Rights: Exploring the New Reproductive Technologies*. New York: Haworth, pp. 217–224.

Saxton, M. (1998). Disability rights and selective abortion. In R. Solinger (Ed.), *Abortion Wars: A Half Century of Struggle, 1950–2000*. Berkeley: University of California Press, pp. 374–393.

Scharff, D. E., & Scharff, J. S. (1991a). *Object Relations Couple Therapy*. Northvale NJ: Jason Aronson.

Scharff, D. E., & Scharff, J. S. (1991b). *Object Relations Family Therapy*. Northvale NJ: Jason Aronson.

Schneider, K. A. (1994). *Counseling About Cancer: Strategies for Genetic Counselors*: available from National Society of Genetic Counselors, 233 Canterbury Drive, Wallingford, PA 19086–6617.

Schneider, K. A., & Kalkbrenner, K. J. (1998). Professional status survey 1998. *Perspectives in Genetic Counseling*, 20(3 supplement):S1–S8.

Schneider, K. A., & Marnane, D. (1997). Cancer risk counseling: How is it different? *J Genet Counsel*, 6:97–109.

Schneider, K. A., Stopfer, J. E., Peters, J. A., Knell, E., & Rosenthal, G. (1997). Complexities in cancer risk counseling: Presentation of three cases. *J Genet Counsel*, 6:147–167.

Schuette, J. L., & Bennett, R. L. (1998). Lessons in history: Obtaining the family history and constructing a pedigree. In D. L. Baker, J. L. Schuette, & W. R. Uhlmann (Eds.), *A Guide to Genetic Counseling*. New York: Wiley-Liss, pp. 27–51.

Seiffge-Krenke, I. (1998). *Adolescents' Health: A Developmental Perspective*. Mahwah NJ: Lawrence Erlbaum.

Seligman, M. (1991). Family systems and beyond: Conceptual issues. In M. Seligman (Ed.), *The Family with a Handicapped Child*. (2nd ed.) Boston: Allyn and Bacon, pp. 27–53.

Seligman, M., & Darling, R. B. (1989). *Ordinary Families, Special Children: A Systems Approach to Childhood Disability*. New York: Guilford.

Seller, M., Barnes, C., Ross, S., Barby, T., & Cowmeadow, P. (1993). Grief and midtrimester fetal loss. *Prenat Diagn*, 13:341–348.

Shapiro, C. H. (1993). *When Part of the Self Is Lost: Helping Clients Heal After Sexual and Reproductive Losses*. San Francisco: Jossey-Bass.

Shapiro, E. R. (1994). *Grief as a Family Process: A Developmental Approach to Clinical Practice*. New York: Guilford.

Shiloh, S. (1994). Heuristics and biases in health decision making: Their expression in genetic counseling. In L. Heath, R. S. Tindale, J. Edwards, E. J. Posavac, F. B. Bryant, E. Henderson-King, Y. Suarez-Balcazar, & J. Myers (Eds.), *Applications of Heuristics and Biases to Social Issues*. New York: Plenum, pp. 13–30.

Shiloh, S. (1996). Decision-making in the context of genetic risk. In T. Marteau & M. Richards (Eds.), *The Troubled Helix: Social and Psychological Implications of the New Human Genetics*. Cambridge UK: Cambridge University Press, pp. 82–103.

Shiloh, S., & Sagi, M. (1989). Effect of framing on the perception of genetic recurrence risks. *Am J Med Genet*, 33:130–135.

Shiloh, S., & Saxe, L. (1989). Perception of risk in genetic counseling. *Psychology and Health*, 3:45–61.

Simpson, E., Gawron, T., Mull, D., & Walker, A. P. (1994). A Spanish-language prenatal family health evaluation questionnaire: Construction and pilot implementation. *J Genet Counsel*, 3:39–62.

Slotki, I. W. (1936). Yebamoth: Translated into English with notes, glossary and indices. In I. Epstein (Ed.), *The Babylonian Talmud: Seder Nashim*, vol. 11. London: Soncino Press.

Smith, A. C. M. (1998). Patient education. In D. L. Baker, J. L. Schuette, & W. R. Uhlmann (Eds.), *A Guide to Genetic Counseling*. New York: Wiley-Liss, pp. 99–121.

Smith, K. R., West, J. A., Croyle, R. T., & Botkin, J. R. (1999). Familial context of genetic testing for cancer susceptibility: Moderating effect of siblings' test results on psychological distress one to two weeks after BRCA1 mutation testing. *Cancer Epidemiology, Biomarkers and Prevention*, 8:385–392.

Smith, S. C., Warren, N. S., & Misra, L. (1993). Minority recruitment into the genetic counseling profession. *J Genet Counsel*, 2:171–181.

Solnit, A. J., & Stark, M. H. (1961). Mourning and the birth of a defective child. *Psychoanal Study Child*, 16:523–537.

Sorenson, J. R. (1976). From social movement to clinical medicine: The role of law and the medical profession in regulating applied human genetics. In A. Milunsky & G. J. Annas (Eds.), *Genetics and the Law*. New York: Plenum, pp. 467–485.

Sorenson, J. R. (1993). Genetic counseling: Values that have mattered. In D. M. Bartels, B. S. LeRoy, & A. L. Caplan (Eds.), *Prescribing Our Future: Ethical Challenges in Genetic Counseling*. New York: Aldine de Gruyter, pp. 3–14.

Sorenson, J. R., & Culbert, A. J. (1977). Genetic counselors and counseling orientations—unexamined topics in evaluation. In H. A. Lubs & F. de la Cruz (Eds.), *Genetic Counseling*. New York: Raven, pp. 131–156.

Sorenson, J. R., Scotch, N., Swazey, J., Wertz, D. C., & Heeren, T. (1987). Reproductive plans of genetic counseling clients not eligible for prenatal diagnosis. *Am J Med Genet*, 28:345–352.

Sorenson, J. R., Swazey, J. P., & Scotch, N. A. (1981). Reproductive pasts reproductive futures: Genetic counseling and its effectiveness. *Birth Defects*, 17(4).

Spector, R. E. (1996). *Cultural Diversity in Health and Illness*. (4th ed.). Stamford CT: Appleton & Lange.

Spencer, S. J., Josephs, R. A., & Steele, C. M. (1993). Low self-Esteem: The uphill struggle for self-integrity. In R. F. Baumeister (Ed.), *Self-Esteem: The Puzzle of Low Self-Regard*. New York: Plenum, pp. 21–36.

Spinetta, J. J. (1980). Disease-related communication: How to tell. In J. Kellerman (Ed.), *Psychological Aspects of Childhood Cancer*. Springfield IL: C. C. Thomas, pp. 257–269.

Stacey, M. (1997). About genetics: Aspect of social structure worth considering. In A. Clarke & E. Parsons (Eds.), *Culture, Kinship and Genes: Towards Cross-Cultural Genetics*. New York: St. Martin's, pp. 231–244.

Statistical Abstract of the United States (1998). (118 ed.). Washington DC: U.S. Department of Commerce.

Sue, D. W., & Sue, D. (1990). *Counseling the Culturally Different: Theory and Practice*. (2nd ed.). New York: John Wiley.

Suslak, L., Scherer, A., & Rodriguez, G. (1995). A support group for couples who have terminated a pregnancy after prenatal diagnosis: Recurrent themes and observations. *J Genet Counsel*, 4:169–178.

Swinford, A., Phelps, L., & Mather, J. (1988). Countertransference in the counseling setting. *Perspectives in Genetic Counseling*, 10(3):1, 4.

Tafoya, N., & Del Vecchio, A. (1996). Back to the future: An examination of the Native American holocaust experience. In M. McGoldrick, J. Giordano, & J. K. Pearce (Eds.), *Ethnicity and Family Therapy*. (2nd ed.) New York: Guilford, pp. 45–54.

Telfair, J., & Nash, K. B. (1996). African American culture. In N. L. Fisher (Ed.), *Cultural and Ethnic Diversity: A Guide for Genetics Professionals*. Baltimore: Johns Hopkins University Press, pp. 36–59.

Tervalon, M., & Murray-García, J. (1998). Cultural humility versus cultural competence: A critical distinction in defining physician training outcomes in multicultural education. *Journal of Health Care for the Poor and Underserved*, 9:117–125.

Thompson, R. J. J. (1985). Coping with the stress of chronic childhood illness. In A. N. O'Quinn (Ed.), *Management of Chronic Disorders of Childhood*. Boston: G K Hall, pp. 11–41.

Tibben, A., Frets, P. G., van de Kamp, J. J. P., Niermeijer, M. F., der Vlis, M. V., Roos, R. A. C., Rooymans, H. G. M., van Ommen, G.-J. B., & Verhage, F. (1993). On attitudes and appreciation 6 months after predictive DNA testing for Huntington disease in the Dutch program. *Am J Med Genet*, 48:103–111.

Toupin, E. S. W. A. (1980). Counseling Asians: Psychotherapy in the context of racism and Asian-American history. *Am J Orthopsychiatry*, 50:76–86.

Trad, P. V. (1993). The ability of adolescents to predict future outcome. Part II: Therapeutic enhancement of predictive skills. *Adolescence*, 28:757–780.

Turk, J. (1964). Impact of cystic fibrosis on family functioning. *Pediatrics*, 34:67–71.

Tuttle, L. C. (1998). Experiential family therapy: An innovative approach to the resolution of family conflict in genetic counseling. *J Genet Counsel*, 7:167–186.

Tversky, A., & Kahneman, D. (1974). Judgment under uncertainty: Heuristics and biases. *Science*, 185:1124–1131.

Tversky, A., & Kahneman, D. (1981). The framing of decisions and the psychology of choice. *Science*, 211:453–458.

Tversky, A., & Kahneman, D. (1982). Judgment under uncertainty: Heuristics and biases. In D. Kahneman, P. Slovic, & A. Tversky (Eds.), *Judgment Under Uncertainty: Heuristics and Biases*. Cambridge UK: Cambridge University Press.

U. S. Bureau of the Census (1992). *Population Projections of the United States by Age, Race, Sex and Hispanic Origin 1992–2050*. Washington, DC: U.S. Government Printing Office.

U. S. Bureau of the Census (1998). *Current Population Reports, Series P23-194, Population Profile of the United States: 1997*. Washington, DC: U.S. Government Printing Office.

Van Spijker, H. G. (1992). Support in decision making processes in the postcounseling period. *Birth Defects*, 28(1):29–35.

Varekamp, I., Suurmeijer, T., Bröcker-Vriends, A., & Rosendaal, F. R. (1992). Hemophilia and the use of genetic counseling and carrier testing within family networks. *Birth Defects*, 28(1):139–148.

Vetrano, M. A., & Siegel, B. (1987). Clergy liaison groups. *Birth Defects*, 23(6):206–213.

Viviano, F. (1988). Bay Area in 1990s—preview of big changes. *San Francisco Chronicle*, Dec. 5: A1, A6–A7.

Vlek, C. (1987). Risk assessment, risk perception and decision making about courses of action involving genetic risk: An overview of concepts and methods. *Birth Defects*, 23(2):171–207.

Wachtel, E. F. (1994). *Treating Troubled Children and Their Families*. New York: Guilford.

Walker, A. P. (1998). The practice of genetic counseling. In D. L. Baker, J. L. Schuette, & W. R. Uhlmann (Eds.), *A Guide to Genetic Counseling*. New York: Wiley-Liss, pp. 1–20.

Walsh, F. (1993a). Conceptualization of normal family processes. In F. Walsh (Ed.), *Normal Family Processes*. (2nd ed.) New York: Guilford, pp. 3–69.

Walsh, F. (Ed.). (1993b). *Normal Family Processes*. (2nd ed.). New York: Guilford.

Walsh, F. (1998). Beliefs, spirituality, and transcendence: Keys to family resilience. In M. McGoldrick (Ed.), *Re-visioning Family Therapy: Race, Culture, and Gender in Clinical Practice*. New York: Guilford, pp. 62–77.

Wang, V. (1993). *Handbook of Cross-Cultural Genetic Counseling*: available from Vivian Ota Wang, Division of Psychology in Education, College of Education, Arizona State University, P.O. Box 870611, Tempe, AZ 85287–0611.

Wang, V., & Marsh, F. H. (1992). Ethical principles and cultural integrity in health care delivery: Asian ethnocultural perspectives in genetic services. *J Genet Counsel*, 1:81–92.

Weil, J. (1991). Mother's postcounseling beliefs about the causes of their children's genetic disorders. *Am J Hum Genet*, 48:145–153.

Weil, J., & Mittman, I. (1993). A teaching framework for cross-cultural genetic counseling. *J Genet Counsel*, 2:159–170.

Wertz, D. C. (1992). How parents of affected children view selective abortion. In H. B. Holmes (Ed.), *Issues in Reproductive Technology I. An Anthology*. New York: Garland, pp. 161–189.

Wertz, D. C., & Fletcher, J. C. (1988). Attitudes of genetic counselors: A multinational survey. *Am J Hum Genet*, 42:592–600.

Wertz, D. C., & Fletcher, J. C. (1993). Feminist criticism of prenatal diagnosis: A response. *Clin Obstet Gynecol*, 36:541–567.

Wertz, D. C., Janes, S. R., Rosenfield, J. M., & Erbe, R. W. (1992). Attitudes toward the prenatal diagnosis of cystic fibrosis: Factors in decision making among affected families. *Am J Hum Genet*, 50:1077–1085.

Wertz, D. C., Sorenson, J. R., & Heeren, T. C. (1986). Clients' interpretation of risks provided in genetic counseling. *Am J Med Genet*, 39:253–264.

Wexler, N. S. (1979). Genetic "Russian roulette": The experience of being "at risk" for Huntington's disease. In S. Kessler (Ed.), *Genetic Counseling: Psychological Dimensions*. New York: Academic Press, pp. 199–220.

Whipperman, L., & Perlstein, M. (1987). The professional as a person: Enhancing the former by supporting the latter. In N. J. Zellers (Ed.), *Strategies in Genetic Counseling, Vol. 2: Tools for Professional Advancement*. New York: Human Sciences Press, pp. 27–66.

White, M. T. (1997). "Respect for autonomy" in genetic counseling: An analysis and a proposal. *J Genet Counsel*, 6:297–313.

Wills, T. A. (1985). Supportive functions of interpersonal relationships. In S. Cohen & S. L. Syme (Eds.), *Social Support and Health*. Orlando: Academic Press, pp. 61–82.

Wolff, G., & Jung, C. (1995). Nondirectiveness and genetic counseling. *J Genet Counsel*, 4:3–26.

Wortman, C. B., & Silver, R. C. (1989). The myths of coping with loss. *J Consult Clin Psychol*, 57:349–357.

Yamoto, G. (1988). Something about the subject makes it hard to name. In J. W. Cochran, D. Langston, & C. Woodward (Eds.), *Changing Our Power: An Introduction to Women's Studies*. (2nd ed.) Dubuque IA: Kendall-Hunt, pp. 7–10.

Zola, I. K. (1985). Depictions of disability—metaphor, message, and medium in the media: A research and political agenda. *Social Science Journal*, 22(4):5–17.

Zuskar, D. M. (1987). The psychological impact of prenatal diagnosis of fetal abnormality: Strategies for investigation and intervention. *Women Health*, 12:91–103.

INDEX